Therapeutic landscapes

MANCHESTER
1824
Manchester University Press

Therapeutic landscapes

A history of English hospital gardens since 1800

Clare Hickman

Manchester University Press

Published by Manchester University Press
Altrincham Street, Manchester M1 7JA, UK
www.manchesteruniversitypress.co.uk

British Library Cataloguing-in-Publication Data is available

ISBN 978 0 7190 8660 1 *hardback*

First published by Manchester University Press in hardback 2013

This edition first published 2018

Printed by Lightning Source

Contents

Figures and tables

Figures

Table

Acknowledgements

I would like to begin by thanking the GNS Trust, as without their generous scholarship for my original doctoral research, none of this would have been possible, and the Leverhulme Trust for funding my time as a Research Fellow on the Historic Gardens & Landscapes of England Project at the University of Bristol from 2007 to 2011. Special thanks must go to Professor Timothy Mowl for being an inspiring academic colleague, as well as guiding me through the world of garden history as my doctoral supervisor, and Michael Liversidge for his wise advice on all art historical and academic matters. I would also like to thank the peer reviewers of this manuscript for their thoughtful, detailed and very constructive comments, which have undoubtedly improved the text, and the team at Manchester University Press for all their hard work and enthusiasm. Deep appreciation and thanks also go to Laura Mayer, Stephen Soanes and George Campbell-Gosling for commenting on sections, as well as their general encouragement, and very warm thanks to Vicky Long for not only reading nearly the entire manuscript, but also her unfailing support and friendship.

Many people have been generous with their time and encouragement and, in particular, I would like to thank all the Bristol MA and PhD Garden History students who have supported me over the years. Those deserving special mention for their contributions include Angela Nutbrown, Carole Fry, Emma Jones, Caroline Garrett, Diane James, Dianne Barre, Marion Mako, Jane Bradney, Judy Preston, Valerie Joynt, Janet Carter, Kate Felus, Katie Campbell and Elain Harwood.

Numerous archivists and librarians have helped throughout my research but I would particularly like to thank Michael Richardson and

Hannah Lowery of Special Collections at the University of Bristol for all their help and support. Others include Chris Addison (the Historic Environment Record Officer of Northamptonshire County Council), the Wellcome Library, Bristol Record Office, Bristol Central Local Studies Library, Northampton Gardens Trust, Somerset Archives and Local Studies, Borthwick Institute for Archives at the University of York, Tyne & Wear Archives and the archive of St Andrew's Healthcare, Northampton. Thanks go to those who have acted as knowledgeable guides and allowed me access to relevant gardens, including Alex Coulter, Arts Co-ordinator at West Dorset General Hospital, Veronica and Eric Long at Long Fox Manor, Bristol, Bronwen Gray at The Retreat, York and Roger Skipp at The Priory Ticehurst House, Sussex. Every effort has been made to trace the copyright owners of all the images used within this book, however anyone claiming copyright should contact the author.

Warm personal thanks are due to my many friends and colleagues who have supported my research over the last decade – the numbers are too great to name them all, but special thanks go to the Humanities Division Research Team at the University of Oxford, colleagues of the Department of Archaeology & Anthropology at the University of Bristol, Peter Coates, Tim Cole, Chris Pearson, Jonathan Reinarz, Michael Brown, Karen Moore, Naomi Baker, Nikki Horrobin, Stephanie Wynne-Jones, Justine McConnell, Cathy Hume, Cathy Ladds, Jane Weston, John Halliwell, Ariane Magny, Dominic Cote, Catherine Jones, Tamsin Hellier-Hough, Gilly Rendle, Alexandra Harris, Sheila Whitcombe, David McCarthy and Mike Race; and to the Hawthorns crowd of Jan Cox, Chris Gibson, Victoria Meir, Tricha Passes, Rachel Flynn, Louise Gray and Jo Kear for cheering me on. Exceptional levels of gratitude are due to Rose White and Rachel Pick for offering support and encouragement on all aspects of my life.

Finally, the ultimate thanks go to my mother, Carol, and brother, Guy, for their unstinting support and encouragement throughout my life. This book is dedicated to them both.

1

The hospital garden as a space for health

> A man of rank comes in, ragged and dirty, and unshaven and with the pallor of a dungeon upon him; wild in aspect, and as if crazed beyond recovery. He has passed months in a lonely apartment, looking out on a dead wall; generally fastened in a chair . . . Liberty to walk at all hours of the cheerful day in gardens or fields, and care and attention, metamorphose him into the well dressed and well bred gentleman he used to be.
>
> John Connolly, 1856[1]

> [Patients] assigned to rooms with windows looking out on a natural scene had shorter postoperative hospital stays, received fewer negative evaluative comments in nurses' notes, and took fewer potent analgesics.
>
> Roger Ulrich, 1984[2]

The views of these writers are separated by over 100 years but they both portray the perceived therapeutic value of the natural environment for patients, whether it is through the view out of a window or a walk in a garden. As well as being found in written accounts, the material traces of gardens associated with medical establishments can be found on maps, in photographs and engravings, and sometimes by physically walking the site or conducting archaeological excavations. They are materially present and yet have often been overlooked by historians. The central aim of this work is to draw on detailed site-specific research to explore the medical and cultural significance of a variety of therapeutic landscapes created over the past 200 years.

Therapeutic Landscapes considers the term therapeutic in its broadest definition. In 1839, the *Lexicon Medicum; or Medical Dictionary* defined therapeutics as including the 'healing powers of nature'.[3] The author goes on to state that 'many diseases are cured by attention merely to the air we breathe, the food we eat, the state of the mind, the rest and exercise of the body; and many are naturally removed as life advances, and by alteration of habits, change of temperature, clothing and climate, without the aid of medicines'.[4] It is this wider concept of the environment as an agent that can affect the maintenance of health and the recovery from disease which will be explored primarily in this text. The explanations for the mechanisms by which the environment might affect patient recovery have changed over time, but the notion that the landscape can act as a therapeutic agent is as valid now as it was in previous centuries. In fact, the late twentieth century has witnessed a renewed interest in the therapeutic role of the environment. This has been informed by the work of behavioural psychologists such as Roger Ulrich, who has demonstrated that recovery from surgical procedures may speed up if patients are given natural views from their hospital windows.[5]

The landscapes under scrutiny are all located in England, simply in order to make the scope of the book manageable. They can be defined as the immediate gardens and wider open spaces which can be accessed or viewed from institutions whose primary concern is related to medical practice. The text will focus on the relationship between the institution and its external setting which includes designed hospital gardens as well as the wider landscape; whether viewed from inside the building, from within the gardens or experienced directly by patients through exercise, recreational activity or physical work such as gardening. The research does not intend to establish how successful the use of such landscapes were as therapeutic agents, but rather to uncover the cultural and medical concepts that led to their inclusion and consideration in hospital designs. Equally, given the broad time span and inclusion of contemporary accounts, this text does not interrogate the conceptual arguments regarding these landscapes in depth, offering instead an account of the rhetoric used to describe such landscapes.

The aim of this book is to highlight the existence of the hospital garden and encourage future researchers to consider it as an important space in its own right; one which was intentionally included as part of the overall design of institutions. As it currently stands scholars have, in the most part, either overlooked these spaces or viewed them as an unimportant addition to the more obviously medically oriented spaces within the institution. By utilising garden history methodologies, it is hoped that this approach will offer new insight into medical processes and beliefs.

My approach also reflects new methodologies in garden history. As Michel Conan has written: 'Asking ... "How did garden making or garden forms play an instrumental role in historical changes?" allows us to discover how gardens have offered the arena or the medium for the negotiation of social issues. It allows us to show how garden changes have contributed to cultural developments as much as they built up on them.'[6] Gardens can, therefore, be seen as agencies of cultural change as well as representatives of such developments.

In the case of hospital gardens they can fulfil a number of different roles which relate to wider cultural concerns. Often the gardens can be read as a complicated mix of different ideas and beliefs. In the case of the elite lunatic asylums of Ticehurst Place, Sussex and Brislington House, Bristol, images of the gardens are included in promotional literature and so the ornamented landscapes can be viewed as a marketing tool for the recruitment of clients, as well as an integral part of the therapeutic regime. Gardens were also used to attract donations to voluntary hospitals, particularly those gardens that were at the front of buildings and in clear view of the public, such as that near the entrance of Leeds General Infirmary. The gardens at the Homeopathic Hospital, Bristol, perhaps best demonstrate the overlay of several different meanings. The gardens reflected the design style preferred by the donor family, were used as a tool to promote the regime of homeopathy, were often described in civic pride terms as beautifying the city, and yet they also contained revolving chalets that were used by patients.

The use of garden history methodology with its focus on the close reading of individual sites through site walking, maps and primary research can, therefore, complement and add new dimensions to our understanding of the role and use of space surrounding medical institutions. The use of hospital gardens as broader cultural signifiers has been explored by Harriet Deacon. She has argued that 'ideas about the importance of gardens and the right sort of natural environment were . . . associated with particular visions of cure and rehabilitation and with particular visions of ethnic or group identity'.[7] It is this approach to gardens as more than aesthetic spaces that will be utilised within this study.

The garden history approach means that the text is built around a number of detailed case studies. These sites have been chosen for a variety of reasons: they are high-profile institutions, demonstrate a specific contemporary design principle or illustrate a particular idea that was prevalent at the time. Some fall into more than one of these categories. It is, however, not intended to be a comprehensive gazetteer and chooses instead to present detailed analyses of a small number of sites. A table on page 11 attempts to map these case studies to definitions of garden styles and features used by garden historians to describe domestic gardens and public parks. In this way it is hoped that hospital gardens can be set within the wider garden historical context.

Wherever possible images have been used to accompany the text and depict the wide range of garden styles. However, given the scarceness of original visual sources and the low-quality reproduction techniques of the earlier periods under discussion, there have been issues reproducing images for use in this publication and some that have been invaluable in conducting the research could not be successfully reproduced.[8] Other images have been used, even though the quality of the image is low by twenty-first-century standards, simply because the author believes they are a valuable historic resource and will hopefully add to the reader's understanding of the subject.

When I began researching this subject for my doctorate I was unaware of the rich resources available and so the case studies were developed on a rather ad hoc basis as I began uncovering the wealth of source material. However, there were general criteria that the sites had to reach before more detailed analysis could be undertaken – there had to be archival evidence available, they needed to represent a particular approach to treatment and they had to be of interest from a garden history perspective. A number of the institutions chosen were at the forefront of new medical ideas in their field. These include Brislington House, St Thomas's Hospital, Hailey Open-Air Sanatorium and the King Edward VII Sanatorium, Midhurst. Others illustrate the use of cutting-edge technology in relation to their garden design, such as the glass-roofed winter garden at Leeds General Infirmary which was influenced by the Crystal Palace, and the roof-top garden created using newly invented asphalt at Bristol General Hospital. The King Edward VII Sanatorium where Gertrude Jekyll was employed, the Homeopathic Hospital, Bristol, which commissioned the Pulham firm, and contemporary planned gardens by Dan Pearson's Studio for two London hospitals have been chosen because of their involvements with important garden designers. The comparative study of three asylums in Northampton was conducted to complement the work of Sarah Rutherford, whose thesis, *The Landscapes of Public Lunatic Asylums in England, 1808–1914*, explored the design and use of gardens associated with one major type of asylum.[9] As the institutions were aimed at a different clientele, the analysis also offered the opportunity to explore issues concerning the perceived therapeutic effect of hospital landscapes in relation to the social class of the patient.

Some institutions are much less well known and have been chosen because the archival sources are particularly good, such as the Winford

Orthopaedic Hospital, Bristol, with its minute books of the Garden Committee. Alternatively they offer an unusual perspective. In the case of Blackwell Convalescent Home, Bromsgrove and Abington Abbey Retreat, Northampton, postcards or letters sent by patients have survived and they give a rare glimpse of how the gardens were experienced by them. Similarly, Brislington House was described by John Perceval during his time there, and this contemporary source provides an unusually detailed account of how the landscape of an early nineteenth-century asylum was perceived and used by a patient.[10] These accounts often suggest a mixed experience of hospital gardens and landscapes. The forced regimen of being outside, particularly in the psychiatric institutions and open-air hospitals, during all weathers led to patient complaints, and may even have harmed those undergoing these treatments. However, the intention of those in power remained that time spent outside in garden settings was beneficial for a range of conditions.

This interest in space, place and material cultures also speaks to recent trends in medical history. Texts that have addressed these issues include: Ann-Marie Adams, *Medicine By Design: The Architect and the Modern Hospital, 1893–1943* (Minneapolis: University of Minnesota Press, 2008); Carla Yanni, *The Architecture of Madness: Insane Asylums in the United States* (Minneapolis: University of Minnesota Press, 2007); and Leslie Topp, James Moran and Jonathan Andrews (eds), *Madness, Architecture and the Built Environment: Psychiatric Spaces in Historical Context* (London and New York: Routledge, 2007). Much of their research has so far been confined to life within the walls of institutions and the aim of this research is to extend those modes of enquiry in order to analyse the external spaces.

Geographers have also taken an interest in the role of place in relation to science, particularly David Livingstone with *Putting Science in its Place* (Chicago and London: University of Chicago Press, 2003). A recent collection of essays reflects this growing concern in relation to health and medicine. *Locating Health: Historical and Anthropological Investigations of Place and Health* edited by Erika Dyck and Christopher Fletcher (London: Pickering and Chatto, 2011) utilised historical and anthropological perspectives to tackle the 'dynamic relationship between health and place'. Similarly a recent conference at Exeter University[11] and a workshop at the University of Bristol[12] took medicine and place as their themes. This demonstrates a growing interest in this area. By using garden history methodologies this research aims to add to this discourse by looking at material hospital gardens as both the generic spaces that surround institutions and as individual places with specific meanings. As Kerry Davies has asserted in her analysis of interviews conducted with mental health users in Oxfordshire 'both physically and poetically, the most significant patient spaces have tended to be hospital grounds'.[13]

This research explores a specific area and time period that has previously been neglected. The only substantial work that has surveyed the gardens associated with a single type of hospital is Rutherford's unpublished thesis on the landscapes of English public lunatic asylums. This research has also informed her book, *The Victorian Asylum*[14] but this is not specifically dedicated to the use and design of the gardens. There have been passages on individual hospital gardens in hospital biographies, such as S.T. Anning's *The General Infirmary at Leeds*, which describes both the old infirmary garden and the new one.[15] These tend only to concentrate on one example and are descriptive rather than analytical. Some medical historians, including Andrew Scull and Linda Bryder, have discussed the hospital landscape in relation to issues such as economics and national efficiency.[16] Such references have generally only been brief and have omitted any consideration of the aesthetic role of the landscape in relation to the therapeutic regime.

Several architectural historians have also touched on gardens in their work on hospitals, namely Jeremy Taylor, Christine Stevenson, Harriet Richardson and Margaret Campbell, but gardens and designed landscapes have not been the main focus of their work.[17] Similarly, some cultural geographers have taken an interest in the concept of therapeutic landscapes. Indeed, this notion was first developed in geographical terms in 1992 by Wil Gesler.[18] However, research in this field has generally concentrated on studies of a specific group of people in relation to the landscape or a particular site, or has concentrated on wider issues concerning landscape and well-being, and has rarely considered the role of hospital gardens.[19] Exceptions to this rule include the work of Chris Philo on asylums, Hester Parr on mental health and space and the work by Gesler.[20] In particular, Philo's work on the historical geography of asylums gives an in-depth account of the relationship between place, space and therapeutic rationale and does give attention to the design, role, use and experience of gardens. This text aims to build on such work, widening the context to include a range of medical institutions and expanding the time period.

Given the recent interest in contemporary gardens as therapeutic places, it is perhaps no surprise that landscape architects, in particular those based in the United States, have taken an interest in the historical background of these spaces. Therefore, summaries of the history of hospital gardens can be found within the introductory chapters of such texts as *Healing Gardens: Therapeutic Benefits and Design Recommendations*, edited by Clare Cooper Marcus and Marni Barnes, and Nancy Gerlach-Spriggs, Richard Enoch Kaufman and Sam Bass Warner Jr.'s *Restorative Gardens: The Healing Landscape*.[21] However these texts provide only an overview of the area as their focus is elsewhere, and are, again, more descriptive than analytical.

This book attempts to follow an original line of argument focusing solely on the relationship between medical institutions and their gardens and surrounding landscape. It presents a wide range of primary source material as well as utilising traditional methods of field walking where possible. Additionally it discusses developments in design, use and philosophy in a variety of types of hospital over 200 years. In contrast to the often descriptive and narrowly taxonomical approach used by other researchers, this study also takes a broader multi-disciplinary approach to the subject, combining evidence from medical history, garden history, literary studies, art history, political history, philosophy and social history. Although evidence of the physical existence of these gardens can be found from maps and visual sources, there is a scarcity of written documentation of the reasons for their origins and uses. This book will use conjectural arguments from a wide range of associated sources to reconstruct why these gardens were created and how they may have been utilised.

Overview

The book is primarily concerned with landscapes that were designed specifically for purpose-built medical institutions, so the time period under consideration begins at the end of the eighteenth century. Before this date there were only about thirty general hospitals in England, but this number rapidly increased during the nineteenth century.[22] In relation to the care of those suffering from insanity, the purpose-built asylum, which emerged as a new architectural form at the end of the eighteenth century, became the norm for psychiatric treatment during the nineteenth century. The term 'asylum' will be used as it was the contemporary description for these buildings. Whether they were intended for the treatment of physical or mental illness, many of these purpose-built establishments seem to have included gardens in their design. For example, in 1863 John Syer Bristowe and Timothy Holmes described at least forty-six general hospitals as having some kind of external grounds.[23]

The governors of these institutions, particularly those dealing with psychiatric cases, also appear to have believed that the wider landscape was a vital element of the therapeutic regime. The notion that hospital gardens could play a therapeutic role continued through the open-air movement and its associated institutions during the Edwardian period and was taken up at the end of the twentieth century by a number of influential organisations, including the British Medical Association. This study traces these developments over the past 200 years and places these new contemporary approaches within their wider historical context.

Given the constraints of this research, there has not been space or time to investigate the gardens associated with every type of medical institution, resulting in some, inevitably, being omitted from this study. These include workhouse infirmaries, military hospitals, fever hospitals, lying-in hospitals and general children's hospitals. These institutions are all in need of further research. This work concentrates on hospitals which were either the most prevalent form of institution at the time of activity, such as the general hospital and the psychiatric asylum, or those that followed a therapeutic regime that relied heavily on the external environment, such as the open-air institution.

The findings of this research are organised into three main sections: firstly psychiatric institutions, secondly institutions dealing with physical illnesses, such as general hospitals and tuberculosis sanatoria, and thirdly contemporary hospital gardens. Chapters 2 and 3 are concerned with the rise of the nineteenth-century asylum as a specific method for treating the insane, and concentrate on the factors that influenced the design and use of landscapes associated with these institutions. Chapter 2 focuses in detail on the examples of Ticehurst Place and Brislington House. These landscapes are placed within the context of prevailing theories concerning madness and its treatment, as well as fashions in garden and architectural design.

Later Victorian asylums were generally based on the models of these early rural institutions. Chapter 3 explores nineteenth-century concepts of the countryside as a place of health, the therapeutic power of landscape, the perceived relationship between God and the landscape, and how these concerns relate to developments in the design and location of Victorian asylums. It demonstrates how the gardens and grounds around the institution remained important therapeutic tools into the twentieth century. It also looks at the specific example of asylums based in and around Northampton, a county town in the East Midlands. Rutherford has already conducted a national study of landscapes associated with public asylums in England.[24] Within her thesis she briefly discussed the landscapes of private asylums but, apart from one small mention, she does not discuss any of the asylums in Northampton. Therefore this section compares these neglected examples and by looking in detail at one town it will be possible to see how complex issues concerning the role of gardens and the wider landscape are applied in practice. In addition to its neglected status, Northampton was chosen because the town contained examples of the three main types of asylum found nationally during the nineteenth century: a charitably founded institution, a private institution and a publicly funded pauper asylum. This allows comparisons to be made between asylums aimed at different classes of society, in terms of the design and use of the landscape. Developments over time can also be traced, as the period of operation of the Northampton General Lunatic Asylum spans from 1838 to the present. By looking at one specific town in detail it is possible to determine to what extent wider beliefs and ideas were influential.

The number of hospitals dramatically increased during the nineteenth century. The Victorian period saw the creation of hospital gardens that used new technologies, such as the roof-top garden at Bristol General Hospital and the winter garden at Leeds General Infirmary, as well as gardens that complemented the popular pavilion plan hospitals, such as St Thomas's Hospital. Chapter 4, therefore, focuses on general hospitals and their gardens.

Aside from the general hospital, there were specialist hospitals for individual physical ailments, workhouse infirmaries, convalescent homes and dispensaries that provided outpatient facilities for the sick poor. The gardens associated with specialist hospitals and convalescent homes are described in chapter 5. The late Victorian period saw a proliferation in the number of specialist hospitals for a variety of conditions, but this chapter focuses on those that specifically employed open-air therapies, and therefore included the landscape as part of their therapeutic regime. By the start of the twentieth century, the number of convalescent homes and specialist hospitals, particularly those for chronic conditions such as tuberculosis, had grown considerably and many were practising the new open-air therapies developed in Germany at the end of the nineteenth century. These therapies were designed around the idea that the patient should spend as much time in the open air as possible, to the extent of sleeping in shelters that were open to the elements.

Within conventional medical treatment three main types of institution seem to have developed open-air treatments. These were convalescent homes, orthopaedic hospitals and tuberculosis sanatoria. The landscapes and gardens associated with these are explored in detail through the examples of the Blackwell Convalescent Home for Birmingham and the Midland Counties, Bromsgrove and the Winford Orthopaedic Hospital, Bristol. A comparison of two tuberculosis sanatoria is conducted through an investigation of the landscapes associated with Hailey Open-Air Sanatorium, Wallingford and the King Edward VII Hospital, Midhurst. Alternative and complementary medicines were also popular at the start of the twentieth century, and the Bristol Homeopathic Hospital has provided an example of how conventional and alternative medicines crossed over in terms of their use of open-air therapeutic methods. Each of these had specific landscapes, which are explored in terms of their design in relation to the therapeutic regime as well as their rhetorical role.

In the final chapter on the situation of hospital gardens at the end of the twentieth century, the relationship between nineteenth- and early-twentieth-century ideas concerning the therapeutic role of such gardens will be explored in relation to more recent thinking. Contemporary scientific evidence in relation to gardens will be discussed and there will also be an analysis of hospital garden designs in relation to historical examples through the detailed exploration of a number of themes. These themes include views, light, the size and accessibility of the landscape, the therapeutic use of the landscape and contemporary design.

The overall aim of this text is to confirm that gardens and the wider landscape have been perceived as playing a therapeutic role almost continuously over the past 200 years, apart from a brief period in the middle of the twentieth century when hospitals became inward-looking and largely concerned with internal spaces and processes. The scientific underpinning for the therapeutic mechanism which is expressed in the rhetoric arguing for the inclusion and use of such gardens has certainly changed over time, but the idea that recovery can be improved if there is a natural scene, rather than a blank wall, for a patient to look at, is still as prevalent today as it was in the Regency period.

Early therapeutic landscapes

To fully comprehend the importance of the landscapes surrounding medical institutions of the nineteenth and twentieth centuries, it is worth considering the preceding long history of the natural environment in relation to the prevention and cure of disease. According to Gesler, 'we know that many, if not most, societies around the world believe that nature has healing powers'.[25] In the Western medical tradition the concept

Table 1: Dominant garden styles and features found within selected hospital gardens.

Type of institution	Name of institution	Dominant garden styles	Main garden features	Decade of initial garden development
Psychiatric	York Retreat	Landscape garden; agricultural; walled gardens	Walks; summer houses; cottages; recreation grounds; agricultural land	1790s
Psychiatric	Ticehurst Place	Landscape garden; picturesque	Walks; Chinese gallery; aviary; pagoda; moss house; hermitage; bowling green	1790s
Psychiatric	Brislington House	Landscape garden; picturesque; walled gardens	Grotto; ornamental cottages; walks including cliff-top walk; walled gardens with mounds; recreation areas	1800s
General	Derby Infirmary	Villa; parkland	Gardenesque flowerbeds;	1810s
Psychiatric	Northampton General Lunatic Asylum	Parkland; walled gardens	Walks; shelters; ornamental cottage; croquet lawn; agricultural land	1830s
Psychiatric	Abington Abbey Retreat	Parkland; walled gardens	Walks	1840s
General	Old Leeds Infirmary	Villa	Walks; Gardenesque flowerbeds	1840s
General	Bristol General Hospital	Roof-top garden	Flowerbeds; trees	1850s
General	Leeds Infirmary	Public park; winter garden	Victorian civic flowerbeds; glass-covered courtyard	1860s
Psychiatric	Northampton County Lunatic Asylum	Parkland; public park; walled gardens	Walks including woodland walks; recreation areas; bandstand; agricultural land	1870s
General	St Thomas's Hospital	Courtyards	Grassy courts; flowerbeds; colonnade walks; sculpture	1870s

Table 1: (*Con'd*)

Type of institution	Name of institution	Dominant garden styles	Main garden features	Decade of initial garden development
Convalescent	Blackwell Convalescent Home	Terraced; parkland	Terraces; sun lounge; orchard	1870s
TB Sanatorium	Hailey Sanatorium	Garden rooms; parkland	Shelters; flower-beds; vegetable garden; pine trees; orchard	1890s
TB Sanatorium	Edward VII Sanatorium	Arts and Crafts; garden rooms	Walled areas; terraces; pine woods	1900s
General	Homeopathic Hospital	Pulhamite artificial rock; Arts and Crafts; garden rooms	Rock garden; planted walls; pond; shelters; rose garden; tennis court	1920s
Orthopaedic	Winford Orthopaedic	Parkland	School flowerbeds; rose gardens	1930s
Convalescent	Kewstoke Convalescent Home	Modernist	Grassy terraces; minimal planting	1930s
General	Charing Cross Hospital	Courtyards; water	Moat-like pond; grassy court	1970s
General	Dorchester Hospital	Courtyards	Sculpture; bird bath; waterfall; dry stone-wall; naturalistic planting	1990s
Cancer Care	Maggie's Centre, Charing Cross, London	Japanese; courtyards	Minimal planting; natural sculpture	2000s

Note: Given the development of gardens, over sometimes long periods of time, only a general indicator of the date the garden was first developed is given. The gardens selected are all from within the text.

of the environment as an active agent is generally traced back to Ancient Greece. The site of Epidauros, a Greek temple dedicated to the god of healing, Aesclepius, had a sacred spring, groves of trees and far-reaching views.[26] Similarly the Hippocratic text of *Airs, Waters, Places*, described the relationship between geography, climate and health. This was a concern that continued for many centuries and health advice books produced in early modern England were concerned with the effect of environment on health.

Andrew Wear has suggested that 'the large number of "itineraries" and descriptions of England, parts of Europe and lands further afield, such as America, routinely mentioned the healthiness of the places they were describing, and provide evidence of lay beliefs about the relationship between places and health'.[27] Although the underlying theories might be anything from Galenic, humouralism, alchemy, iatrochemistry or chemistry to iatromechanism, the idea that good health was closely related to the environment was retained.[28] In practice, this generally meant that cities were considered bad and the countryside was good – a concept preserved by the Victorians and Edwardians and upheld to some extent today. This idea of medical topography continued throughout the eighteenth century and was a major concern of colonialists. It is also related to the idea of travelling for the good of one's health – a change in the environment could achieve relief from ill-health or even prevent diseases occurring. This can be seen in the development of spas, seaside resorts, travel for health and health tourism. These concepts similarly affected the siting of hospitals so that suburban or even rural settings were often viewed as healthier and more likely to encourage the recovery of patients than more urban, inner-city locations.

Gardens, as designed natural spaces, can be seen to reflect these wider ideas about the agency of the physical environment. Andrew Boorde in his *Dyetary of Helth* insisted that a person's house should have a prospect or view in order to avoid ill-health and that there should also be 'a garden with sweet herbs, a fish pond and parkland for deer'.[29] The garden, if one could afford to build on this scale, was therefore an essential singular feature for good health. The role of gardens as physical spaces can be viewed as part of the well-known tradition of retaining plants for their use in remedies, and as foodstuffs necessary for a healthy diet. However, new research is shedding light on the extent to which there was an intertwined human–plant relationship in the early modern period.[30] A long relationship between gardens and medicine can also be demonstrated through the creation and use of botanical gardens. A primary example of this is the Chelsea Physic Garden in London, founded in 1673 as, amongst other things, 'a site for the growing of plants used in medicines for correct identification by the [Worshipful Society of Apothecary's] apprentices'.[31] The medical usage of plants is illustrated by the fact that the educational curriculum for the Apothecaries Society as late as 1835 included courses on 'Materia Medica and Therapeutics' and 'Botany and Vegetable Physiology' alongside 'Dissection', 'Clinical Medicine' and 'Practical Chemistry'.[32]

The earliest botanic gardens of the seventeenth century, those encyclopaedic collections of plant material from around the world, have also been interpreted as the 're-creation of the earthly Paradise, or Garden of Eden'.[33] These botanical collections represented an attempt to bring together as many plants as possible so that each illness could be cured; 'there would be no hurt without a heal'.[34] This was related to the idea that Nature, or God through Nature, had provided a remedy for every ailment. In early hospitals, God was considered to be 'the supreme physician'.[35]

There was a spiritual element and a clear relationship between earthly gardens and the Garden of Eden. In 1661 John Evelyn outlined an early garden city scene whereby 'a mass of sweet smelling trees, bushes and plants would be planted to surround and vivify London'.[36] Andrew Wear has argued that such urges to bring the 'rural' into the urban centres was related to the belief in 'the paradisical garden where the smells of the plants were most fragrant and where there was neither death nor disease. In a sense, paradise was the absolute measure against which all other environments were measured.'[37] Although Eden itself was lost, gardens were perhaps the next best thing to an earthly paradise. Richard Austen discussed the benefits of creating orchards in part through an admiration for the work of God – 'the spirituall use of an orchard' – but also for their health benefits: 'Health is preserved by fresh and wholesome Ayres which in the heat of the summer is found in Arbors, Seats, and Walks in the garden of Fruit-trees.'[38] This concept of wholesome healthy air is of continual concern from the Ancients to the Edwardians with their open-air therapies. Austen wrote that 'An orchard of Garden of Fruit-trees, and imployment therein, worke upon the spirits for their refreshing two waies: First by the Organs of the Body. Secondly, by the Affections of the Minde. Touching the first, The operation upon the spirits through the Organs of the body, bee at large in the pleasure of the five senses.'[39] The use of gardens themselves, rather than just the individual plants within them, as therapeutic spaces is less well discussed. A recent article by Carole Rawcliffe has highlighted the healing power of the late medieval and early modern garden through the senses, particularly smell and sight.[40]

Given the healing powers associated with plants and gardens in the period, it is perhaps not surprising that early hospital precincts also included gardens: 'Monastic infirmaries invariably cultivated them for the production of medicinal herbs and scented plants. But it also provided a natural extension of the infirmary space which would be used in a similar way to the ward itself.'[41] At St Giles' Hospital in Norwich, the surrounding landscape was utilised in a variety of different ways: there was the cemetery; trees, which could be used for fuel as well as fencing and building materials; meadows, including one named the 'paradyse'; an orchard and gardens.[42] Rawcliffe describes how the gardens not only provided useful materials such as food, fuel and botanical plants for medicaments but how they also engendered 'a sense of spiritual and psychological well-being'.[43]

The relationship between the economic and therapeutic benefits of a garden is summed up in this quote from 1625. The master of the Long Alley almshouses in Abingdon describes the improvements that had been made in 1590:

> the Masters and Governors, since the foundation of the hospital (1580) have enclosed and annexed a garden plot to the said almshouses on the west side thereof . . . This plot they have cleansed, manured, dressed and made it fruitful ground and new ditched it about and caused fair sweet water to run by it, they fenced it with a quick mound and planted the borders with fruit trees and allotted each of the almsfolk a portion of the ground to bear them herbs for their use and flowers for their pleasure, and so, the place that was offensive and noisome before is now become healthy and profitable for them.[44]

In this period gardens played an especially important role in leper hospitals and almshouses. According to Rawcliffe, 'in accordance with the *regimen sanitatis*, these activities offered a healthy type of outdoor exercise, while also combating the sins of idleness and depression to which the leprous, in particular were reputedly prone'.[45]

Robert Burton, in his *Anatomy of Melancholy* of 1621, wrote that, 'the most pleasant of all outward pastimes is that of *Aretus, deambulatio per amaena loca*, to make a petty progresse, a merry journey now and then with some good companions'.[46] Within his list of cures for melancholy he included visiting friends, cities, castles, towns, fields and a variety of garden features:

> To walke amongst Orchards, Gardens, Bowres, Mounts and Arbors, artificiall wildernesses, greene thickets, Arches, Groves, Lawnes, Rivulets,

> Fountains and such like pleasant places, like that Antiochian Daphne, Brooks, Pooles, Fishponds, betwixt wood and water, in a faire meadow, by a river side, ubi variae avium cantationes, florum colores, pratorum frutices, &c. to disport in some pleasant plaine, parke, run up a steep hill sometimes, or sit in a shady seat, must needs be a delectable recreation.[47]

He also suggested that designed landscapes could improve the mental health of an individual by their sheer beauty as well as having beneficial physical effects through walks made within them. To illustrate this he included a quote, which he claims to be from St Bernard:

> A sicke man (saith he) sits upon a greene banke, and when the dog-starre parcheth the Plaines, and dries up rivers, he lies in a shadie bowre . . . and feeds his eyes with variety of objects, hearbes, trees, to comfort his misery, hee receaves many delightsome smels, and fills his ears with that sweet harmony of Birds.[48]

The concept of the garden as a place of health, particularly for active recreation, continued over the centuries and can be located in the domestic setting of the eighteenth-century country house. In *Clean*, Virginia Smith describes how the 'romantic English parkscape that developed in the first half of the eighteenth century had long informal paths that rambled around the estate towards newly-built plunge pools, cricket pitches, stables, and carriage rides, fishing lakes, archery butts, boatsheds, and carefully placed picnic pavilions'.[49] These are generally viewed as ornamentations for the landscape but she has argued that they were places for strenuous physical activity, and were in turn related to a growing market in medical advice books. According to Smith, a 'personal regimen had become a constant topic of conversation, like the weather, when there was little else to say: some eighteenth-century diaries and journals often recorded little else but their owner's non-natural health regime'.[50] By copying this domestic model in the nineteenth century early park designers, such as Joseph Paxton, translated the elite healthy landscapes of the gentry into promenading, fishing and places for carriage rides for the general public.

Joan Lane has stated that 'many eighteenth-century voluntary hospitals bear a striking external resemblance to the great country houses of the period'.[51] These hospital buildings were often the first purpose-built establishments for institutions that had originally utilised existing houses. Christine Stevenson has suggested that these hospitals had often begun as hospitable houses, which were almost by definition, 'big old houses . . . which had grown up piecemeal over the years as need dictated, but not by plan'.[52] In fact 'many new eighteenth century hospitals started off in houses that needed little more refurbishment than a boarding house would',[53] which was in part related to the therapeutic regimen these hospitals offered. Generally, this was centred on food and time for convalescence, which required little in the way of physical structure that differed from a large domestic house. Therefore, it is difficult to distinguish whether the gardens associated with these institutions were remnants of their previous domestic history or specifically designed and used by patients when they were utilised as hospitals.

As the medical profession became more involved with hospitals towards the end of the eighteenth century, doctors began to suggest that hospitals should be purpose-built. In 1758, Edward Foster, an Irish physician, wrote that 'in general, Houses have been rented for Hospitals, which are as fit for the Purposes, as Newgate for a Palace'.[54] The idea of building general hospitals fit for purpose ran alongside the discussion relating to lunatic asylums and the same kind of desire to build them specifically for their role rather than using generic buildings.

In terms of provision for those classed as insane, the lack of charitable hospitals meant that during this period a combination of private madhouses, forms of care in the community (often provided by the afflicted person's family) and a system of boarding-out were the main sources of care.[55] Following the 1714 Vagrancy Act, which distinguished for the first time between poverty-stricken lunatics and 'rogues, vagabonds, sturdy beggars and vagrants', parishes had a duty to pay for the treatment of the lunatics in their care.[56] This meant that although private madhouses were generally associated with wealthy patients, until the widespread building of county lunatic asylums in the nineteenth century, they also treated the poor in return for payment from the patient's parish.

Given their lack of regulation (a later Act in 1774 only brought in restricted regulatory powers) and the variety of their clientele, the madhouses varied greatly in their standards of treatment and care.[57] However, the fate of patients incarcerated within them was not always as desperate as many reformers from the end of the eighteenth century onwards have suggested. As Andrew Scull and others have commented: 'The very existence of a free trade in lunacy, essentially untrammelled by outside intervention, supervision or control, created a social space within which therapeutic experimentation could proceed; and while neglect may indeed have been the norm, individual madhouses seem to have made genuine efforts to secure their inmates' well-being and comfort.'[58] It is in fact this 'free trade in lunacy', described in detail by William Parry-Jones, that appears to result in the building of the first asylums, such as the York Retreat, York, and Brislington House, where new theories of treatment were developed in which the environment was a key element.

In *Mind Forg'd Manacles*, Roy Porter commented that little evidence remains from this time of privately operated madhouses. This was in part because there was no real regulation, and therefore no legal requirement to keep records, and, as he also states, because they were 'in the business of preserving discreet silences'.[59] This means that it is hard to know what relationship existed, if any, between the patients and the landscapes surrounding these establishments. However, it is likely that the surrounding land was not designed specifically from the outset to be therapeutic, in contrast to the landscapes surrounding the purpose-built asylums at the end of the eighteenth and beginning of the nineteenth centuries. This was because private madhouses often made use of buildings that had originally been designed for other purposes, and it was only with the development of 'moral therapy' at the end of the eighteenth century (see Chapter 2) that gardens and the wider landscape developed a new level of therapeutic importance.

This book will explore the later developments in the nineteenth and twentieth centuries that led to the creation of designed gardens and landscapes around mainly purpose-built medical institutions. In this way it is hoped that these often overlooked spaces that exist as material features, and are depicted in visual sources and written descriptions, can be placed within their wider cultural context and be considered as a significant landscape type with their own specific historical narrative.

Notes

1 John Connolly, *Treatment of the Insane Without Mechanical Restraints* (1856), ed. with an introduction by Richard Hunter and Ida Macalpine (Folkestone and London: Dawsons of Pall Mall, 1973), pp. 154–5.

2 Roger S. Ulrich, 'View through a window may influence recovery from surgery', *Science*, 224:4647 (1984), 420–1, p. 420.

3 Robert Hooper, revised by Klein Grant, *Lexicon Medicum; Or Medical Dictionary*, seventh edition (London: Longman Orme & Co, 1839), p. 1287.

4 *Ibid.*

5 Ulrich, 'view through a window'.

6 Michel Conan, ed., *Bourgeois and Aristocratic Cultural Encounters in Garden Art, 1550–1850* (Washington: Dumbarton Oaks, 2002), p. 24.

7 Harriet Deacon, 'Landscapes of exile and healing: climate and gardens on Robben Island', *South African Archaeological Bulletin*, 55:172 (2000), 147–54, p. 152.

8 In particular this includes the images reproduced in the *British Journal of Tuberculosis* in the 1900s and 1910s, and the images in the prospectus for Hailey Sanatorium: Charles Reinhardt, *Hailey Open Air Sanatorium for the Treatment of Consumption and Other Tuberculosis Diseases* (Stratford: Cole and Clark Printers, c.1900).

9 Sarah Rutherford, *The Landscapes of Public Lunatic Asylums in England, 1808–1914*, PhD Thesis, 3 vols (Leicester: De Montfort University, 2003).

10 John Perceval, *Perceval's Narrative: A Patient's Account of his Psychosis, 1830–1832*, ed. Gregory Bateson (London: Hogarth Press, 1962).

11 *The Importance of Place in Medical Practice*, hosted by the Centre for Medical History at the University of Exeter and sponsored by The Wellcome Trust and The Society for the Social History of Medicine, 18–19 September 2006.

12 Workshop funded by the Wellcome Trust and co-organised by Clare Hickman and Alexander Bird at the University of Bristol, *Putting Medicine in its Place: Exploring the Role of Place in Relation to Medical Practice, Health and Disease*, 8 July 2011.

13 Kerry Davies , 'A small corner that's for myself: space, place and patients' experiences of mental health care, 1948–98', in Leslie Topp, James E. Moran and Jonathan Andrews, eds, *Madness, Architecture and the Built Environment* (London and New York: Routledge, 2007) 305–20, p. 314.

14 Sarah Rutherford, *The Victorian Asylum* (Oxford: Shire, 2008).

15 Stephen T. Anning, *The General Infirmary at Leeds*, 2 vols (Edinburgh and London: E. & S. Livingstone, 1963/66).

16 Andrew Scull, *The Most Solitary of Afflictions: Madness and Society in Britain 1700–1900* (New Haven and London: Yale University Press, 1993) and Linda Bryder *Below the Magic Mountain: A Social History of Tuberculosis in Twentieth-century Britain* (Oxford: Clarendon Press, 1988).

17 Jeremy Taylor, *The Architect and the Pavilion Hospital: Dialogue and Design Creativity in England, 1850–1914* (London and New York: Leicester University Press, 1997) and *Hospital and Asylum Architecture in England, 1840–1914: Building for Health Care* (London: Mansell, 1991); Christine Stevenson, *Medicine and Magnificence: British Hospital and Asylum Architecture, 1660–1815* (New Haven and London: Yale University Press, 2000); Harriet Richardson, ed., *English Hospitals, 1660–1948: A Survey of Their Architecture and Design* (Swindon: RCHME, 1998); and Margaret Campbell, 'What tuberculosis did for modernism: the influence of a curative environment on modernist design and architecture', *Medical History*, 49:4 (2005), 463–88.

18 Wil Gesler, 'Therapeutic landscapes: medical issues in light of the new cultural-geography', *Social Science & Medicine*, 34:7 (1992), 735–46.

19 K. Wilson, 'Therapeutic landscapes and first nations peoples: an exploration of culture, health and place', *Health & Place*, 9:2 (2003), 83–93; Allison Williams *Therapeutic landscapes: The Dynamic Between Place and Wellness* (Lanham: University Press of America, 1999); Gavin J. Andrews, '(Re)Thinking the dynamics between healthcare and place: therapeutic geographies in treatment and care practice', *Area*, 36:3 (2004), 307–18.
20 Chris Philo, *A Geographical History of Institutional Provision for the Insane from Medieval Times to the 1860s in England and Wales: The Space Reserved for Insanity* (Lewiston and Queenston, USA and Lampeter, Wales: Edwin Mellen Press, 2004); Hester Parr, *Mental Health and Social Space: Towards Inculsionary Geographies?* (Malden: Blackwell, 2008) and Wil Gesler et al., 'Therapy by design: evaluating the UK hospital building program', *Health & Place*, 10:2 (2004), 117–28.
21 Clare Cooper Marcus and Marni Barnes, eds, *Healing Gardens: Therapeutic Benefits and Design Recommendations* (New York and Chichester: John Wiley and Sons, 1999) and Nancy Gerlach-Spriggs, Richard Enoch Kaufman and Sam Bass Warner, *Restorative Gardens: The Healing Landscape* (New Haven and London: Yale University Press, 1998).
22 Richardson, *English Hospitals*, p. 16.
23 John Syer Bristowe and Timothy Holmes, 'Report on the hospitals of the United Kingdom', appendix 15 to the sixth report of the Medical Officer of the Privy Council, 1863, *British Parliamentary Papers*, xxviii (1864).
24 Rutherford, *The Landscapes*.
25 Wil Gesler, *Healing Places* (Lanham: Rowman & Littlefield, 2003), p. 8.
26 *Ibid.*, pp. 21–41.
27 Andrew Wear, *Knowledge and Practice in English Medicine, 1550–1680* (Cambridge: Cambridge University Press, 2000), p. 185.
28 Andrew Wear, ed., *Medicine in Society: Historical Essays* (Cambridge: Cambridge University Press, 1992), p. 137.
29 Wear, *Knowledge and Practice*, p. 195.
30 See in particular Peter Dendle and Alain Touwaide, eds, *Health and Healing From the Medieval Garden* (Woodbrige: Boydell, 2008). Also Barbara Griggs, *Green Pharmacy: A History of Herbal Medicin*e (London: Jill Norman and Hobhouse, 1981).
31 Sue Minter, *The Apothecaries' Garden: A New History of the Chelsea Physic Garden* (Stroud: Sutton, 2000), p. 1.
32 Charles Newman, *The Evolution of Medical Education in the Nineteenth Century* (London: Oxford University Press, 1957), pp. 107–8.
33 John Prest, *The Garden of Eden: The Botanic Garden and the Re-creation of Paradise* (New Haven and London: Yale University Press, 1981), p. 6.
34 *Ibid.*, p. 57. For more on this subject see Griggs, *Green Pharmacy*.
35 Sylvia Landsberg, *The Medieval Garden* (London: British Museum Press, 2002), p. 38.

36 Wear, *Medicine in Society*, p. 138.

37 *Ibid.*, p. 139.

38 Ralph Austen, *A Treatise of Fruit Trees Together With the Spirituall Use of an Orchard* (Oxford: Printed for Thomas Robin, 1653) (reprinted New York and London: Garland Publishing, 1984), p. 23.

39 *Ibid.*, p. 25.

40 Carole Rawcliffe, '"Delectable sightes and fragrant smelles"': gardens and health in late medieval and early modern England', *Garden History*, 36:1 (2008), 3–21.

41 *Ibid.*, p. 15.

42 Carole Rawcliffe, *Medicine for the Soul: The Life, Death and Resurrection of an English Medieval Hospital, St Giles's, Norwich, c.1249–1550* (Stroud: Sutton Publishing, 1999), pp. 49–50.

43 *Ibid.*, p. 51.

44 Quoted in Elizabeth Prescott, *The English Medieval Hospital 1050–1640* (Melksham: Seaby, 1992), p. 100.

45 Rawcliffe, 'Delectable sightes', p. 16.

46 Robert Burton, *The Anatomy of Melancholy* (1621), ed. T.C. Faulkner, N.K. Kiessling and R.L. Blair (Oxford: Clarendon Press, 1990), pp. 72–3.

47 *Ibid.*, p. 73.

48 *Ibid.*

49 Virginia Smith, *Clean: A History of Personal Hygiene and Purity* (Oxford: Oxford University Press, 2007), p. 236.

50 *Ibid.*, pp. 239–40.

51 Joan Lane, *A Social History of Medicine: Health, Healing and Disease in England 1750–1950* (London: Routledge, 2001), p. 83.

52 Stevenson, *Medicine and Magnificence*, p. 17.

53 *Ibid.*, p. 3.

54 Edward Foster, *An Essay on Hospitals, or, Succinct Directions for the Situation, Construction, and Administration of Country Hospitals* (Dublin: Printed for the author by W.G. Jones, 1768), pp. 22–3.

55 Roy Porter, *Mind Forg'd Manacles: A History of Madness in England from the Restoration to the Regency* (London: Penguin Books, 1987), p. 119.

56 12 Anne c.23, 1714 Vagrancy Act. The Statute was laid down in 1713 (Bristol Central Local Studies Library – hereafter BCLSL).

57 See William Llewellyn Parry-Jones, *The Trade in Lunacy: A Study of Private Madhouses in England in the Eighteenth and Nineteenth Centuries* (London: Routledge and Kegan Paul, 1972).

58 Scull, *The Most Solitary of Afflictions*, p. 23. This free trade in lunacy has also been described by Parry-Jones (*The Trade in Lunacy*) and by Porter (*Mind Forg'd Manacles*).

59 Porter, *Mind Forg'd Manacles*, p. 137.

2

Cliff-top walks, summerhouses and pagodas: picturesque garden features and the elite private asylum

> The views . . . from the windows, embrace flower-beds and shrubberies, beautiful landscapes, or the grand park, according to the divisions from which they are seen. Whilst the range of view from the windows of the restless and maniacal patients is narrow and uniform, that from the windows of the melancholy patients is wide and variegated, surprising and delighting the eyes by the multitude of beautiful objects presented to it.
>
> Maximilian Jacobi, 1841[1]

Nineteenth-century private lunatic asylums that catered predominantly for wealthy clients were often surrounded by vast tracts of designed gardens and pleasure grounds. In a reflection of wealthy country house estates, these contained a wide range of ornamental features, from ornate thatched cottages to aviaries, and Gothic summerhouses to ornamental pagodas. Two famous examples of this type of elite institution, which will be explored in detail here, are Ticehurst Place, Sussex (opened in 1792), and Brislington House, Bristol (opened 1804–6). These were by no means representative of the majority of institutions catering for those categorised as insane but their overt interest in the design of the gardens indicates the significance attached to the physical environment at the time. This chapter will concentrate on these early nineteenth-century private institutions which were at the forefront of developments in treatments of mental illness while Chapter 3 will concentrate on later asylums aimed at a wider variety of clientele.

One element that sets nineteenth-century asylums apart from most of their predecessors is that they were generally purpose-built institutions. Many institutions have been given the accolade of being the first purpose-built asylum. For example, Barry Edginton claims that the York Retreat (1796) was the first purpose-built asylum and that before its construction 'lunatic asylums were not purpose-built but rather made up of existing buildings'.[2] Brislington was also, according to the English Heritage listing description, the 'first purpose-built establishment in England'.[3] However, given that the dictionary definition of 'purpose-built' is that it is something 'built or made for a specific purpose', a more worthy recipient of this coveted title might be the well-known Bethlem Hospital, which was built to Robert Hooke's designs in 1676. This building was constructed specifically as a hospital for people diagnosed with insanity. Although this was not representative of institutions for the insane before the nineteenth century, it is worth briefly considering the design of Bethlem's landscape as it differs considerably from later asylums.

Hooke's Bethlem Hospital, better known as Bedlam, was built in Moorfields, London. It replaced the priory of the Order of St Mary of Bethlehem, which had housed lunatics since 1377. According to Christine Stevenson, the popular story that Hooke had based the building on a palace in France, either the Louvre or the Tuileries, is based on myth rather than fact. She suggests that the rumour appeared in 1700 without any documentary evidence.[4] However, the fact that this came to be widely believed, by the public and historians alike, illustrates the way in which the building has been received. It is, therefore, possible to view Bethlem as palatial in style, if not as a direct copy of a French palace.

Although the architecture resembled a palace, the landscape surrounding it certainly did not. In Robert White's engraving of the hospital (1677) the only external spaces shown appear to be flat, bare and enclosed by high walls.[5] These are known as 'airing courts', enclosed areas designed so that the patients could exercise and take the air, and were a generic feature of asylum garden design. In the case of the engraving of Bethlem (Figure 1), the unornamented airing courts not only contrast with the architecture but also with the public park of Moorfields, which can be seen in the foreground. This visual evidence is given weight by written accounts which suggest that the airing courts available to the patients of Bethlem were covered with either gravel or grass: 'Separate yards for both sexes at either end of the Hospital comprised of grass and gravel plots of 120 feet each.'[6] By 1719 benches had been constructed for the use of patients, but these appear to have been the only form of ornamentation. This is in stark contrast to the lavish formal gardens created in this period for grand buildings, the most famous example of which is the Jardin de Tuileries in Paris designed by André Le Notre in the 1660s.

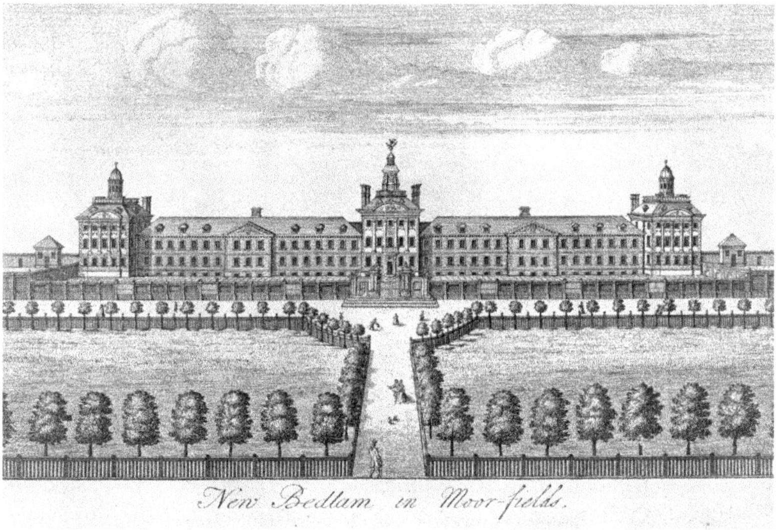

Figure 1 Engraving of Bethlem hospital showing Moorfields park in the foreground and the bare airing courts surrounding the palatial building designed by Robert Hooke.

These had elaborate parterres and ornamental fountains rather than plain grass or gravel plats.

Within the airing courts there were small buildings that Rutherford has described as being similar in style to the eighteenth-century summer-houses found on many contemporary country house estates.[7] However, she also made the point that their purpose at Bethlem was likely to have been as watchtowers to enable surveillance by the staff rather than as buildings designed to be enjoyed by the patients. This again suggests that there was a dichotomy between the palatial style of the building and the surrounding landscape.

In the period between the building of Hooke's Bethlem and the York Retreat (1796), there were only six such hospitals built in England, excluding private madhouses. Those that were built were heavily influenced by the design of St Luke's Hospital, London. One of the reasons for the desire to copy St Luke's was the influential work published in 1758 by William Battie, the doctor in charge of St Luke's. In his *Treatise on Madness*, Battie claimed that it was possible to treat the insane within asylums using methods other than the restraints and medicaments used at the rival institution, Bethlem.[8] As Roy Porter has written, 'Battie touted the curability of insanity, and the St Luke's annual reports seemed to support him'.[9] Whether his success rate was all it seemed is open to discussion, but it is possible that the well-publicised idea that insanity could be cured through treatment in asylums was an impetus for the building of similar establishments in the provinces.[10] Engravings of St Luke's and the Leicester Asylum suggest that these institutions would have had the same basic airing courts that appear to have existed at Bethlem. According to Leonard Smith, the driving force behind the Leicester Asylum was Dr Thomas Arnold, who 'had highlighted how the building was too much exposed to public view . . . His solution was a high and forbidding brick wall that surrounded the asylum, insulating it both from the parent hospital and from the outside.'[11] This type of forbidding, prison-like situation with little outdoor space was something that later asylums attempted to move away from.

Moral therapy and the asylum

Unlike Bethlem, the York Retreat, Brislington and Ticehurst all appear to have encouraged patients to spend as much time as possible in the gardens, which were anything but plain plots of grass. In these asylums, the architecture was generally less palatial in style and bore more of a resemblance to the domestic gentry houses of the time. The gardens were similarly also more akin to gentry landscape design, so the architecture and landscape in these examples can be seen as forming a whole, related environment, in contrast to the disconnect in styles seen in the example of Bethlem. This shift can be viewed as a reflection of the introduction of a new mode of treatment, 'moral therapy'.

The increasing importance of the asylum environment was closely related to changes in the therapeutic approaches advocated. In contrast to the plethora of physical remedies popular in the eighteenth century, there arose a relatively new idea of 'management'.[12] Rather than madness being viewed as primarily a physical or spiritual disease, it came to be seen as predominantly a psychological illness. Philosophical treatises, such as John Locke's 1690 *Essay Concerning Human Understanding*, looked at the human mind and the way it functioned in a relatively new way. Locke believed that thought developed through the association of ideas, and therefore insanity could be seen as the incorrect association of these ideas. Madmen, he suggested 'do not appear to me to have lost the faculty of reasoning: but having joined together some ideas very wrongly, they mistake them for truths; and they err as men do that argue right from wrong principles'.[13] He went on to say that 'a man, who is very sober, and of right understanding in all other things, may in one be as frantic, as any in Bedlam; if either by any sudden very strong impression, or long fixing his fancy upon one sort of thoughts, incoherent ideas have been cemented together so powerfully, as to remain united'.[14]

This concept of the mis-association of ideas as a cause of madness became popular during the eighteenth century and by the end of the period it was generally accepted as a common philosophical explanation of how madness might be caused.[15] It removed any remaining notion that madness was a permanent condition, as Locke suggested that insanity could be developed in anyone at any time. Towards the end of the eighteenth century, ideas such as Locke's were gradually integrated into the therapies used by doctors for treating the insane. If, after all, madness was simply caused by problems in the train of thought, then some doctors began to think that the insane might be cured if they were taught the correct association of ideas. This idea influenced many people, including William Battie at St Luke's, London, William Tuke at the York Retreat, York, and Dr Edward Long Fox at Brislington, Bristol.[16]

One of the results of the incorporation of Locke's philosophy into medicine was the development of moral therapy or 'moral management'. Moral therapy as pioneered and popularised by Samuel Tuke at the York Retreat (opened in 1796), can be briefly described as a mild regimen centred around the placement of the patient in a carefully designed environment, and one that tried to minimise the use of physical forms of restraint.[17] This form of therapy led to the idea that the institution itself could play a part in the re-education of the patient and became so popular that many nineteenth-century psychiatrists said that they 'confidently expected the asylum itself to be therapeutic'.[18]

However, this change did not automatically mean that restraints were abandoned all together. John Perceval was a patient at Edward Long Fox's establishment at Brislington in the 1830s and in his account of his time there he does describe being restrained. However, this was generally done in the communal area of the day room rather than in isolation, which may be indicative of the introduction of new techniques.[19] In other ways the change brought about by the development of moral therapy is more obvious. From Perceval's writings it is clear that a dramatic change had occurred in terms of physical medication. In contrast to his description of the medicine he was given in Dublin before his confinement, he complains that he was not given any medication during his stay at

Brislington: 'I do not recollect at any time medicine being given to me; neither to purify the blood; neither as tonics; except on two occasions. No! The cheap and universal nostrum was to be ducked in the cold bath; in the depth of winter or not.'[20] This demonstrates a move away from medicaments and other physical treatments, although the remedy of the cold bath remained popular.[21] This is not to say that restraints, purgatives or other treatments were completely absent, but there seems to have been an attempt to limit them.

As the physical environment of the asylum was considered crucial for the successful application of 'moral therapy', it is perhaps unsurprising that its surrounding landscape became a significant feature. However, it is striking how prominent images of the gardens were within the promotional literature produced to advertise both Ticehurst and Brislington. In the case of Ticehurst, Charlotte MacKenzie has noted that in the prospectus produced in 1827–28, 'all the engravings are of the asylum's exterior and grounds rather than the interior'.[22] In fact, apart from a number of letters of recommendation, the prospectus for Ticehurst consisted mainly of etchings of the extensive grounds.[23] Perhaps even more surprisingly there is no explanation about the type of treatments available.

The prospectus depicts a pagoda, aviary or pheasantry, mosshouse (Figure 2), Vineyard cottage, a highly fashionable Gothic summerhouse, hermitage, bowling green and another castellated summerhouse.[24] An account of the institution in Thomas Horsfield's *History, Antiquities and Topography of Sussex* includes engravings of the grounds similar to those in the prospectus and one which shows the Chinese Gallery, shrubbery planting and main house (Figure 3). The Chinese Gallery (Figure 4) seems to have been a reasonably substantial building as he describes it as being 'fitted up with much taste and affords to the invalids a secure retreat in wet weather'.[25] He also states that there are several buildings connected with the establishment, which from 'their ornamented appearance, possess claims to architectural distinction' (Figure 5).[26] From this and the engravings in the prospectus it is possible to argue that these were fashionable garden buildings that one would expect to find in any English landscape garden owned by the upper classes. The significance of this will be discussed below.

In contrast to the Ticehurst images, the first Brislington prospectus, which was probably produced some time between 1804 and 1809 at the time the asylum opened, includes only one etching of the main asylum building but includes detailed accounts of the treatment and

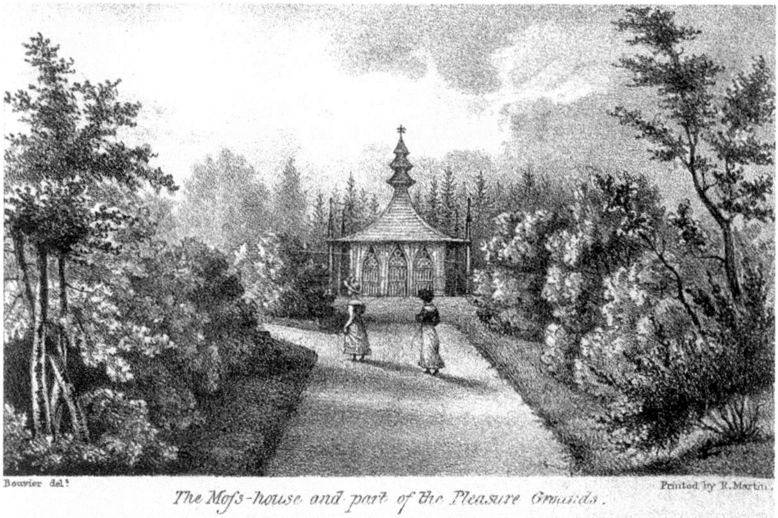
Bouvier del.t
Printed by R. Martin.
The Moss-house and part of the Pleasure Grounds.

Figure 2 The mosshouse and shrubbery planting in the grounds at Ticehurst Place, as depicted in the asylum's prospectus.

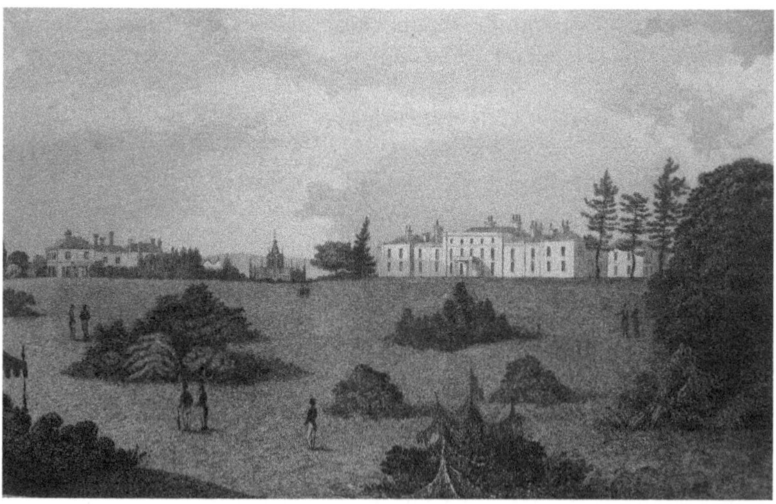

Figure 3 View of Ticehurst Place from Thomas Horsfield's *History, Antiquities and Topography of Sussex* (1835) with the Chinese Gallery pictured in the centre at the back of the image.

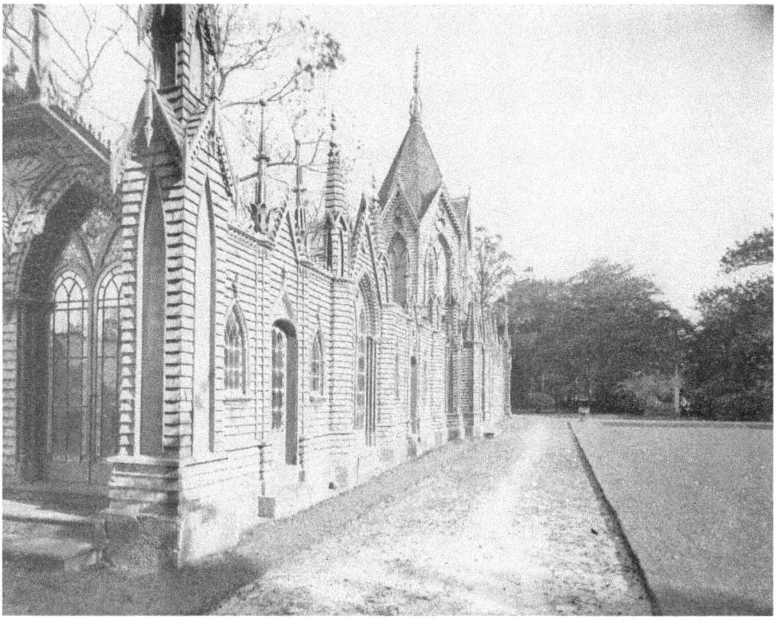

Figure 4 Photograph of the Chinese Gallery at Ticehurst which demonstrates the ornate and occasionally oriental style of the garden buildings.

Fox's philosophy.[27] By 1836 the textual element of the prospectus had been expanded further and included more detail. It was now also illustrated by etchings of the airing courts and the cottages situated in the grounds around the main asylum, which were used for the confinement of the more wealthy and upper-class patients. One wonders whether the Ticehurst prospectus influenced that produced by Brislington.

As the owners of elite private establishments aimed mainly at an affluent clientele, both the proprietors of Ticehurst and Brislington hoped that their prospectuses would attract the upper classes. For example, the sum of 300 guineas was paid for the fourteen months that Perceval was looked after at Brislington between 1831 and 1832, which was no small sum.[28] It is worth noting at this point that Brislington did admit pauper patients along with those from more affluent backgrounds, but the prospectus would not have been aimed at this category of patient. Therefore it seems plausible that the gardens were seen as one of the main selling

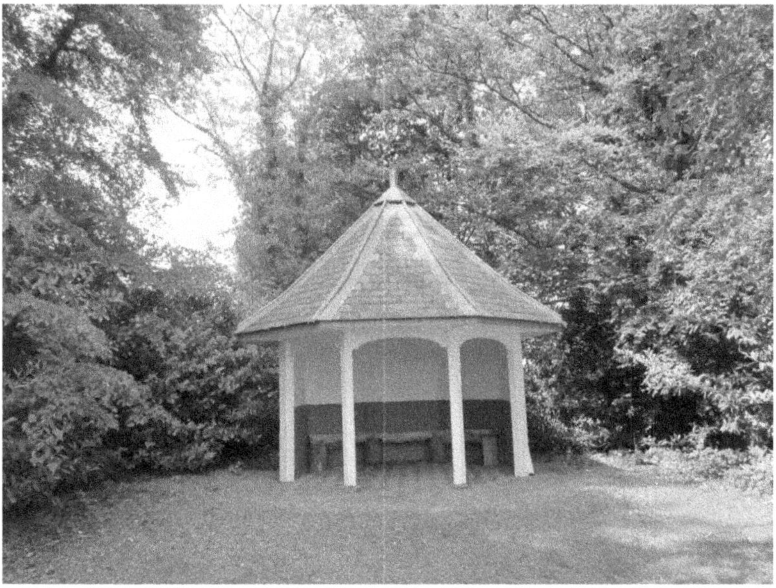

Figure 5 One of the recently restored garden buildings at Ticehurst. The estate is now part of the Priory Group.

points for relatives, and that the physical environment was seen, by the proprietors and the families alike, as an important consideration.

Location, location, location

The choice of location seems to have been an important factor for both Ticehurst and Brislington. In the case of Ticehurst, which was officially opened by Samuel Newington in 1792,[29] the immediacy of Tunbridge Wells seems to have been a factor: 'The chalybeate springs of Tunbridge Wells had been renowned in the seventeenth century for their reputed medicinal properties, notably the treatment of infertility and (of particular interest in this context) melancholia.'[30] Brislington was also located on the road between Bristol and Bath (now the A4), which meant it was close to the famous Roman spa town. However, whereas the Newingtons adapted an existing house, Fox built a new house designed specifically for its purpose as an asylum.

Dr Edward Long Fox was a well-respected doctor in the Bristol area, even before he opened his own asylum at Brislington.[31] He was attached to the Bristol Royal Infirmary from 1784–1816 and ran a private asylum at Cleve Hill from 1794, which he subsequently purchased. From the advertisement below, which appeared in the *Exeter Flying Post* in 1795, it would appear that Fox already believed that the external environment could be beneficial – an idea which was to be expressed more fully in his designs for Brislington:

> Asylum for Lunatics at Cleve Hill, near Bristol. Dr Edward Long Fox, having enlarged and improved his house at Cleve Hill for the reception of insane persons, takes this opportunity of announcing to the public that he can accommodate a greater number of patients now than heretofore, when, added to the advantage of a pure air, they will benefit of a quiet, retired, and pleasant situation, free from the risk of dangerous accidents.[32]

In 1799 Fox purchased an area of land that had previously been part of Brislington Common. According to Fox's sons, Dr Francis Ker Fox and Dr Charles Fox, who ran the institution alongside him until his death and became the joint proprietors thereafter:

> The situation which was selected for this building was in the centre of a recently enclosed common, nine miles from Bath and three miles from Bristol; where the proprietor could not be incommoded by neighbours, and to which his taste gave an imposing appearance, having laid it out in diversified walks and extensive plantations that afford shelter and security from intrusion.[33]

When Rev. Kilvert visited in 1874 he also commented on the location: 'Brislington Asylum is . . . very beautifully situated on the high ground between Keynsham and Bristol, and the grounds are large and well kept.'[34] This is similar to the description of the slightly earlier York Retreat (Figure 6), which undoubtedly influenced Fox, as it was 'situated on an eminence, at the distance of about half a mile from the eastern gate of the city of York. It commands a very delightful prospect, extending, on the south, as far as the eye can reach, over an area of wooded, fertile plain; and terminating on the north and east, by the Hambleton Hills and the Wolds; which are seen, in some places, at the distance of about twenty-five miles.'[35] Ticehurst, although a house that was adapted for its new purpose, was similarly placed on an eminence with extensive views across the Sussex countryside.

The choice of an elevated position for an asylum with views over the surrounding landscape was not only confined to Britain. According to Dr Maximilian Jacobi (the proprietor of an asylum at Siegburg), a private asylum at Vanves, near Paris, was situated, 'upon a tract of elevated

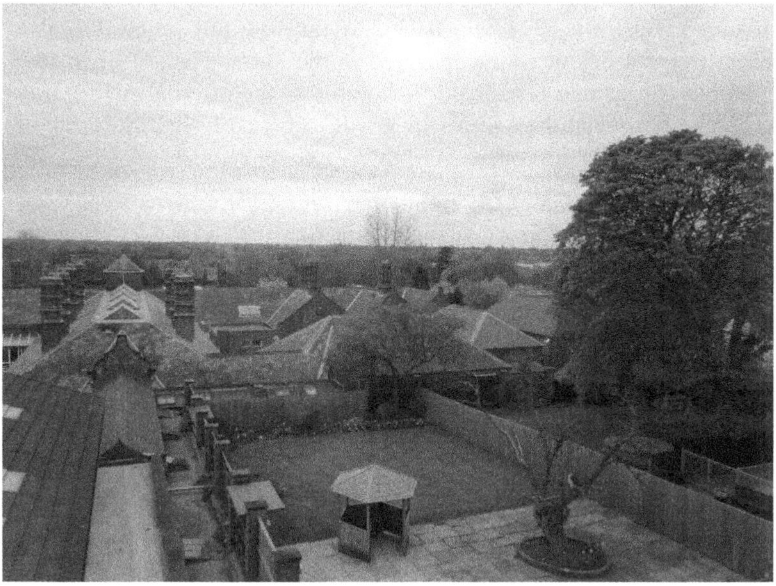

Figure 6 View from inside the York Retreat, encompassing the modern courtyards and showing the extensive views of the wider landscape.

ground, which offers, in its extent, the greatest diversity of scenery, and would, without any artificial assistance, present many strikingly beautiful prospects'.[36] He went on to suggest that Dr Falret, who had designed Vanves, had done so in order to place the patients 'in a situation which should agreeably affect both eye and mind'.[37] In relation to the York Retreat, Rutherford has suggested that the '"borrowed" views not only acted as a "reward" for the patient's existing condition, but were also intended to modify it beneficially'.[38] This use of views reflects the appropriation of the wider landscape by domestic parks and town gardens that had become common during the eighteenth century. As Rutherford has argued, the design of the landscape also 'incorporated elements of design of the typical landscape park surrounding the fashionable country house'.[39]

This concept seems to have derived from the view prevalent in the early nineteenth century that nature had curative powers. This is demonstrated by the fact that the proprietors of these asylums believed it was fundamentally important that patients should be able to interact with the landscape. According to Barry Edginton:

> The features of these asylums were that they were soundly built, located in pleasant rural surroundings and were designed to afford patients a close relationship with nature. The focus of the treatment was not the patient but the attachment of the patient to the healing ability of natural and social environments. These principles can be seen in the great window space, verandas, large day rooms, galleries, gardens, greenhouses, sports facilities and farms.[40]

This is a description that could be applied to nearly all nineteenth-century asylums.

The location seems to have been a factor in the decision to send patients to Brislington. John Perceval wrote that, 'my family chose the situation for me partly on account of the beautiful scenery'.[41] However, he goes on to say that he felt that the scenery had the opposite effect on him: 'Their kindness was ill-judged; for I have no doubt the noble view excited my spirits, awakened by imagination, and redoubled every blow of affliction, reminding me of my former health and force of mind, and liberty.'[42] Rutherford has suggested that this response 'directly contradicted the reasoning for the provision of just such views for lunatics ever since the 1808 Lunatics Act'.[43] However, it could be argued that this was exactly the kind of effect that the proprietors hoped the landscape would have on the mind of the patient. This disconnect will be discussed in more detail below.

The idea of nature as a healing force, particularly for the mind, is one that Romantic poets such as William Wordsworth and Samuel Taylor Coleridge explored. For Wordsworth the important factor in developing these associations was a close relationship with the natural world. In 'The Prelude' (published posthumously in 1850, but begun in the 1790s), he described how his own mind was formed:

> thus from my first dawn
> Of childhood didst thou intertwine for me
> The passions that build up our human soul;
> Not with the mean and vulgar works of man,
> But with high objects, with enduring things –
> With life and Nature, purifying thus
> The elements of feeling and of thought[44]

Coleridge also believed that nature could have an important impact on the formative mind. In 'The Nightingale' (1798), he narrates the story of a child who wakes in tears during the night. The child is then taken into an orchard, where according to the poem, the sight of the moon hushes him and makes him laugh. Towards the conclusion of the poem he writes that:

> his childhood shall grow up
> Familiar with these songs, that with the night
> He may associate joy.[45]

In the same way that the Romantic poets believed nature could play a role in the formation of the minds of children, Wordsworth also suggested that it could help heal the adult mind. He viewed the relationship between nature and the human mind as one of 'mutual dependence' according to Ronald Gaskell.[46] Similarly, Louis James has suggested that in 'Lines Composed a Few Miles Above Tintern Abbey', 'landscape becomes more than a giver of heightened sensations: it is an active element working on the individual, a "medicine" for the soul suffering from the effects of weariness, doubt, and the pressures of an increasingly urbanised society'.[47] This idea concerning nature's therapeutic powers appears to have been popular during the great urbanisation of the nineteenth century. Evidence of this popularity is provided in the private diary of Lord Macaulay. On reading 'The Prelude', which was published posthumously in 1850, Macaulay recorded that 'there are the old raptures about mountains and cataracts; the old flimsy philosophy about the effect of scenery on the mind'.[48]

Whether or not the idea of the healing power of nature had become a bore to Macaulay, the Quakers at the York Retreat were still applying the theory of the association of ideas in the middle of the nineteenth century. In 1841, Samuel Tuke wrote that 'the cultivation and extension of the remaining healthy feelings and associations forms one of the most important parts of moral management'.[49] As the landscape was of great importance to the workings of the York Retreat, it can be assumed that it was expected to play a part in cultivating and extending feelings in the way Wordsworth described.

Similarly, W.A.F. Browne described how his utopian asylum should be placed upon a hill or summit so that patients could obtain therapeutic benefits from being exposed to the surrounding scenery:

> If the building is placed upon the summit or the slope of a rising ground, the advantages are incalculable. To many of those whose intellectual avenues to pleasure are forever closed, the mere extent of country affords delight; to some the beauty of wood and water, hill and dale, convey grateful impressions.[50]

In this description the scenery itself appears to be important. This is illustrated by the fact that the view from within the house could be considered as important as the patient spending time outside in the landscape. The *Cambridge Chronicle* described the Cambridgeshire Asylum (opened in 1858) as 'giving command of view of all places, as well in the house as out of doors'.[51] This suggests that the aesthetic aspects of the scenery were important in their own right as a form of therapy.

This does not mean that mental illness was seen solely as a mental disturbance during the nineteenth century. It could also be seen as a physical condition, or at least as having physical dimensions, which could then be treated with traditional purges, emetics, breedings and other physical remedies. According to Showalter, 'even when there was brain disease, and even when madness had set in, sanity might be restored by a regime that encouraged and supported the will'.[52] She has also suggested that asylum superintendents struggled to separate physically caused illnesses from moral ones. For example:

> Out of 411 men admitted to Colney Hatch [Middlesex, opened in 1851] in its first six months . . . 'physical' causes were identified for 140, including intemperance, masturbation, head injury, epilepsy, and fever. 'Moral' causes were indicated for 89 cases; these included domestic grief, unemployment, loss of property, jealousy, and 'over-excitement at the Great Exhibition'.[53]

An example of this medico-moral discourse can be found in the 1860 *Annual Report* of St Andrew's Hospital. The superintendent, Edwin Wing, suggested that efforts for the recovery and amelioration of patients was directed towards three general purposes:

> First, to promote a sound state of bodily health, by placing the patients under such circumstances as are most favourable to the correct performance of the function of the various organs of the body, such as appropriate diet, good clothing and lodging, pure air, exercise and judicious medical treatment. The first step to sound mind is a sound body. Second, comfort and ease, both of body and mind by the removal, as far as possible, of all sources of discomfort and irritation. Third, to divert the mind from a morbid train of thought and feeling, and prevent it preying upon itself by directing it into new and more healthful channel . . . in short by the employment of the various means ranged under the general heading of moral treatment.[54]

This shows how closely the medical and moral aspects of insanity and its treatment were intertwined. Similarly this discourse was used in relation to decision-making concerning where an asylum should be located and the design and use of the surrounding landscape. However, as Philo argues, much of the medical discourse in relation to location was not specifically concerned with madness but was related to the physical health of patients.[55] For example, Browne's description of the medical reasons for a rural location can be compared with the rhetoric used in relation to general hospitals of the same period:[56]

> It certainly is indispensable that the situation chosen should be healthy, that it should possess the advantage of a dry cultivated soil and an ample supply of water, that it should be so far in the country as to have an unpolluted atmosphere.[57]

The 'unpolluted atmosphere' described here is one free of miasmata – corruptions of the air which were thought to cause disease.[58]

For most of the nineteenth century it was believed that urbanisation brought with it an unhealthy polluted atmosphere, so in order to improve or maintain the physical health of the patients a rural location was essential: 'The chief medical emphasis in this respect was on basic conditions of hygiene, healthiness, "sanitation" and "salubriousness" that could only properly be maintained in the woods, hills and rivers of natural *milieux* beyond the polluted "close spaces" of the city.'[59] There were also considerable outbreaks of diseases such as cholera, which in the first part of the century were believed to be caused by miasmata. However, even after the miasma theory of disease causation was replaced by that of germ theory (the anthrax bacillus was identified by Robert Koch in 1876), rural situations were still seen as important, as Rutherford's research on the increasing size of asylum estates into the twentieth century testifies.

Environment and classification

While both Ticehurst and Brislington had similar ornamented landscapes and rural locations with far-reaching views, the architecture of the two main buildings and the designs of the gardens closest to them were entirely different. Ticehurst was adapted from an earlier estate so 'ground plans of the asylum which appeared in a prospectus in 1828 suggest the layout of a country mansion, with no system of classification'.[60] However Brislington (Figure 7) was purpose-built and the main asylum building embodied in physical form Fox's ideas on the therapeutic effect of the environment.[61] According to one of his descendants, Annie Fox, 'when first built, the Asylum consisted of the main central block with three

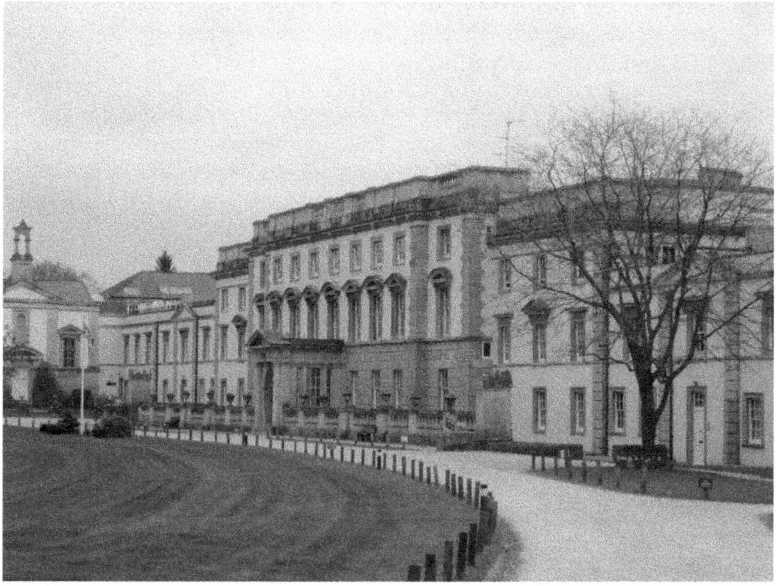

Figure 7 Photograph of Brislington House – now converted into flats and known as Long Fox Manor. Like the York Retreat, the approach to the house used to terminate at a circular grass area and the general impression was that of a Regency gentry house.

detached blocks on either side, connected on the basement'.[62] The arrangement of the house in three central blocks is clearly depicted on the etching which was used as an illustration in an early prospectus for the asylum dating from the mid-1800s.[63] This plan was related to Fox's belief in a therapeutic regime based on segregation and classification by gender, medical symptoms, and the patients' social and financial backgrounds.[64] There appear to have been several ideas converging here, which were being expressed through the design of the building and grounds.

Segregation by gender was already common in many institutions and reflected current moral sensibilities. However, segregation on the basis of disease diagnosis reflected the changes that had taken place in medicine during the eighteenth century. The Scientific Revolution of the seventeenth century heavily influenced medicine during the following period. One outcome was the desire to create a nosology, or classification of diseases, and this resulted in texts such as Karl Von Linné Linnaeus's pioneering *Genera Morborum* (Types of Diseases) published in 1763.

From the description of the 1815 Parliamentary Committee, and Fox's own prospectus, it seems that Brislington was a physical extension of this same desire to classify disease:

> Sept 21st, 1815, I called at Dr Fox's, a house near Bristol. Dr Fox has laid out a very large sum of money upon building an establishment, this being a series of houses for the purpose of classification . . . Three different houses are devoted to three different classes of female patients. To the left are three houses for the male patients.[65]

In the prospectus Fox describes this in more detail in relation to the separation of those patients presenting with a physical disease alongside their mental illness from those suffering solely from insanity:

> The smallest house on either side is for such persons of the respective sex, who, having some bodily disease superadded to the mental affection, require different accommodation as to quietness and regimen, or demand an exclusive treatment to prevent contagion.[66]

The organisation by social and financial factors relates to the idea of the asylum as a place that maintained a similar domestic setting to that in which the patient was exposed in everyday life outside the asylum. According to Fox:

> The individuals of one class never see or have intercourse with those of another. As the accommodations vary in proportion to the class, this arrangement prevents invidious comparisons. It is grateful by humouring the prejudices of men in respect to rank in society, and it is useful by preventing persons of rank and quality from an indiscriminate association with those of inferior manners and condition; which, otherwise might lead to inconvenient, if not detrimental acquaintance.[67]

Although this reflects a general awareness of class and its social conventions, it also appears to be related to the idea that in order for the asylum to be a therapeutic place it needed to reflect the domestic world outside. John Perceval describes the domestic arrangements of the house in some detail and from his descriptions it is possible to suggest that the domestic setting provided by Fox for wealthy patients was similar to that which they would expect in any residence outside the asylum. Perceval even recognises this as such himself, when he writes that, 'my dinner in this room was served on a tray, with a napkin, silver forks, decanters, &c. &c., and in these respects, such as was fitting for a gentleman'.[68] Similarly, Rutherford has written that at the York Retreat the use of a hedge as a boundary, as well as specially adapted window frames, was 'to prevent the estate appearing to be a place of confinement'.[69] She goes on to say that 'this exemplifies the introduction of a domestic theme in the scale and character of asylum building'.[70]

The segregation within the house was also extended to the gardens outside. Originally the airing courts consisted of six walled areas to the east (garden front) of the house.[71] These were accessed directly from the patients' day rooms. They were segregated in the same way as the building, so that, according to Fox, 'each class inhabits a distinct house, detached from the others by an interval of eighteen feet, with a separate court for the exercise of the patients'.[72] These courts were originally terminated 'to the east by a continuous range of cells to accommodate the refractory patients'.[73] Similarly the gardens at the private Charenton Hospital on the outskirts of Paris were organised by the classification of patients: '[Jean Etienne Dominique] Esquirol provided a summary division as follows: the violently insane, to be accommodated in two yards; senile patients also in two yards, epileptics, in one or two yards; monomaniacs and melancholics in one yard; convalescents in one yard, undisturbed patients in one yard.'[74]

Fox also wrote that the patients were allowed to exercise in the courts 'whenever they please', and that the courts themselves had elevated ground so that the patients could 'view the surrounding country, while a border sloping towards the wall secures them from escape'.[75] The elevated ground within the courts was not necessarily just a simple raised area in the centre. From the detailed plans made in 1843 (Figure 8) it seems that one of the courts contained a 'snail mount', a mound whose summit would be reached by a path winding around it in a spiral. This use of mounts was consistent with the original purpose of their design. Dating from the Tudor period, raised ground was often used to 'provide a view over the wall'.[76]

Mounts had generally gone out of fashion by the eighteenth century, probably because walls had been removed and replaced with ha-has on country estates.[77] However, they solved the asylum problem of combining security with curative views of nature.[78] The boundary wall that separated the courts from the countryside beyond was graduated so that it was lower across the central section of the courts than at either end. This reduction in height also increased the ease with which patients could view the surrounding landscape. Each of these courts also had 'a walk round it under the Walls'.[79]

Another interesting development at this time was the use of birds to amuse the patients. At Brislington there was a 'distinct and separate yard;

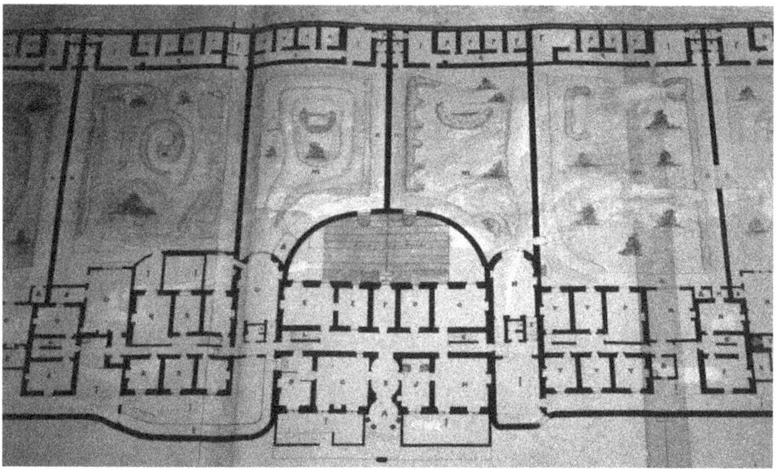

Figure 8 This detail from an 1843 plan of Brislington House shows the design of the airing courts. Paths and shrubberies are clearly depicted and a snail mount can be seen in the airing court on the left.

in these yards were silver pheasants and doves with which the patients amuse themselves'.[80] Similarly the York Retreat had a collection of birds and the following description explains why they were considered to be an important part of the patients' therapy:

> The superintendent has also endeavoured to furnish a source of amusement, to those patients whose walks are necessarily more circumscribed, by supplying each of the courts with a number of animals; such as rabbits, sea-gulls, hawks, and poultry. These creatures are generally very familiar with the patients: and it is believed they are not only the means of innocent pleasure; but that the intercourse with them, sometimes tends to awaken the social and benevolent feelings.[81]

As late as 1902, the *York Retreat Annual Report* noted that: 'An aviary, 30 feet by 21 feet, for the golden pheasants has been erected . . . The damage done to the garden by the pheasants was considerable, and though it used to be very pleasant to see when running about amongst the patients, it was felt that flowers would be generally more attractive.'[82] This suggests that the therapeutic effect of the birds could also be somewhat problematic.

There is a description of the courts at Brislington dating from 1874, which indicates that they were small walled gardens rather than the bare courts described at Bethlem in the previous century. The Rev. Kilvert wrote:

> Mrs Hopton [the matron] accompanied us out on to a nice large lawn, in which stood a magnificent weeping willow. There was a high ivied wall running round three sides of this lawn and the house bounded it on the fourth. Aunt Emma was sitting on a low seat in a sunny corner doing some work, with a cat or two cats on her lap.[83]

By the time this observation was made the courts had been amalgamated so that rather than three airing courts for each gender there were just two, and the original ornamental layout of snail mounts and walks had been simplified.[84]

Later developments in the layout of the airing courts also include an arcade. This was built some time before 1836 and the Drs Fox described how 'an arcade extends throughout the length of these courts, affording exercise in wet weather'.[85] This reinforces the notion that they considered exercise to be curative and that they encouraged their patients to walk as much as possible. An impression of the courts with their associated planting can also be obtained from the engraving used in the 1836 prospectus.[86]

Airing courts, however, were never intended to be the patients' sole place of outdoor recreation, except in the most severe cases.[87] Tuke described the limitations of the airing courts at the York Retreat:

> I cannot, however, forbear observing, that the courts appear to be too small, and to admit of too little variety, to invite the patient to take exercise. The boundary of his excursion is always before his eye; which must have a gloomy effect on the already depressed mind. This might be considered a serious defect, if it was not generally compensated, by taking such patients as are suitable, into the garden; and by frequent excursions into the city or the surrounding country, and into the fields of the Institution.[88]

Similarly, Brislington and Ticehurst had a variety of pleasure grounds, fields and shrubberies.

Use of the wider landscape

The importance of having green space outside the asylum for the use of patients, particularly for walking and recreation, developed through the first decades of the nineteenth century to such an extent that, in 1847, the Commissioners in Lunacy stated in their rules for new asylums that:

> The airing courts, pleasure grounds, gardens and fields annexed to an asylum, should be of such an extent as to afford the patients ample means of exercise and recreation, as well as the healthful employment out of doors: and should, as far as possible, be in the ratio of at least one acre to ten patients.[89]

By this time the Commissioners also believed that having grounds of a suitable size and diversity actually reduced the need for mechanical restraint within the asylums. For example, they criticised Hoxton House, London, as it had been run in 1815, because it was 'deficient in the extent and number of its airing grounds, and, as a consequence, the use of mechanical restraint has prevailed here more than in many other establishments'.[90] It would seem that at this time they believed that the grounds surrounding an asylum were the key to the effectiveness and implementation of moral therapy.

The idea of employment, entertainment and amusement in the open air was particularly important in relation to the idea of moral treatment. According to the Lunacy Commissioners in 1847, 'employment in agricultural labour and in gardening; and recreation in the open air, are most advantageous as they tend not only to occupy the mind but to improve the bodily strength and promote a healthy state of the natural functions'.[91] In fact they believed in this so strongly that they proposed the following rule for the government of lunatic asylums:

> That, during the day, the patients of both sexes be employed as much as practicable out of doors; the men in gardening and husbandry, the women in occupations suited to their ability; and that, as a principle in treatment, endeavours be continually used to occupy the minds of the patients, to induce them to take exercise in the open air, and to promote cheerfulness and happiness amongst them.[92]

These rules may have been influenced by the practical experiences at the York Retreat. In the 1839 *Annual Report* Samuel Tuke stated that:

> The employment of the patients has always been deemed an object of great importance in the Retreat. It has from the commencement of the Establishment, been extensively introduced amongst the women; and a considerable number of the men, have also been from time to time engaged in the garden and other occupation. Particular care has been exercised to endeavour to lead the convalescent patients into some regular employment, adapted to their taste or former habits; and there can be no doubt that these engagements have been highly salutary, but the attempts to introduce

a *general system* of employment amongst the men patients, have heretofore proved unsuccessful. These experiments have usually been made more with reference to mechanical and agricultural work; but the Committee, encouraged by the success of several other Establishments, determined to make an effort to induce a number of the men, heretofore wholly unemployed, to engage in gardening and agricultural labour.[93]

Rutherford argues that this use of the wider landscape 'was the most innovative development of the asylum estate . . . its novel purpose being specifically for the therapeutic use of patients'.[94]

It should be noted that even institutions such as the York Retreat, which admitted Quakers from various backgrounds, did not employ a great number of people in agricultural work – John Thurnam, the resident surgeon in 1842 wrote that concerning employment:

The proportion, it will be seen, is almost the same as in preceding years; and the advantage which has accrued to such of the men as have been occupied in the open air, has been quite as decided; both as regards the improvement in the general health, and in some cases as promoting the more complete restoration of the convalescent. The proportion of men who are employed, though less than in many of the larger asylums, is perhaps nearly as large as could be expected, when the previous habits and circumstances of many of the patients at the Retreat, (and particularly the greater average age to which the patients attain in our establishment) are considered.[95]

So employment rates seem to have been dependent upon age, class and gender, even when outdoor labour was seen as an important therapeutic tool.

Finding outdoor employment for patients other than walking and games does not appear to have been particularly easy during the early years of Brislington. In 1815 the Parliamentary Committee reported that 'the Doctor does all he can to lead them to employ themselves, but he [Fox] remarked that it is difficult to give employment to gentlemen'.[96] In his 1804–9 prospectus, Fox stated that 'the more useful employments of Agriculture and Mechanism are preferred for those who are willing to undertake them'.[97] However, this probably only refers to the pauper and lower-class patients as an English Heritage report, related to the heritage listing of the landscape, describes these patients as being 'employed on manual work' while 'those of middle and upper class backgrounds [took] walks and exercise in the grounds under supervision'.[98]

By the 1830s, changes had occurred which appear to have reflected wider social changes outside the walls of the asylum. Perceval, son of a former prime minister and in receipt of a considerable private fortune, described how he became involved in practical gardening and helped to cut a walk through the shrubbery during his time at the asylum:

> Soon after liberty of limb had been restored to me, my mother, to whose exertions I owe, after all, whatever was likely to restore me to sound reason whilst under the care of Dr. F., begged that I might be allowed to work in his garden; this was indeed beneficial, as it gave me occupation and more privacy. Later in the year I was employed with two gentlemen and a keeper, to cut out a small path in the shrubbery. I was entrusted with the mattock and the spade.[99]

It is clear that the younger Drs Fox believed strongly that this type of exercise had curative properties as they state that 'many of the most favourable results which have occurred in their practice ought to be mainly attributed to the constant succession of bodily exercise, and to the variety of mental recreation which is provided for their patients'.[100]

This idea was not reserved solely for those suffering from psychiatric disorders. The garden writer, John Claudius Loudon, believed that gardening was beneficial to everyone's health:

> Thus, it is not only a condition of our nature, that, in order to secure health and cheerfulness, we must labour; but we must also labour in such a way as to produce something useful or agreeable. Now, of the different kinds of useful things produced by labour, those things, surely, which are living beings, and which grow and undergo changes before our eyes must be more productive of enjoyment than such as are mere brute matter; the kind of labour, and other circumstances, being the same.[101]

Although, by 1836, gardening was considered suitable employment for gentlemen at Brislington, the doctors still struggled to find suitable employment for ladies:

> It is more difficult to engage the females in much bodily exercise; but, besides a daily promenade and the regulated use of musical instruments, it is found easy to interest this portion of patients in mechanical occupations, which, next to muscular exertions in the open air, may be considered as the most favourable employment for the insane.[102]

However, given the class of patients at Ticehurst and Brislington, the patients would have been more likely to be engaged in gentle recreational pursuits such as bowling rather than agricultural employment.

Herman Merivale described how his time as a patient was occupied while at Ticehurst, 'with carriages to take me out for drives, closed upon wet days, open on fine; with cricket and bowls and archery for the summer, and a pack of harriers to follow across country in the winter'.[103] To the front of Brislington there was a bowling-green which was created when the house was opened by Fox, and somewhere within the grounds there was also a fives court.[104] By 1836 other forms of exercise included 'grounds for cricket, foot-ball and other athletic amusements; and in the proper season, parties with greyhounds extend their walks round the neighbouring country in search of game'.[105] The flat area directly in front of the house was later used for croquet.[106]

This use of the asylum landscape, particularly for cricket, continued throughout the nineteenth century and has been discussed in detail by Steven Cherry and Roger Munting.[107] It seems that the patients were not always keen on the emphasis on exercise and recreation. Merivale wrote that:

> Of the cricket I had enough on my first visit, and would not run the gauntlet again. To some sort of distraction I was often driven by despair; for the constitutionals round the mile-circuit of the grounds, or along the lanes and roads, were maddening. The Sunday walks were the worst, when the British villager was out on holiday, and gaped and wondered at us. In the winter months I made occasional attempts to follow the pack of harriers which was kept for our benefit – which at all events amused the warders and country-siders a good deal.[108]

Notwithstanding such complaints, the concept that accessible outdoor space was essential certainly increased amongst those running the asylums. When the York Retreat opened in 1796 the *Annual Report* stated that 'about eleven acres of ground, in a very eligible situation near York, have been purchased, and a House erected'. However by 1839, more ground was being purchased at the Retreat, partly to reflect the growing size of the institution but also to extend the amount of land available for activities:

> A purchase has been recently made of nine acres of land, on the western side of the property belonging to the Institution, and almost immediately adjoining the buildings allotted to the women patients . . . It will allow of an increase of the women's airing courts, or gardens, which has long been thought desirable, and will afford the opportunity of a greater extension of the walks within the boundary of the establishment. The buildings are now surrounded by about 27 acres of excellent land, adding much to the adaptation of the place, to the wants of its inmates, by the variety and employment which it affords.[109]

By 1841 Tuke could report that:

> The fields recently purchased adjoining the women's wing, have afforded the opportunity of improved and more select airing grounds and gardens for that department – a long terrace walk within the inclosure, commands and extensive view of the city and surrounding country . . . They afford also the opportunity of ample and agreeable walks within their own inclosure, which is a point of great importance as a means of treatment and of enjoyment to the patients.[110]

The improvements continued so that by 1870:

> The Ladies' pleasure grounds have been enlarged and beautified by throwing down the fences between them and Laurel Hill, giving the Patients access at all times to the winding paths leading round it to the Summerhouse upon it. The Committee have sanctioned the erection of a covered alcove to reach from the Western porch to the first arbour, by which the female patients will be enabled to walk under shelter both from the rain and from the heat of the sun, without losing enjoyment either of the fresh air or the garden.[111]

This establishes that the provision of spaces in which walking could take place, both covered and open, and with objects of interest to walk to, such as a summerhouse, were of continual, and even increasing, importance throughout the nineteenth century.

At Ticehurst, 'perhaps emulating the varied walks advocated as therapeutic by Samuel Tuke in 1813, Charles and Jesse employed men who had been demobilized after the battle of Waterloo to landscape and ornament over forty acres of grounds in 1816. Over two miles of footpaths led through plantations, orchard and gardens, past summer houses.'[112] The ornamented landscape reflected trends in gardening fashions, particularly the interest in the Chinese and the Gothic which developed in the mid-eighteenth century. According to Horace Walpole in 1750, 'everybody is improving their places . . . I mean temples bridges etc., are generally Gothic or Chinese and give a whimsical air of novelty that is very pleasing'.[113] This popularity for exotic irregularity in both buildings and planting, as well as the desire to surprise visitors within the garden, led to a number of pattern books being created so that owners could choose a style of garden building. These included William Halfpenny's *Rural Architecture in the Chinese Taste* (1750), William and John Halfpenny's *Chinese and Gothic Architecture Properly Ornamented* (1752) and William Chambers' *Designs of Chinese Buildings* (1757). This encouraged an eclecticism of garden design, which was still influential in the Regency period. This is demonstrated by the building of the oriental-influenced Royal Pavilion in Brighton (1822), and, in 1826, designs for Vauxhall Gardens in London, depicted a 'Chinese entrance reflecting a renewed interest in Chinese architecture among the wealthy and fashion conscious'.[114] The garden buildings at Ticehurst can be seen to be part of this trend and to be similarly fashionable.

Similarly, at Brislington the doctors also created a range of diverse walks within the estate. There appear to have been wooded walks running through the shelter belt plantations around the edge of the main grounds surrounding the house. Walking south from the front of the house there were a number of walks including a serpentine, raised promenade.[115] The importance of walking as part of the therapy cannot be underestimated. The patients were even taken for walks further afield than the immediate estate. While at Brislington, Perceval described how 'very often we walked out in the fields, and to farm-houses in the neighbourhood . . . I walked for usually one hour before dinner, sometimes for an hour after dinner. After some time, I accompanied the other patients, who walked out in a body, with two or three keepers, and we went through the villages.'[116] Similarly, during his time at Ticehurst walking was advocated even after he had attempted to abscond; 'the centrality of at least moderate exercise to the regimen practiced at Ticehurst may be inferred from the fact that the day after his escape attempt, Perceval was allowed to go out for a walk, although accompanied by two attendants rather than one'.[117]

Within the pleasure grounds, and offering points of interest on the walks, there were a number of garden features. As mentioned above, the York Retreat landscape contained a summerhouse placed on top of a mound. This rustic summerhouse had wide-ranging views and was approached by a winding path (Figure 9). At Ticehurst the array of garden features was in line with the gardens created by the landed gentry. According to Mackenzie, the profits obtained from the patients 'were ploughed back to improve the attributes of the asylum'. As one 'obituarist rather laconically expressed it: there was always some new conservatory or aviary, some pagoda or flower garden, some evergreen alley or artificial fountain, to construct, in order to make the place more attractive and comfortable'.[118]

However, as Philo has discussed in detail, all these attractions may not have been viewed as entirely therapeutic by the inmates.[119] In a discussion of Mabel Etchell's fictitious account, *Ten Years in a Lunatic Asylum*, a text which he convincingly argues is based on the author's personal knowledge

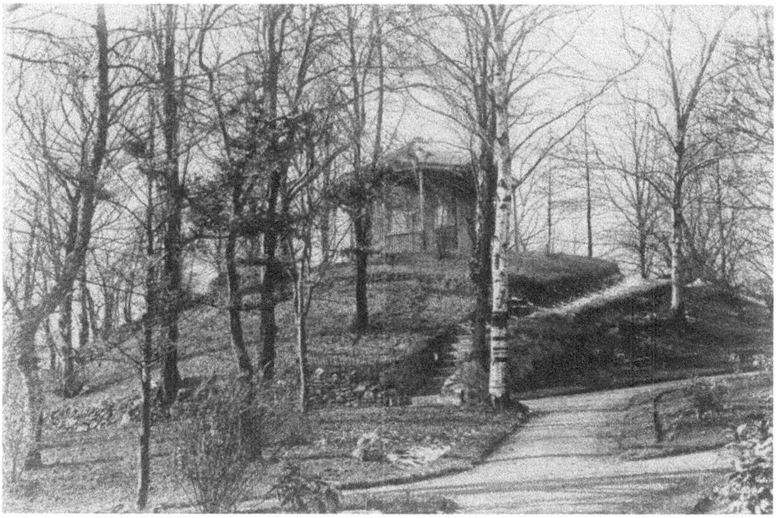

Figure 9 The summerhouse at the York Retreat, which was built on the top of an existing hill and reached by way of a winding path, rather like the snail mount at Brislington. From an album of photographs, c.1900.

of the asylum system, Philo explored the darker side of the asylum landscape. In relation to the private madhouse in Etchell's book, known as Hygeria Lodge (a play on Hygeia, the goddess of health perhaps), he states that 'it is salient to consider the rural angle in more depth and to underscore that Hygeria Lodge is painted as lost in rural surroundings cut off from the sights, sounds and smells of the urban realm'.[120] As Philo eloquently discusses, this is of course a problem of the rural asylum – it is disconnected from the urban world. Etchell describes how:

> the garden of Hygeria Lodge might in some respects be called itself a sepulchre, its high walls and dark foliage scarcely concealing the occupants within; who, amid its silence and seclusion, buried the hopes and joys of their former existence in one common grave, half-hidden in the leaves and flowers that grew upon its margin.[121]

This is a much darker image of the asylum garden than the one projected by superintendents, doctors and others involved in the business of treating those classed as mad. Etchell also argues that:

> The costly buildings, the enchanted pleasure-grounds, beautiful strains of music, and the well-dressed inmates and dependants with their autocratic

lord (even the doctor himself) at the head, are often the only visions presented to the minds of those who trouble to associate the poor lunatic even for a few moments in their minds, without looking behind the scenes, or recollecting that the traces of the serpent which once lurked in the beauteous shrubs and flowers of the primal Eden are printed here in burning-fire.[122]

The gardens here are depicted as gilded cages surveyed and monitored by the autocratic doctor. As a contrast to the usual positive imagery of the garden of Eden with its lack of disease and death, Etchell instead sees it as a place containing the serpent, hidden amongst the shrubberies and ornate pleasure grounds. This is a very different impression of the garden but one that is equally powerful.

Philo also utilises the example of the poet William Cowper, known for his love of the natural world, to argue that the poem 'The Shrubbery' illustrates the ineffectiveness of nature as a cure for someone in a state of distress. In these examples the landscape becomes dark, threatening and not all it seems on first glance. Similarly Richard Paternoster, who spent a short time as a patient in William Finch's madhouse in Kensington, wrote a commentary in which he 'he indicates that his time spent walking the gardens of Finch's madhouse were far from uplifting, being instead destined to leave him ever more "forlorn and wretched"'.[123] Philo argues that this is where 'a gulf of sorts hence opens up between the geographical attributes of madhouses as envisaged by the powerful running the system and as perceived by the powerless enduring it'.[124] It is a reminder that the Chinese galleries, ornamental cottages (or *cottages ornées* as they were referred to), aviaries, moss houses and other seductive elements of the picturesque asylum garden may have felt as much of a prison as the bare airing courts of Bethlem in the earlier period. They too could cause isolation and distress.

As the seductive gardens at Ticehurst are depicted in the asylum's prospectus, one can certainly see them as advertising tools and the vision that Etchell suggests people were encouraged to see. However, they also represent the keen gardening talents of the Newington doctors. According to Merivale, the superintendent 'was happier in his own little house, at some distance from the asylum, where he lived, with one of the unfortunates under his immediate eye. He pottered about among a large variety of baby greenhouses, which he had constructed on patterns of his own, or made geological investigations under his fields.'[125] Similarly at Brislington one of the Fox doctors was known for his fashionably Victorian obsession with ferns.[126] By 1870, Ticehurst was apparently renowned for its garden: 'the Commissioners in 1864 state that the grounds and gardens were in a state which "could hardly be surpassed". In the early 1870s an "Italian garden" was laid out, containing ornamental fountains. By 1877, land owned by the Newingtons around the asylum extended over 200 acres, and the asylum's reliable profits were used to subsidise their less profitable farm.'[127]

This fascination with farming and gardening can be read as a particular personal interest of the Newington and Fox families, or even as a significant gentlemanly occupation. In the late eighteenth century, physicians seem to have had an interest in agriculture and gardening. In 1793, Thomas Baird described how the pioneering surgeon, John Hunter, 'is trying many experiments, which may be of considerable service, both to the gardener and the husbandman' at his villa at Earl's Court.[128] He goes on to describe him as 'very curious in plants' and that he 'has in his green-houses and hot-houses a great variety of the most choice and rare productions of nature, in the collection of which he has neither spared pains or expense'.[129] Edward Jenner was also trialling manure experiments at Berkeley in Gloucestershire which he outlined in a letter to Joseph Banks. Michael Brown has discussed this relationship in relation to the York physician, Alexander Hunter. He argues that 'agricultural knowledge was polite knowledge. It was not only aesthetically pleasing, but also morally improving, allowing for deep reflection on the wonders of Providence . . . Such pursuits were, by their very nature, leisured. By taking an active interest in natural history and agriculture, Hunter announced that he had the time, the money and the intellectual freedom becoming a gentleman.'[130] It is possible that some of these elements come into play when analysing the complex estates at both Brislington and Ticehurst, and is an area where further research might be enlightening.

Within the Brislington estate there was also a primitive stone seating area (Figure 10) and a number of cottages. At the edge of the north side of the estate there was a wooded area that formed a separate pleasure garden, which ran along the top of the steep-sided Avon valley. From the Tithe Map there appears to have been a walk that ran along the cliff top past the site of a 'Battery'. We know that the patients were taken along this walk as Perceval describes it, and its dangers, very clearly:

> Dr. F.'s madhouse stood in a very fine and picturesque country, and near a steep and wooded bank that bordered the river. At one elevated spot that commanded a view down the valley, a natural or artificial precipice yawned in the red soil, crowned with a small parapet, in rear of which was a small

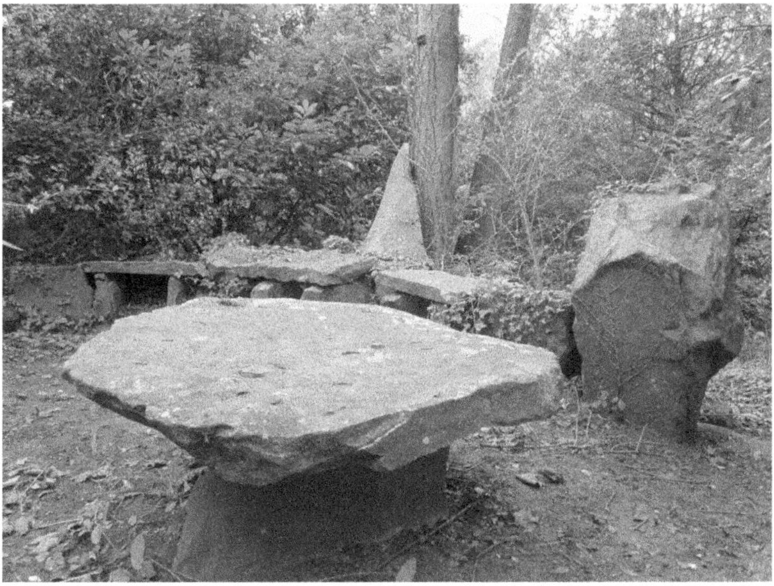

Figure 10 This primitive-looking stone table with benches and standing stones is presumably the Grotto at Brislington mentioned on the 1843 Tithe Map. It is situated on a raised viewing point, from which Lansdown Hill and its Iron Age hill-fort can be seen. There was originally an ornate metal fence (the panels of which were situated in the shelter underneath on this visit).

> terrace and a summerhouse. When I went out with the patients we were often conducted here. They called it the battery. The view was enchanting, but I looked down on the people working and the boats moving in the valley, with feelings that they were dead to me, and I dead to them . . . And after the second visit I did not approach the parapet, but sat in the summerhouse to avoid the temptation. The other patients sat on the battery. I consider it a most imprudent place to take them to.[131]

There is no longer any sign of the parapet or the summerhouse, but a photograph of the summerhouse exists (Figure 11). This is another rustic building, reminiscent of the illustration for a 'rustic thatched hovel, on the summit of a naked brow, commanding views in every direction' in Humphry Repton's *Observations on the Theory of Landscape Gardening* of 1803.[132] There are illustrations of similar rustic shelters in Loudon's *The Surburban Gardener and Villa Companion.*[133]

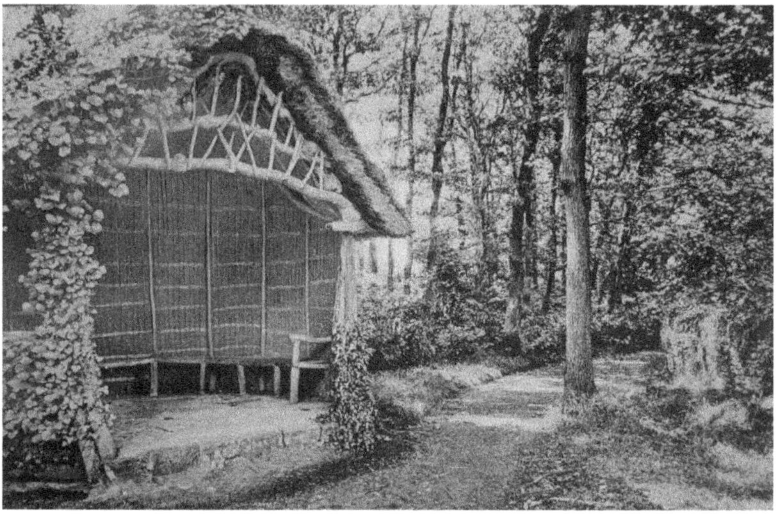

Figure 11 The rustic shelter pictured above is inscribed as being the 'Battery Summer House' in an album of photographs taken of Brislington c.1900. It can be assumed that this is the same summerhouse that Perceval described as being located near the Battery on the cliff-top walk.

The ornamented cottage and the influence of Regency style

Although Fox states that there were separate houses on the estate in his early account of the asylum (1804–9), it appears that most of the estate houses were built over the first twenty years of the asylum's existence.[134] Annie Fox, in her *A Short Account of Brislington House, 1804 to 1906*, states that 'in 1816 the detached cottage called Lanesborough Cottage was built for Lord Lanesborough, and in 1819 Carysfort Cottage was built for a peer of that name'; she also says that Heath House was built by Fox in 1825.[135] This suggests that the estate developed over a period of time and was not necessarily fully formed when the asylum opened in 1804–6.

Other later institutions had similar cottages. At the Northampton General Asylum a picturesque *cottage ornée*, thought to date from around 1858, was described as being for the use of lady patients (Figure 12).[136] Like the cottages at Brislington, the General Lunatic Asylum cottage also had a conservatory, and the garden portrayed in the engraving is laid out in the 'Gardenesque' style, which was fashionable during the first

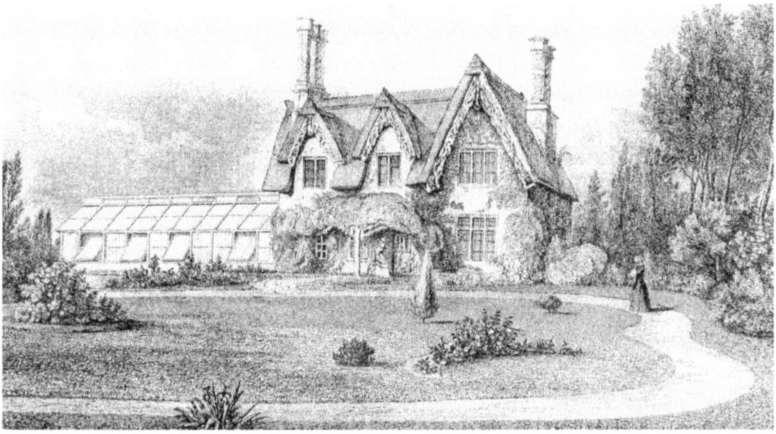

Figure 12 Ornamental cottage at the Northampton General Lunatic Asylum for the use of lady patients, illustrated in a similar picturesque style, with Gardenesque planting, as the cottages at Brislington House. There is also a large conservatory attached to the building, presumably for the use of patients.

half of the nineteenth century. Loudon was the main proponent of the Gardenesque style and described it as:

> the production of that kind of scenery which is best calculated to display the individual beauty of trees, shrubs and plants in a state of culture; the smoothness and greenness of lawns; and the smooth surfaces, curved directions, dryness and firmness of gravel walks; in short, the gardenesque style is calculated for displaying the art of the gardener.[137]

This can be seen in photographs of the gardens associated with the cottages at Brislington.[138] The sole use by lady patients of the Northampton cottage reflects the classification of the patients within the hospital, which was also practised at Brislington.

The use of cottages reflected a growth in the popularity of the cottage as a residence suitable for classes other than the poor. James Malton's *British Cottage Architecture* of 1798 attempted to portray cottages as being as picturesque as castles: 'These picturesque vernacular cottages could be built, not only for peasants and farmers but as "retreats for gentlemen".'[139] Jane Austen described the use of a cottage as a gentleman's residence in *Sense and Sensibility* through the character of Mr Robert Ferrars: '"For my own part," said he, "I am excessively fond of a cottage; there is always so much comfort, so much elegance about them . . . I advise everybody who is going to build, to build a cottage".'[140] Austen, who was always very acute in her observations, was responding to the Regency trend for building cottages as residences for the upper classes. However, it is possible that she did not entirely approve of such ideas as her heroine, Elinor, agrees with Ferrar's overwhelmingly enthusiastic monologue on cottages only because 'she did not think he deserved the compliment of rational opposition'.[141] According to Giles Worsley, inspirations for this fashion included 'the vernacular architecture of the South of England, and in particular cottages portrayed by contemporary painters', such as Thomas Gainsborough.[142]

A number of cottages were built on the Brislington estate. These had a variety of uses. The Beeches was built to house the Fox family, the Lodge or Wheelhouse contained the mechanism for opening the gates and four other cottages were built, of which at least two were designed to house upper-class patients. Fox's sons ran the asylum from the 1830s and they wrote that, although they generally believed in the efficacy of social interaction between the patients:

> There are some cases is which it may be more judicious to avoid the former, and to place the patient at some distance from scenes that may engage too much of his attention. For such persons there are upon the estate houses . . . some of which are at present inhabited by members of the nobility, who are accommodated with servants from the institution; and are allowed to pursue any style of living and expense as to carriages, horses, &c. most suitable to their former habits, and not inconsistent to their present situation.[143]

Although the Brislington cottages are classed as 'houses' in both the prospectuses, Annie Fox states that at least two of them were originally called cottages, Carysfort Cottage and Lanesborough Cottage.[144] Carysfort Cottage (Figure 13) also appears to have become known as the Swiss Cottage by 1827, as in a pencil and sepia wash of the cottage of this date by T.L.S. Rowbotham it is given this name.[145] It may be that, given the variety of buildings on the estate, the term 'cottages' rather than 'houses' was used, thereby conferring on them the added status of picturesque objects in the landscape.

This reflected the growing interest in cottages as picturesque residences designed for the upper classes. According to Edmund Bartell in 1804:

> A Cottage, to use the word in its literal sense, means a house of small dimensions, appropriated to the use of the lower class of people; but to buildings of this description, the fashion of the present day has added one which bears a distinct character, and is known as by the appellation of the

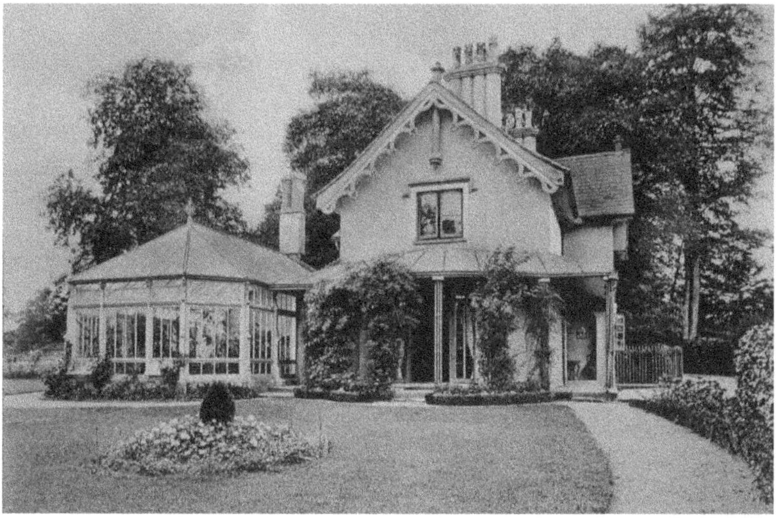

Figure 13 The Swiss (or Carysfort) Cottage at Brislington with conservatory and Regency style verandah, from an undated album thought to be c.1900.

> ornamented, or adorned cottage . . . As a retreat from the hurry of a town-life, the ornamented cottage is rational and elegant . . . Of late, the ornamented cottage has frequently become the residence of people of fortune.[146]

This view was held well into the nineteenth century, as in 1832 J.B. Papworth suggested that 'the cottage orné is a new species in the building of domestic architecture, and it is subject to its own laws of fitness and propriety. It is not the habitation of the laborious, but of the affluent, of the man of study, of science, or of leisure.'[147]

The design of the cottages at Brislington, with their trefoil patterned barge-boards and verandas, suggests that they were intended to form part of the picturesque landscape and provide interest during walks – although in this case, the cottages also allowed extra privacy for the titled and gave them the option of being accompanied by their own servants while they were resident at Brislington. Other influences of Regency style can be seen in the canopies projecting from the rear of the main building at Brislington, the training of plants up the external walls of the cottages and the conservatories attached to both the main house and the cottages. Regency blinds are also shown in a photograph of one of the cottages.

Both the engravings from the 1836 prospectus and some of the undated photographs show plants, which appear to be mainly ivy, trained in

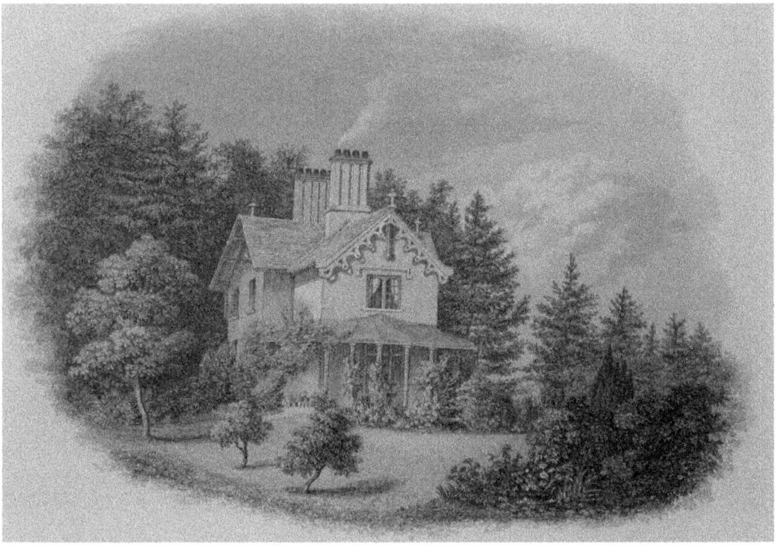

Figure 14 The picturesque Swiss Cottage depicted almost being subsumed by the garden in true Regency style, reproduced in the prospectus. Note also the ornamental barge-boards on the house and the verandah with climbing plants.

picturesque fashion up the walls (Figure 14). At the York Retreat ivy was encouraged to grow up the front of the building and as late as 1896 the *Annual Report* stated that ivy should be planted to cover blank walls wherever possible.[148] According to Batey, 'many pattern books for cottages ornées showed walls "adapted to receive trained foliage"'.[149] The attractive iron verandas were also used as supports for plants. According to Repton, 'there are many plants, such as jasmine and creepers, requiring the support of a wall, which so clothed, forms a luxurious decoration to a garden in summer; and by ivy, and other evergreens, may partly be extended through the year'.[150] This reflected the Regency love of the picturesque, including buildings that were secluded and half-hidden by plants, and the movement to blur the boundaries between the house and the garden.

The therapeutic role of the gardens and landscape

Given the lack of documentary evidence, particularly for Brislington, it is difficult to determine exactly why the gardens were designed in the way they were and why picturesque elements were included within the landscape. Before looking at the various roles this type of landscape played within the asylum setting, it should be noted that the cost of creating complex landscapes would have restricted such designs to institutions with a wealthy clientele. This is likely to have been the most important factor linking them to elite private asylums. Picturesque features such as grottos, ornate aviaries, pagodas and ornamental cottages would also have helped to create a setting that 'wealthy patients and their relations would at once recognise and be able to relate to as a typical domestic setting of their own socio-economic class'.[151] This was of great importance at the time, as the establishment of a familiar domestic setting was required for the successful implementation of moral therapy.[152]

It is possible to speculate that the picturesque elements would have performed a rhetorical function in convincing members of the upper classes that Brislington and Ticehurst were suitable locations for their mentally ill friends and relatives. As Rutherford has said in relation to Brislington, 'all this high ornament, which was exceptional in its lavishness, was provided because Fox aimed at a wealthy clientele of the highest social standing'.[153] The fact that the cottages played an important part in illustrating the early nineteenth-century prospectus also provides evidence to suggest that this was the case. This is further emphasised by comparing the illustrations with photographs as this demonstrates that the cottages were depicted in the prospectus as being more picturesque than they were in reality. This use of artistic licence suggests that the Drs Fox felt this setting would attract a wealthy clientele.

The link between paying clientele and the agency of the landscape is perhaps more complex than initially appears. In the *Description of the Retreat*, Tuke described how he tried to take a patient on long walks and draw him out with conversation but that these did not work as effectually as labour in the garden. He went on to say that 'had his [the patient's] education enlarged his curiosity, and encouraged a taste and observation respecting the objects of nature and art, he might have derived much greater advantage, as many patients obviously do, from variety of conversation and scenery'.[154] This appears to draw on eighteenth-century debates concerning taste and the need for education or a high level of morality in order to appreciate art and nature fully.[155]

The idea that a well-educated person, or at least a person of higher social status, might be more receptive to the therapeutic benefits of nature is also suggested in this example of the benefits of moral therapy given by John Connolly: 'A man of rank comes in . . . as if crazed beyond recovery . . . Liberty to walk at all hours of the cheerful day in gardens or fields, and care and attention, metamorphose him into the well dressed and well bred gentleman he used to be.'[156] The suggestion here is that as he was previously a 'well bred' gentleman it took very little moral therapy to revert him back to this state. So perhaps the fact that picturesque elements are only found in private asylums relates to the idea that only the well educated could derive some therapeutic benefit from them. This appears to have been the case at Germany's first purpose-built asylum, Schleswig Asylum. According to Christine Stevenson, 'patients of the "educated" class could enjoy a plantation of trees, a lawn, a "hermitage", and a bowls alley. The poor and quiet insane had their own flower beds.'[157] That said, it is of course impossible to disentangle education from wealth at this time.

The investment in the design of the grounds and the amount of time patients were expected to spend outside also suggest that the doctors considered these elements to be a part of the therapeutic regime of the asylum. Stevenson has suggested that in the case of architecture in Denmark there was a belief that 'emotional responses could be manipulated through the presentation of calculated visual stimuli'.[158] Similarly, gardens were expected to provoke emotional responses. Horsfield, in his description of Ticehurst, wrote that 'the pleasure which these combined beauties of nature and art are calculated to give, is greatly enhanced by the reflection that they are set apart for the comfort and improvement of those who labour under such a distressing malady, and we have reason to believe that they materially tend to promote the recovery of the patients'.[159] This suggests there was understood to be a connection at the time between the role of art and nature, and the recovery of a patient, and that the ornamented gardens were viewed as materially relevant.

The elite private hospital at Vanves, near Paris, can be considered to be analogous to Brislington and Ticehurst, and according to Dr Jacobi the grounds there had been designed to have specific effects upon the emotional state of the patients:

> Whilst the range of view from the windows of the restless and maniacal patients is narrow and uniform, that from the windows of the melancholy patients is wide and variegated, surprising and delighting the eyes by the multitude of beautiful objects presented to it; in order, as M. Falvret says, to soothe the former by uniformity and quietude, and to rouse the latter to a sense of pleasure, and withdraw them from their gloomy abstractions.[160]

It is impossible to know if similar thinking affected the designs of the gardens in England. However, Fox's sons mention that their father had visited the best asylums in Europe, so he is likely to have known of the asylum at Vanves.[161] He, and Newington, would also no doubt have read the work of the pioneering French doctor, Philippe Pinel, who was most famous for removing the chains restraining insane patients in the infirmaries at Bicêtre, Paris, at the end of the eighteenth century. The removal of the chains was the application of a 'moral (psychological) treatment initiated by Pinel' which was similar to the moral therapy practised by Fox at Brislington.[162] In 1801 Pinel advocated that 'patients be situated in "locations most appropriate to counteract their delusions" and proposed that melancholics in particular should be placed in agreeably planted surroundings'.[163]

Similarly the essays by Rev. Archibald Alison, first published in 1790, related the theory of associations, as expounded by Locke, to ideas concerning the effect of the sublime and the beautiful on human states of mind: 'When any object, either of sublimity or beauty, is presented to the mind, I believe that every man is conscious of a train of thought being immediately awakened in his imagination, analogous to the character or expression of the original object.'[164] He continued to suggest that 'Picturesque Objects' could produce a chain of associations which could, in turn, increase the emotions that they naturally produced: 'They are, in general, such circumstances, as coincide, but are not necessarily connected with the character of the scene or description, and which at first affecting the mind with an emotion of surprise, produce afterwards an increased or additional train of thought.'[165] Although it is not possible to state definitely whether asylum proprietors would have known of Alison's ideas, his book was undoubtedly a popular text at the start of the nineteenth century. According to Michael Liversidge, *Essays on the Nature and Principles of Taste* was reprinted in 1811, 1812, 1815, 1830 and 1853 so it is likely that educated men would have at least been aware of it.[166]

The evidence outlined in this chapter indicates that the picturesque elements in garden design were conceived in the hope that gardens would inspire particular emotions in the patients and not simply be places for the patients to engage in recreational activities, take exercise or be employed in some form of work. If, as is likely, Fox and Newington believed in the Lockeian idea that madness was caused by the mis-association of ideas, then the grottos, aviaries, picturesque cottages and surrounding scenery were designed to inspire the correct associations of thought and awaken a variety of emotions within the patients. The idea of the effect the sublime could have on the mind, as discussed by Alison, seems to have been shared by others and, therefore, to have contemporary currency. He quoted heavily from *Observations on Modern Gardening* (1770) by Thomas Whateley, who wrote:

> It suffices that the scenes of nature have power to affect our imagination and sensibility: for such is the constitution of the human mind, that if once it is agitated, the emotion often spreads beyond the occasion: when the passions are roused, their course is unrestrained, when fancy is on the wing, its flight is unbounded, and quitting the inanimate objects which first gave them spring, we may be led by thought above thought, widely differing in degree but still corresponding in character, til we rise from familiar subjects up to the sublimest conceptions, and are rapt in the contemplation of whatever is great or beautiful, which we feel in nature, feel in man or attribute to the Divinity.[167]

Within institutions where the basis of moral therapy was the re-education of the mind of the insane person, it seems likely that the physicians consciously employed the external environment as a vital part of this process because of its perceived effect on the imagination and emotions.

Religion was another factor that was relevant to the relationship of the picturesque elements of the gardens and moral therapy. Church of England services were seen as playing a vital role in the treatment of patients at Brislington. It is, therefore, possible that the doctors hoped that religious thoughts would be inspired within the patients by the landscape itself. Whateley attributed the great and the beautiful to God and Alison wrote that, 'nothing is more sublime than the form of Rocks, which seem to be coeval with Creation'.[168]

The religious influence, at the beginning of the nineteenth century, on the medical understanding of insanity cannot be underestimated. When, in 1819, William Lawrence, a surgeon at Bethlem Hospital, suggested that insanity was a solely physical illness and 'thus possessed "the same relation to the brain, as vomiting, indigestion, heartburn to the stomach; cough, asthma to the lungs; or any other deranged functions to their corresponding organ"',[169] he was condemned as being an atheist and a menace to social order.[170] Scull has suggested that it was only later in the century, after medical men had developed the idea of a Cartesian duality of the mind and body, that a more somatic understanding could be developed.[171] Fiona Godlee has argued that 'the techniques of moral therapy bring the patients to attempt to conceal their antisocial tendencies'.[172] In fact it was precisely the patient's outward appearance that formed the criteria by which superintendents would judge the level of insanity.

These were ideas that were not only used in relation to asylum patients, but also in regard to the general population, in particular the poor, in the Victorian period. Bound up in ideas of Victorian respectability were the concepts of cleanliness and order.[173] In giving evidence to Edwin Chadwick's *Report on the Sanitary Condition of the Labouring Population of Great Britain* (1842), Mr Monck of Reading described how he discriminated between his tenants on the basis of external morally correct behaviour:

> 'The care taken of these cottages and gardens,' said he, 'afford an excellent criterion of the character of the labourers. I have paid especial attention to those labourers who have displayed cleanliness and order; and I pay the most respect to those who have achieved a situation of the greatest comfort, and keep themselves and their houses, cleanly, and their children tidy'.[174]

In a similar way Connolly believed that the practice of moral management within the asylum could bring about the same degree of order, cleanliness and decency amongst the patients as was expected from society generally:

> Calmness will come; hope will revive; satisfaction will prevail. Some unmanageable tempers, some violent or sullen patients, there must always be; but much of the violence, much of the ill-humour, almost all the disposition to meditate mischievous or fatal revenge, or self-destruction will disappear . . . Cleanliness and decency will be maintained or restored; and despair itself will sometimes be found to give place to cheerfulness or secure tranquillity.[175]

Dr Thomas Octavius Prichard at the Northampton General Lunatic Asylum also considered it important that the patients led an 'ordered and disciplined life'.[176] Through moral management he and Connolly hoped asylums could bring about what Showalter has described as 'general social peace'.[177]

Similarly, wider nineteenth-century views concerning the behaviour of the population can be found in the reasons given for the importance of creating public walks and parks. In Chadwick's *Report* those giving evidence on the importance of developing public open spaces gave essentially moral reasons. One such example was the evidence given by the committee of physicians and surgeons in Birmingham: 'There are no public walks in or near this town; no places where the working-people can resort for recreation. The consequence is that they frequent the ale-houses and skittle alleys for amusement.'[178] In this example the green spaces are seen as a means of distracting people from immoral behaviour. Similarly the gardens and landscapes around asylums were intended to provide distractions from the patients' internal 'immoral' thoughts. Browne, in his 1837 treatise, suggested that the role of the landscape was to give the patients 'new and pleasing and yet unexciting impressions conveyed to their minds, all calculated to suggest healthy trains of thought, all foreign to their morbid feelings, and furnishing some materials for reflection more allied to sanity than the ravings of their fellow-prisoners, or the glare of a dead wall'.[179]

There are possibly further moral aspects to the landscape, beside its perceived ability to provide a distraction. The York Retreat and Brislington were both established by men who were practising Quakers, and it can be argued that the Quaker idea of moral order was reflected in the surrounding landscape (Figure 15). From the asylum the patients could see open countryside, which can be understood as symbolic of the retreat's

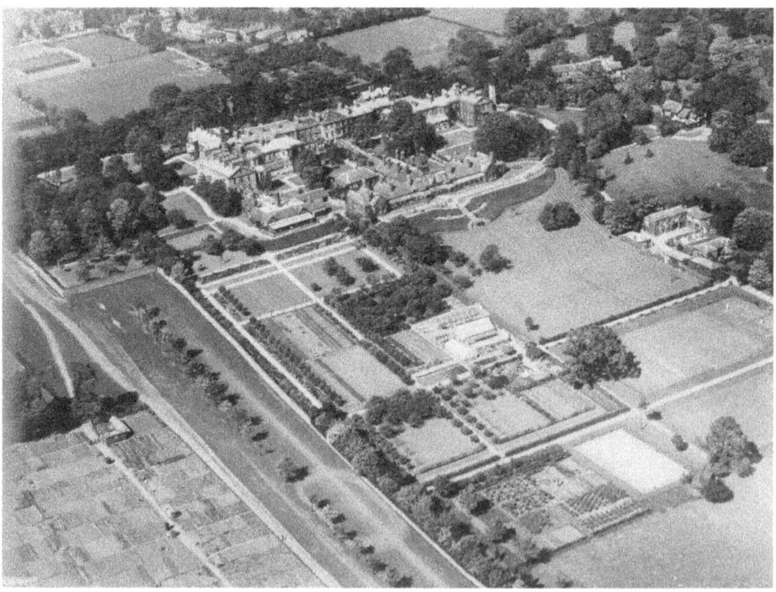

Figure 15 This early twentieth-century aerial photo of the York Retreat demonstrates the orderliness and regularity of the gardens.

acceptance of a natural moral order,[180] or as Klaus Doerner has written, specifically 'the curative power of pure romantic nature'.[181] He also suggests that 'nature was to heal insanity like all the other problems caused by chaotic social progress'.[182] However, Anne Digby qualifies the spiritual element inherent in this relationship between order and the landscape by arguing that it 'is important to emphasize that this was a natural order which was divinely ordained. The significance that was attached to country walks in the Retreat's moral treatment was as much because of the spiritual as the physical benefits derived from them.'[183] Theological and scientific changes during the eighteenth century went hand in hand according to Peter Coates. He suggests that they both 'promoted feelings of awe for physical creation as an ordered system whose perfection mirrored that of its creator and overshadowed man's works'.[184]

These interpretations are naturally of a speculative nature but the fact remains that the proprietors of Brislington and Ticehurst invested large amounts of money and time in their gardens. The importance they, and the Tukes at the Retreat, placed upon the external environment became the pattern for later asylums built throughout Britain in the nineteenth century. The large numbers of asylums built during the Victorian and Edwardian periods were certainly designed with airing courts, parks, shrubbery walks and farms and undoubtedly influenced by these early examples.

Notes

1 Dr Maximilian Jacobi, *On the Construction and Management of Hospitals for the Insane with a Particular Notice of the Institution at Siegburg*, translated by John Kitching and with introductory observations by Samuel Tuke (London: John Churchill, 1841), p. 43.
2 Barry Edginton, 'Moral architecture: the influence of the York Retreat on asylum design', *Health and Place*, 3:2 (1997), 91–9, p. 92.
3 English Heritage, 'Draft description: Brislington House, Gd3397', *Register of Parks and Gardens of Special Interest*, May 2001.
4 Stevenson, *Medicine and Magnificence*, p. 300.
5 These enclosed areas were known as airing courts and were designed so that the patients could exercise and take the air – hence the term 'airing' court.
6 Jonathan Andrews et al., *The History of Bethlem* (London: Routledge, 1997), p. 208.
7 Sarah Rutherford discussed this in a paper she gave at the *Space, Psyche and Psychiatry* conference at Oxford Brooks University, Oxford, in December 2002.

8 William Battie M.D., *A Treatise on Madness by William Battie, M.D. and Remarks on Dr. Battie's Treatise on Madness by John Monro M.D.* (1758), introduced and annotated by Richard Hunter and Ida Macalpine (London: Dawsons of Pall Mall, 1962).

9 Porter, *Mind Forg'd Manacles*, p. 131.

10 *Ibid.* See also Philo, *A Geographical History* on this geographical movement.

11 Leonard Smith, 'The architecture of confinement: urban public asylums in England, 1750–1820', in Topp et al., *Madness*, 41–61, p. 48.

12 Much has been written on this subject. In particular see Porter, *Mind Forg'd Manacles.*

13 John Locke, *An Essay Concerning Human Understanding* (1690), ed. Roger Woolhouse (London: Penguin, 1997), p. 157.

14 *Ibid.*

15 Porter, *Mind Forg'd Manacles*, pp. 191–2.

16 *Ibid.*, p. 192.

17 For a detailed study of the York Retreat and its use of moral therapy, see Anne Digby, *Madness, Morality and Medicine: A Study of the York Retreat, 1796–1914* (Cambridge: Cambridge University Press, 1985).

18 Porter, *Mind Forg'd Manacles*, p. 222.

19 Perceval, *Perceval's Narrative*, p. 94. It is worth noting that at least once he is placed in the cells situated at the bottom of the airing courts as a punishment, but it seems to have been considered to be part of his re-education and only lasted for a short while.

20 *Ibid.*, p. 107.

21 When Dr Charles and Dr Francis Ker Fox (sons of Edward Long Fox) reported to the Commissioners in Lunacy in 1847 they stated that hot and cold baths were effective methods of treatment, amongst other factors: *Further Report of the Commissioners in Lunacy to the Lord Chancellor* (London: Shaw and Sons, 1847). Also accounts in the *York Retreat Annual Report* for 1797 record costs of building work including the construction of a cold bath. This suggests that cold baths may have been an integral part of early moral therapy. For more on cold baths and plunge pools in the eighteenth century see Clare Hickman, 'Taking the plunge: eighteenth-century bath houses and plunge pools', in *Historic Gardens* (a supplement to the Building Conservation Directory; Cathedral Communications, 2010).

22 Charlotte Mackenzie, *A Family Asylum: A History of the Private Madhouse at Ticehurst in Sussex, 1792–1917*, PhD Thesis (London: University of London, 1986), p. 90.

23 *Ticehurst Private Asylum for Insane Persons*, c.1828 (Wellcome Library Archives: MS.6783).

24 Two of these buildings have recently been restored and are located at the termination of wooded walks within the grounds at Ticehurst.

25 Thomas W. Horsfield, *The History, Antiquities and Topography of the County of Sussex*, 2 vols (Lewes: Sussex Press, 1835), i, pp. 590–1.

26 *Ibid.*
27 *Brislington House, An Asylum for Lunatics Situated near Bristol on the Road from Bath and Lately Erected by Edward Long Fox M.D.: An Account of the Establishment*, c.1804–9 (Somerset Archives and Local Studies: T/PH/fx\2). The exact date of this early prospectus is unknown. Somerset Archives suggest that it is c.1809 but it could have been written any time after the completion of the asylum building in 1804.
28 Introduction to Perceval, *Perceval's Narrative* written by the editor, Gregory Bateson, p. v.
29 According to Charlotte Mackenzie, Samuel Newington may have been treating patients at his home, The Vineyards, since the 1760s: Mackenzie, *Psychiatry for the Rich: A History of Ticehurst Private Asylum, 1792–1917* (London and New York: Routledge, 1992), p. 37.
30 *Ibid.*, pp. 35–7.
31 For more on Fox see Leonard Smith, 'Gentleman's mad-doctor in Georgian England: Edward Long Fox and Brislington House', *History of Psychiatry* 19:163 (2008), 163–84.
32 Quoted in Annie Fox (assisted by Dr C.H. Fox and Dr A.W.P. Fox), 'A short account of the history of Brislington House', *Brislington House Quarterly* (Centenary Edition), c.1906 (Bristol Record Office 36924 3–5), 4–13, p. 4.
33 *History and Present State of Brislington House near Bristol. An Asylum for the Cure and Reception of Insane Persons: Established by Edward Long Fox M.D. A.D. 1804, and Now Conducted by Francis and Charles Fox. M.D.D.* (Bristol: Light and Ridler, 1836), p. 4.
34 Francis Kilvert, *Kilvert's Diary: Selections from the Diary of the Reverend Francis Kilvert 1870–1879*, ed. with an introduction by William Plomer (London: J. Cape, 1944); diary entry of Monday 2 November 1874, pp. 103–4.
35 Samuel Tuke, *Description of The Retreat: An Institution Near York for Insane Persons of the Society of Friends* (1813), reprinted with an introduction by Richard Hunter and Ida Macalpine (London: Dawsons of Pall Mall, 1964), p. 93.
36 Jacobi, *On the Constriction and Management of Hospitals*, p. 43.
37 *Ibid.*
38 Rutherford, *The Landscapes*, i, p. 121.
39 *Ibid.*, p. 128.
40 Edginton, 'Moral architecture', p. 94.
41 Perceval, *Perceval's Narrative*, p. 117.
42 *Ibid.*
43 Rutherford, *The Landscapes*, i, p. 176.
44 William Wordsworth, *The Prelude: A Parallel Text* (1850), ed. with an introduction by J.C. Maxwell (New Haven and London: Yale University Press, 1971), p. 59, lines 405–11.

45 Samuel Taylor Coleridge, 'The Nightingale', in *Selected Poems*, ed. with an introduction by Richard Holmes (London: Penguin Books, 1996), p. 58, lines 107–9.
46 Ronald Gaskell, *Wordsworth's Poem of the Mind: An Essay on the Prelude* (Edinburgh: Edinburgh University Press, 1991), p. 36.
47 Louis James, 'Landscape in nineteenth-century literature', in G.E. Mingay, ed., *The Victorian Countryside*, 2 vols (London: Routledge and Kegan Paul, 1981), i, 150–65, p. 153.
48 Quoted in W.J. Harvey and Richard Gravil, eds, *Wordsworth, The Prelude: A Casebook* (London: Macmillan, 1972), p. 11.
49 Quoted in Anne Digby, 'Moral treatment at the Retreat, 1796–1846', in William. F. Bynum, Roy Porter and Michael Shepherd, eds, *The Anatomy of Madness: Essays in the History of Psychiatry*, 3 vols (Cambridge: Cambridge University Press, 1985), ii, 52–72, p. 59. Taken from Samuel Tuke's Introduction to Jacobi, *On the Construction and Management of Hospitals*, p. xix.
50 W.A.F. Browne, *What Asylums Are, Were and Ought To Be* (1837), ed. with an introduction by Andrew Scull in *The Asylum as Utopia* (London and New York: Routledge, 1991), p. 182.
51 Quoted in Stephanie Patricia Skene, 'The development of the gardens at the Cambridgeshire pauper lunatic asylum, Fulbourn' in Twigs Way, ed., *Picturing Paradise: Studies in Eighteenth to Twentieth-Century Gardens and Garden Design* (Cambridge: University of Cambridge, 2003), 31–6, p. 32. This concept is discussed in more detail in relation to the Northampton asylums in Chapter 3, pp. 82–3 of this book, where mounds in the airing courts that allowed patients to see over the high walls were seen as problematic because they blocked the view from inside the building.
52 Elaine Showalter, *The Female Malady: Women, Madness and English Culture, 1830–1980* (London: Virago Press, 1987), p. 30.
53 *Ibid.*
54 NGLA, *The Report of the Northampton General Lunatic Asylum for 1860* (Northampton: printed by JAS Butterfield, 1861) (St Andrew's Healthcare Archive).
55 Philo, *A Geographical History*, p. 588.
56 See Chapter 4 for the debate concerning the location of the new St Thomas's Hospital.
57 Browne, *What Asylums Are*, p. 181.
58 See Chapter 4 of this book on general hospitals and Stevenson, *Medicine and Magnificence*, pp. 158–9.
59 Philo, *A Geographical History*, p. 586.
60 Mackenzie, *Psychiatry for the Rich*, p. 39.
61 It is also worth mentioning that although the title of first purpose-built asylum is debatable in relation to Brislington House it was, however, probably

the first asylum designed to be fireproof. Fox recognised the fire risk caused by 'the restricted circumstances of maniacal patients' and in order to counter this he designed the building 'on a plan calculated effectually to obviate this contingency. With the exception of a few doors and windows in the centre house, all the parts usually constructed of wood, are, in this, made with iron or incombustible materials.' From *Brislington House: An Account of the Establishment.*

62 Fox, 'A short account', pp. 4–5.

63 This is held in Somerset Archives and Local Studies, T\PH\fx/2.

64 *Brislington House: An Account of the Establishment.*

65 1815 Committee of the House of Commons, quoted in Fox, 'A short account', p. 4. This represents evidence collected as part of the 1815 Parliamentary Inquiry, which took nearly two years and looked at the treatment of the mad in charity hospitals, county asylums, private madhouses and work-houses. Scull, *The Most Solitary of Afflictions*, pp. 115–22.

66 *Brislington House: An Account of the Establishment.*

67 *Ibid.*

68 Perceval, *Perceval's Narrative*, p. 63.

69 Rutherford, *The Landscapes*, i, p. 120.

70 *Ibid.*

71 Acccording to Rutherford, similar walled enclosures were created in the 1790s for nine medical officers' residences at the Royal Naval Hospital, Haslar, Gosport. *Ibid.*, p. 131.

72 *Brislington House: An Account of the Establishment.*

73 English Heritage, 'Draft description: Brislington House'.

74 Quoted in Pierre Pinon, *L'Hospice de Charenton/Charenton Hospital* (Brussels: Mardaga, 1989), p. 108.

75 *Brislington House: An Account of the Establishment.*

76 Patrick Goode, 'Mounts', in Sir Geoffrey Jellicoe et al., *The Oxford Companion to Gardens* (New York: Oxford University Press, 2001), 382, p. 382.

77 According to Rutherford they were used in terraced town-house gardens in the eighteenth century, some of which were embellished with purely ornamental 'risings, swellings, mounts and irregularities' as referred to by Joseph Spence in 1851. Rutherford, *The Landscapes*, i, p. 131.

78 As Rutherford has suggested there was always a conflict between the need for confinement and the retention of a domestic appearance. *Ibid.*, p. 121.

79 *The Ground Plan of the Asylum for Lunatics at Brislington House near Bristol* from the Huntington Library, c.1809, quoted in English Heritage, 'Draft description: Brislington House'. These walks can be seen on the same plan of the courts.

80 1815 Committee of the House of Commons, quoted in Fox, 'A short account', pp. 4–5.

81 Tuke, *Description of the Retreat*, p. 96.

82 *York Retreat Annual Report*, 1902 (all annual reports are held at York University, Borthwick Institute of Historical Research RET 1/2), p. 28.
83 Kilvert, *Kilvert's Diary*, entry of Monday 2 November 1874, p. 104.
84 English Heritage, 'Draft description: Brislington House'.
85 *History and Present State of Brislington House.*
86 Summerhouses were also situated in the courts in the late nineteenth century, to designs by S.C. Fripp, but these no longer exist. They can be seen adjacent to the ladies' and gentlemen's sitting rooms on the Ordnance Survey Map of 1881–3.
87 Rutherford, *The Landscapes*, i, p. 125.
88 Tuke, *Description of the Retreat*, p. 95.
89 *Further Report*, Appendix E, p. 323.
90 *Ibid.*, pp. 80–1.
91 *Ibid.*, p. 226.
92 *Ibid.*, Appendix F, p. 334.
93 *York Retreat Annual Report*, 1839, pp. 4–5.
94 Rutherford, *The Landscapes*, i, p. 123.
95 *York Retreat Annual Report*, 1842, p. 15.
96 Quoted in Fox 'A short account', pp. 4–5.
97 *Brislington House: An Account of the Establishment.*
98 English Heritage, 'Draft description: Brislington House'.
99 Perceval, *Perceval's Narrative*, p. 150.
100 *History and Present State of Brislington House*, p. 9.
101 J.C. Loudon, *The Suburban Gardener and Villa Companion* (1838), reprinted in The English Landscape Garden Series (New York and London: Garland Publishing, 1982), p. 2.
102 *History and Present State of Brislington House*, p. 9.
103 Herman Merivale published anonymously, *My Experiences in a Lunatic Asylum by a Sane Patient* (London: Chatto and Windus, 1879).
104 *Brislington House: An Account of the Establishment.*
105 *History and Present State of Brislington House*, p. 9.
106 This is shown on a photograph in an album held at the Bristol Record Office (Ref: 39624/5).
107 Steven Cherry and Roger Munting, '"Exercise is the thing"? Sport and the asylum, c.1850–1950', *International Journal of the History of Sport*, 22:1 (2005), 42–58.
108 Merivale, *My Experiences*, p. 147.
109 *York Retreat Annual Report*, 1839, pp. 4–5
110 *York Retreat Annual Report*, 1841, p. 4.
111 *York Retreat Annual Report*, 1870, pp. 14–15.
112 Mackenzie, *Psychiatry for the Rich*, p. 53.
113 Walpole to Sir Horace Mann on 2 August 1750; quoted in Patrick Conner, *Oriental Architecture in the West* (London: Thames and Hudson, 1979), p. 57.

114 *Ibid.*, p. 156.
115 English Heritage, 'Draft description: Brislington House'.
116 Perceval, *Perceval's Narrative*, p. 87.
117 Mackenzie, *Psychiatry for the Rich* p. 71.
118 Mackenzie, *A Family Asylum*, p. 90.
119 Philo, *A Geographical History*, particularly pp. 292–301.
120 Quoted in Philo, *A Geographical History*, p. 296.
121 *Ibid.*
122 *Ibid.*
123 *Ibid.*, p. 349.
124 *Ibid.*
125 Merivale, *My Experiences*, pp. 73–4.
126 Fox, 'A short account', p. 12.
127 Mackenzie, *A Family Asylum*, p. 183.
128 Thomas Baird, *General View of the Agriculture of the County of Middlesex* (London: J. Nichols, 1793), p. 38.
129 *Ibid.*
130 With thanks to Michael Brown who let me read the proof copy of his *Performing Medicine: Medical Culture and Identity in Provincial England, c.1760–1850* (Manchester: Manchester University Press, 2011).
131 Perceval, *Perceval's Narrative*, pp. 116–7.
132 Humphry Repton, 'Observations on the theory of landscape gardening' (1803), reprinted in *Aesthetics and the Picturesque*, ed. and introduced by Gavin Budge, 6 vols (Bristol: Thoemmes, 2001), vi, p. 255.
133 Loudon, *The Suburban Gardener*, pp. 466–7.
134 *Brislington House: An Account of the Establishment.*
135 Fox, 'A short account', p. 5.
136 Used as an illustration in NGLA, *The Report of the Northampton General Lunatic Asylum* for 1859 (Northampton: Printed by JAS Butterfield, 1860).
137 Loudon, *The Suburban Gardener*, pp. 160–1.
138 Bristol Record Office (Ref: 39624/5).
139 Mavis Batey, *Regency Gardens* (Buckinghamshire: Shire Publications, 1995), p. 9.
140 Jane Austen, *Sense and Sensibility* (1811) (reprinted London: Pan Books, 1972), p. 201.
141 *Ibid.*
142 Giles Worsley, *Architectural Drawings of the Regency Period, 1790–1837* (London: Andre Deutsch, 1992), p. 87.
143 *History and Present State of Brislington House*, p. 6.
144 Fox, 'A short account', p. 5.
145 Sheena Stoddard, *Mr Braikenridge's Brislington* (Bristol: City of Bristol Museum and Art Gallery, 1981), pp. 50–1.

146 Edmund Bartell, *Hints for Picturesque Improvements in Ornamented Cottages and Their Scenery* (1804) (reprinted Farnborough: Gregg International Publishers, 1971), pp. 4–5.
147 J.B. Papworth, *Rural Residences, Consisting of a Series of Designs for Cottages, Decorated Cottages, Small Villas and Other Ornamented Buildings* (London: Sedding and Turtle, 1832) p. 25.
148 *York Retreat Annual Report*, 1896, p. 35.
149 Batey, *Regency Gardens*, p. 11.
150 Humphrey Repton, 'Fragments on the theory and practice of landscape gardening' (1816) in J.C. Loudon, ed., *The Landscape Gardening and Landscape Architecture of the Late Humphrey Repton, Esq* (1839), reprinted in *Aesthetics and the Picturesque*, ed. and introduced by Gavin Budge, 6 vols (Bristol: Thoemmes, 2001), vi, p. 433.
151 Rutherford, *The Landscapes*, i, p. 132.
152 See Edginton, 'Moral architecture'.
153 Rutherford, *The Landscapes*, i, p. 133.
154 Tuke, *Description of the Retreat*, p. 155.
155 See the introduction to Edmund Burke, *A Philosophical Enquiry into the Origin of our Ideas of the Sublime and Beautiful* (London: A. Robertson, 1824) and Anthony Ashley Cooper, 3rd Earl of Shaftesbury, *Characteristicks*, 3 vols (Glasgow: R. Foulis, 1743–45) for more on the moral view of taste.
156 Connolly, *Treatment of the Insane*, pp. 154–5.
157 Christine Stevenson, 'Madness and the Picturesque in the Kingdom of Denmark', in Bynum et al., *The Anatomy of Madness*, iii, 13–47, p. 37.
158 *Ibid.*, p. 15.
159 Horsfield, *The County of Sussex*, i, p. 590.
160 Jacobi, *On the Construction and Management of Hospitals*, p. 43.
161 *History and Present State of Brislington House*, p. 6.
162 James C. Harris, 'Pinel orders the chains removed form the insane at Bicêtre', *Archives of General Psychiatry*, 60:5 (2003), 442, p. 442.
163 Stevenson, 'Madness and the Picturesque', p. 29.
164 Rev. Archibald Alison, *Essays on the Nature and Principles of Taste* (Edinburgh: Printed for J.J.G. and G. Robinson, London, and Bell and Bradgate, Edinburgh, 1790), p. 2.
165 *Ibid.*, p. 29.
166 Michael Liversidge, 'Rome portrayed: "To excite the sensibility, and to awaken the admiration of mankind" ', in Michael Liversidge and Catherine Edwards, eds, *Imagining Rome: British Artists and Rome in the Nineteenth Century* (London: Merrell Holberton, 1996), 38–53, Note 1, p. 52.
167 Thomas Whately, *Observations on Modern Gardening, Illustrated by Descriptions* (London: T. Payne, 1770); quotation in Alison, *Essays*, p. 43.
168 Alison, *Essays*, p. 226.
169 Quoted in Scull, *The Most Solitary of Afflictions*, p. 220.

170 Scull, *The Most Solitary of Afflictions*, p. 220.
171 *Ibid.*
172 Fiona Godlee, 'Aspects of Non-conformity: Quakers and the lunatic fringe', in Bynum et al., *The Anatomy of Madness*, ii, 73–85, p. 75.
173 For more on this relationship see Smith, *Clean.*
174 Edwin Chadwick, *Great Britain Poor Law Commissioners: Report on the Sanitary Condition of the Labouring Population of Great Britain, 1842*, ed. with an introduction by M.W. Flinn (Edinburgh: Edinburgh University Press, 1965), p. 338.
175 John Connolly quoted in Showalter, *The Female Malady*, p. 33.
176 *Second Annual Report of Northampton General Lunatic Asylum*, 1839–40 (St Andrew's Healthcare Archive).
177 Showalter, *The Female Malady*, p. 33.
178 Chadwick, *Great Britain Poor Law Commissioners*, p. 335.
179 Browne, *What Asylums Are*, p. 191. For Victorian and late twentieth-century concerns relating to patients suffering from physical illnesses only having a blank wall to look at, see Chapter 6.
180 Digby, *Madness, Morality and Medicine*, p. 55.
181 Klaus Doerner, *Madmen and the Bourgeoisie: A Social History of Insanity and Psychiatry*, translated by Joachim Neugroschel and Jean Steinberg (Oxford: Blackwell, 1981), p. 80.
182 *Ibid.*
183 Digby, *Madness, Morality and Medicine*, p. 55.
184 Peter Coates, *Nature: Western Attitudes Since Ancient Times* (Cambridge: Polity Press in association with Blackwell, 1998), p. 131.

3

The perfect asylum may appear to be a utopia: the Victorian asylum and its landscape

> Conceive a Spacious Building Resembling the Palace of a Peer. Airy, and Elevated, and Elegantly Surrounded by Swelling Grounds and Gardens.
>
> W.A.F. Browne, 1837[1]

By the time W.A.F. Browne (at that time Medical Superintendent of the Montrose Royal Lunatic Asylum, Scotland[2]) published *What Asylums Are, Were and Ought To Be* in 1837, the asylum was considered to be the pre-eminent place in which a cure for insanity could be effected. From 1808, Wynne's Law, also known as the County Lunatic Asylums Act, allowed counties to set up their own asylums if desired.[3] This was only a permissive act, but in 1845 the Lunatic Asylums Act was introduced, which made it compulsory for counties and boroughs to provide publicly funded provision for their pauper lunatics.[4] Between these acts, and two years after the publication of Browne's seminal work, Northampton established its first purpose-built asylum for the care of the insane. It can, therefore, be seen as part of the growing national concern and great period of asylum building which took place throughout the Victorian period and into the twentieth century.

The designs for these institutions were often based on the models of earlier examples, including the York Retreat and Brislington House. Dr Fox even had a direct influence on the design of the asylum at Nottingham as the magistrates consulted him in 1809 for advice and requested to see plans of Brislington House.[5] The gardens and grounds around these later institutions, as well as the wider landscape, maintained their status as important therapeutic tools with both medical and 'moral' underpinnings. As Philo has suggested, by the mid-nineteenth century the discussions related to asylum-siting embraced both medical and moral theories,[6] as well as economic considerations concerning the cost of land.[7] Philo cites the example of the 1844 Metropolitan Commissioners report, which had 'both a medical component (in stressing the hygienic virtues of good water supply and drainage) and a moral component (in stressing the therapeutic value of "cheerful prospects", ample land for "outdoor employment" and protection from outside disturbances)'.[8] The combined powerful force of these discourses led to the increased ruralisation of asylums during the century and the continued importance of landscape in relation to both the physical and mental health of the patients. It is these ideas and their expression through the location of the institutions and the design of the landscapes which will be explored in this chapter.

The utopian asylum vision, as described by Browne and others, reflected the contemporary artistic and literary representations of the English countryside. Elaine Showalter has described how 'English institutions perched on top of mild hills surrounded by the pastoral details familiar from a Constable painting or a Wordsworth poem'.[9] She goes on to quote from Isaac Ray's *Observations on the Principal Hospitals for the Insane in Great Britain, France and Germany*, which was printed in 1846:

> Many of them are placed on eminences which command an extensive view of the adjacent country, the field of vision embracing hill, and valley, wood and water, in their most agreeable combinations; while fields of grass and tillage, divided by hedges and trees, grazing herds, cottages and country seats, form the nearer features of the landscape reposing in the softened light of an English sun.[10]

In this description, which could as easily be applied to an English country house, the fact that the asylum's landscape reflected the artistic taste of the time shows that there was a crossover from 'aesthetic judgements about what was pleasing to the eye in buildings and landscapes to moral prescriptions about how certain scenes were more likely to soothe and even to cure, the minds of mad people than were others'.[11]

The use and design of the asylum landscape was influenced by members of the medical profession and interested lay people (these included members of the asylums' committees and the Commissioners in Lunacy). Therefore, it is important that general views concerning the landscape, or, more specifically, 'nature' are considered here.[12] The dramatic social and economic changes that had begun in the eighteenth century also affected the perception of nature during the nineteenth century. According to W.J. Keith it is 'impossible to overemphasise the fact that, by half way through Victoria's reign, the majority of the population lived and worked in towns'.[13] He continues to state that 'most urban Victorian readers turned to rural literature for the same reasons as they sought the countryside itself – for refreshment and renewal, as a haven from the wearying pace of city life'.[14] It is probably this concept of the countryside offering both 'refreshment and renewal' in terms of physical, mental and spiritual health that influenced the location and design of asylums during the century, as well as the cheaper cost of land on the outskirts of towns. This chapter will explore these general ideas concerning health and the landscape and look at the interplay between these ideas and design in more detail by focusing on three asylums located in Northampton. They are: Northampton General Lunatic Asylum (1839–present day), which for a brief time was also called the Northampton General Lunatic Asylum for the Middle and Upper Classes before assuming the title it retains today of St Andrew's Hospital; Abington Abbey Retreat (1845–92); and Northampton County Asylum (1876–1995) which changed its name to St Crispin's Hospital in 1947, just before the birth of the NHS.[15]

Country house model

From Browne's quote at the beginning of this chapter it is clear that his vision of the utopian asylum bore strong similarities to a contemporary country house. There appear to be similarities between his polemic description and the reality of the design of the Victorian asylum, although it should be stated that this is no way meant to suggest that life inside the asylum was similarly palatial. The aim of this text is to explore the rhetoric behind the design and use of the landscapes. It is not intended as a defence of the asylum regime or to suggest that the experience of being treated within an asylum was not often traumatic.

In Rutherford's extensive work on the landscapes of pauper lunatic asylums from 1800–1914, she has found a great similarity between asylum design and country house estates.[16] An engraving of the Coton Hill Asylum, Staffordshire built in the 1850s, illustrates this relationship between the country house and the asylum in terms of both garden design and architecture (Figure 16). Again, this was a private asylum, and the class of patient and greater financial resources available, meant that the relationship between the country house and the institution is more evident. The example of Abington Abbey demonstrates the incredibly close relationship that could exist between the country house and the asylum, as like Ticehurst Place, this private institution operated

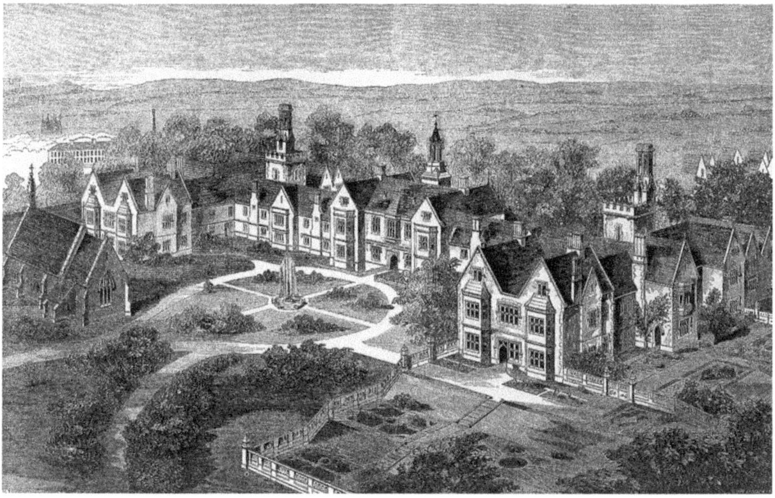

Figure 16 Engraving of the private asylum at Coton Hill, Staffordshire, which is similar in style to domestic country houses of the time. The gardens are depicted as having terraces and a fountain.

within a former country house.[17] Rather than building something new based on the model of a domestic dwelling, it utilised an existing house and its associated landscape.

However, even pauper asylums shared characteristics with the country house. For example, the sale particulars for the estate that was to become the site of the Northampton County Asylum demonstrate the similarity of requirements for both a country house and an asylum:

> Northamptonshire (within two miles of the important town of Northampton) a Freehold Estate of 180 acres of rich land, finely timbered with oaks of good growth and ornamental appearance, lying in a ring fence. Its contiguity to the important town of Northampton, its elevation and position, render it equally desirable as a pure land investment, or as an eligible site wheron to erect a mansion in this famous hunting district. A church almost adjoins the property. There is an abundant supply of water. The land is under drained, and in a high state of cultivation . . . from which site the most charming views of the very pretty surrounding Country are obtained.[18]

Obviously aimed at a private buyer who wished to construct his domestic country mansion, this estate was also exactly what the asylum's Governors desired. The landscape offered the necessary hygiene requirement of an 'abundant supply of water', it was well drained and in a 'high state of cultivation' which would allow patients to work within the landscape tilling the land and make the estate economically viable. It also had the morally important 'charming views of the pretty surrounding Country'. Therefore, the site had both the required medical and moral benefits.

One of the many functions of the landscape was to help create the illusion that the asylum was more of a home than a prison. This can be seen in an entry in the Visitors' Book for Northampton General Lunatic Asylum: these books contain the notes of people appointed from the list of subscribers to act as official visitors. Such visitors were common to voluntary or charitable institutions such as the Northampton asylum. According to Jonathan Reinarz they 'essentially ensured that the charitable funds were carefully spent and the hospital managed efficiently'.[19] On 16 June 1846, one of their concerns was that the front airing courts had unsuitable iron bars that they felt gave the house a 'prison like or menagerie appearance'.[20] As discussed in the previous chapter it was believed that in order for moral therapy to be successful the asylum needed to resemble a home as much as possible.[21] This theory that the asylum should be homely seems to have continued throughout the century so that when the County Asylum extended its open door system in 1887, the *Annual Report* of that year stated that, 'the more the Asylum can be made to resemble a home the greater will be the probability of such cases settling down and deriving benefit from the treatment'.[22] It is possible that the domestic setting sometimes did hide the institutional, particularly in private asylums. Herman Merivale, for example, stated that when he first arrived at Ticehurst he thought he was being admitted to a hotel.[23]

Associated with the provision of a homely environment, there was also an increasing desire for rural locations which was probably influenced by the choice of location made by the private asylums, as discussed in the previous chapter. The choice of rural locations for these institutions has been interrogated eloquently and in great depth by Philo. In the case of Northampton, when the Governors of the General Infirmary arranged to meet in 1789 to 'consider erecting a new, purpose-built hospital, as the original infirmary . . . was no longer large enough to cope with the demand' they proposed that this accommodation should be located next to the General Hospital, which was then on the outskirts of the town.[24] By 1804, £552 10s had been raised by donations to establish a ward at the General Hospital for the purpose of 'treating scientifically the insane'.[25]

It is noteworthy that they suggested that there was a need for the scientific treatment of insanity and that they thought this provision should be located close to the hospital. This statement was made when Brislington House was just being established and nearly a decade after the York Retreat had opened, which implies that the concept of moral therapy was either unknown or not yet seen as important in Northampton. Their intention to 'scientifically' treat the insane is more suggestive of the late eighteenth-century use of medication to treat insanity.[26]

By 1833, donations to the fund had reached £12,038 18s 9d. At this point a sub-committee of the Northampton Infirmary was formed to implement the planned asylum. In July 1834, rather than build adjacent to the hospital, they decided to 'acquire at auction the freehold of 21½ acres of the estate of the late Robert Harding, situated off the Billing Road in an area once occupied by the St Andrew Priory, a Cluniac Foundation from 1100'.[27] In just over forty years it seems that the concept of a rural situation had become more important than the need for close proximity to the infirmary. This is in part due to the increase in popularity of moral therapy for the treatment of the insane and according to Philo, 'by the 1850s . . . virtually all of the public asylums had their own medically-qualified superintendents who were *resident* on the premises'.[28] This combination of an increased interest in moral therapy and on-site medical care meant that there was no longer any great need to be close to the infirmary. This provides evidence for the growing importance of rural locations, which grew in magnitude through the century.[29] The later pauper asylum, Northampton County Asylum, opened in 1876, was located at an even greater distance from the centre of the town.

The growing desire for ruralisation also affected the development of the early General Lunatic Asylum. During the first decades following its establishment the asylum increased the size of its original site by purchasing adjoining land, for example twelve acres were obtained in 1850 and another twenty-eight acres in 1853.[30] As the expanding Northampton town encroached further on the site, the Governors of the General Lunatic Asylum bought 453 acres of farmland further away from the town in 1879, with the intention of moving the hospital to this more rural site.[31] In the event they used the newly acquired farm at Moulton Park to provide produce and livestock for the asylum and the main asylum remained on its original site. However, the Governors created separate accommodation for convalescent patients at the new site and the patients living there were employed on the farm. In what appears to be another attempt to compensate for their more urban environment, they also rented country houses in Wales before purchasing Bryn-y-Neuadd Hall near Llanfairfechan in 1896. Some patients were resident there all year while others were sent for a few weeks in the summer to give them 'a change of scene, and sea air'.[32] This latter example reflected the belief that sea air was particularly therapeutic, along with the provision of a more rural setting and a change of environment.[33]

The desire for rural settings reflected the desire for increased amounts of landscape to surround the asylums as well as economical considerations – rural land was often considerably cheaper. This financial concern was not only confined to mid-nineteenth-century England. In 1818 the French asylum superintendent Esquirol wrote that 'asylums should be built outside of towns. This will be more economical both as regards the initial costs of the establishments and their eventual upkeep, as city tolls will not have to be levied on goods.'[34]

This ruralisation was not without its problems. The building of the Northampton County Asylum (Figure 17) came under fierce local criticism. Along with accusations of the high cost to rate payers of a 'most hideous building',[35] Scull has stated that there were allegations that

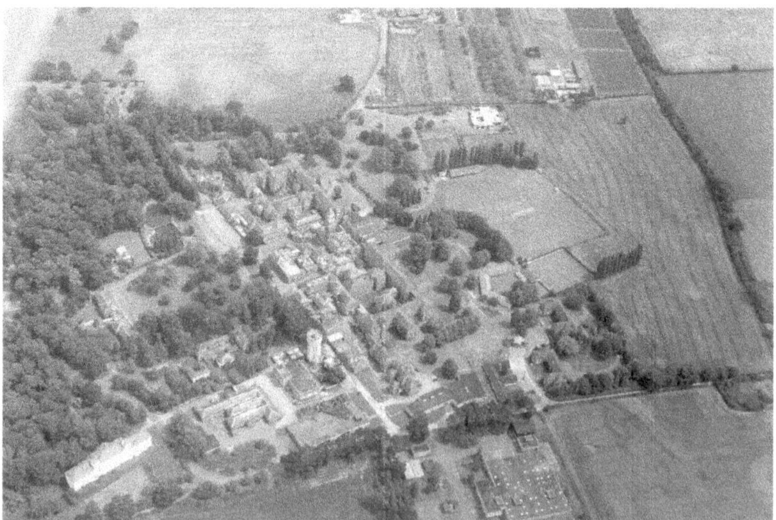

Figure 17 Aerial view of the Northampton County Lunatic Asylum showing the extensive grounds, including areas of woodland.

'behind the high walls and the trees that shielded the asylum from the public gaze, patients were being brutally maltreated'.[36] Using the landscape to separate patients from the civilisation that was thought to be responsible to some extent for their illness, helped to create the frightening asylum of the Gothic imagination. As Scull intimates in the quote above, the extensive landscape that separated the asylum from the rest of civilisation was mainly designed to protect the privacy of the patients. At the County Asylum the perimeter wall, at a height of at least six feet, was also patrolled at weekends to ensure that 'members of the local community did not stray into the grounds'.[37] Rather than seeing rural asylums as a way of protecting society from the patients, it appears that the rhetoric at least suggests that this separation was predominantly for the benefit of the patients, although this is not to say that, in reality, patient benefit was the driving factor.

There was not, however, a consensus that building asylums in the countryside was the ideal solution. As Philo has highlighted, when discussions were taking place in the 1860s regarding the location of the new Bethlem hospital, arguments were made in favour of both rural and urban situations. At a meeting of the Association of Medical Officers of Asylums and Hospitals for the Insane in 1866, W. Wood argued that:

> In London and in its immediate neighbourhood there are many opportunities of amusing, especially the male part of the population, which do not exist in the country . . . There is really no object in going out for picnics when the people are living in a state of picnic. They have no opportunity of going sight-seeing, and their life must necessarily be one of a monotonous character.[38]

In this case an argument is being made for the benefits of an urban location with its variety and opportunities. However, in line with the overall trend, a rural location was decided upon in the end.

The importance of locating asylums in the countryside, as exemplified by the cases in Northampton, became entwined with the idea of order and self-restraint. In his 1855 treatise, John Connolly, who was quoting at length from the 1854 Commissioners in Lunacy Report, condemned the Bristol Lunatic Asylum (known as St Peter's Hospital) for its 'close and confined site, the want of any proper means of separating, classifying, and, when necessary, secluding the patients, and the absence of suitable airing grounds for daily exercise and recreation'.[39] He went on to link this deficiency in the location with what can be expected of the behaviour of the patients: 'It is vain to expect that the good order, tranquillity and repose which are essential to the successful treatment of insanity can ever be permanently maintained within its precincts.'[40]

The descriptive terms of 'good order' and 'tranquillity' appear time and again in relation to patients in asylums. In the Visitors' Books for Northampton General Lunatic Asylum, the description of the patients as tranquil is used on nearly every visit as a positive description to indicate that the asylum is working correctly. The term also reflects Wordsworth's ideas of landscape restoring tranquillity, although for him, even the memory of landscape is restorative:

> These beauteous forms,
> Through a long absence, have not been to me
> As is a landscape to a blind man's eye:
> But oft, in lonely rooms, and 'mid the din
> Of towns and cities, I have owed to them,
> In hours of weariness, sensations sweet,
> Felt in the blood, and felt along the heart;
> And passing even into my purer mind,
> With tranquil restoration[41]

Further extending the idea of nature ordered by man, the concept of cultivated gardens around the asylum might also have reflected a belief in the curative powers of a tamed nature. This may partly explain why, when a group of female patients at the Fisherton Asylum for the criminally insane 'ripped up every flower the minute it showed its head above ground', their action was considered a sign of 'severe psychopathology'.[42] This was presumably the opposite result to the outcome expected by the medical profession, as they believed that the natural setting should have positively influenced the patients. Therefore, it could perhaps only be classed as a form of severe insanity, and it may perhaps have been viewed in such severe terms because the action was executed by female, rather than male, patients.[43] The concept of ordered, tamed nature extended to the concept of work within the landscape where the patient took on the role of taming nature himself or herself.

The gardens of the Victorian asylum

An 1847 map of the General Lunatic Asylum, drawn up ten years into the operation of the institution, depicts quite a plain landscape with what appear to be shrubs bordering the drive running up to the asylum and planted around the area directly in front of the house (Figure 18). The

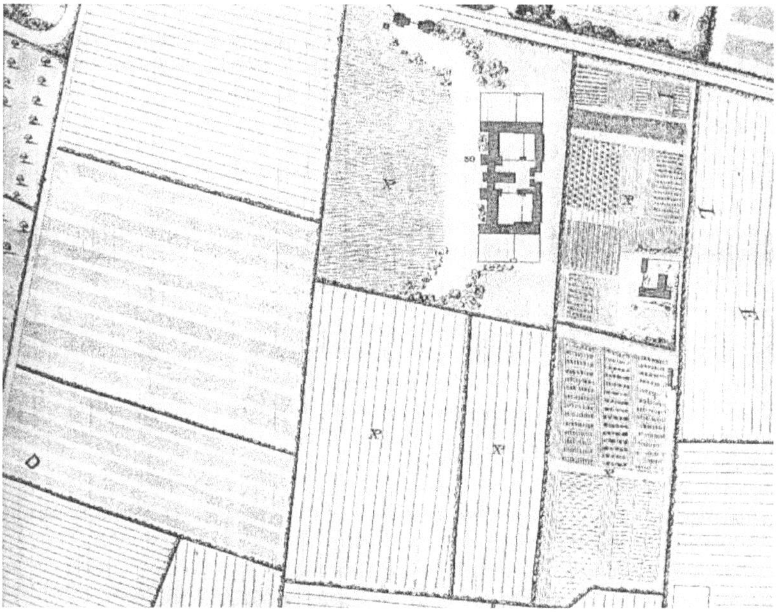

Figure 18 1847 Map of the Northampton General Lunatic Asylum showing limited planting around the asylum and wider agriculturally managed fields. The area to the right of the asylum was a private nursery at this time but was later obtained by the institution.

asylum only owned a small amount of land at this time (the intensively cultivated land shown to the east of the asylum was owned by a nurseryman). However, once the rural farm at Moulton began to be used for agricultural production in 1881, the land adjacent to the General Lunatic Asylum, which had previously been 'used as farm and garden was put down to grass for use not only as grazing land but also for football and cricket'.[44]

The unornamented landscape depicted on the 1847 map is illustrated as such in an early engraving. There are also descriptions of the appearance of the original grounds, as this was often recorded when the Committee decided to alter them. For example, the inner male airing court was described as follows: 'The whole is tiled or gravelled.'[45] This suggests that early on these courts were plain areas without any planting. However, it is likely that there was more planting on the estate than shown on the map and engraving as 'in August 1838, £28 13s 10d was authorised to be paid to John Perkins for eight weeks wages for his foreman, for the use of sixty-five and a half days of his horse and cart and for seeds for the garden which Perkins had undertaken to layout and for which he was later congratulated'.[46]

Apart from the record above of Perkins' involvement at the General Lunatic Asylum there is no other concrete evidence of who was responsible for the design of any of the asylum gardens in Northampton. However, Perkins may well have also been involved in the creation of the landscape of the County Asylum, as he supplied seeds and plants for that estate too.[47] In her research, Rutherford found that designers were often involved in the development of pauper asylum landscapes, and of thirty public asylum sites where designers were identified she found that eleven of them had received a design contribution from a landscape designer of contemporary national renown.[48] In Northampton there is no evidence of any such contribution.

The design of the gardens at the General Lunatic Asylum changed over time. In 1860 one of the projected plans was 'the conversion of the old paved Male Airing Court No. 3 into a garden'.[49] Many of the airing courts seem to have been developed into gardened spaces rather than bare areas during this time. This is demonstrated by the fact that the *Annual Report* of 1864 refers to the 'Women's Airing Garden' rather than an airing court. This change in language suggests that at least some of the courts were viewed as analogous to gardens by this time.

From the introduction of the Visitors' Books in 1846, both the lay Visitors' Committee and the Commissioners in Lunacy are recorded as suggesting improvements to the external facilities. For example the Visitors write that:

> In reference to the observations of the Commissioners respecting the airing courts, we are of the opinion that if the ground was raised in the centre of the courts by removing the soil from the extremities of them the walls might be considerably lowered so as not only to admit the air more freely, but give also an appearance that the courts were not so confined as they appeared to the Commissioners.[50]

This reflects the use of mounds as a way of reducing the feeling of confinement and thereby increasing the homeliness of the asylum – both aims of moral therapy. There are also medical reasons for these alterations, which are reflected in the need to admit the air more freely. Again this shows the close connection between the moral and medical discourses of the time.

The creation of mounds in the airing courts was pioneered by Fox to allow patients to view the landscape while keeping them secure.[51] There is no indication in the quote above as to whether the view of the landscape was held to be important at the General Lunatic Asylum at this time. However, in 1859 the notion that a mound was to be 'raised or perfected in the large female airing Court' was viewed as problematic because the Visitors felt that it would 'obstruct distant views without any internal advantage' which suggests that the view had some value.[52] Similarly at the Charenton Hospital, outside Paris, it was stated that 'one of the essential advantages in the overall layout in the buildings lies in the fact that they do not back onto each other; this allows for an increased number of windows. These can be made sufficiently large to admit constant fresh air and to afford the patient more light and a wider and pleasanter view, so beneficial in their condition.'[53]

According to the *Annual Report* of 1860 a mound was created in one of the female courts, although it is unclear if this is the same mound as discussed above. The report gives more information on the design of the court and records that excavations were 'made to admit of the wall being lowered. The court levelled. A mound, with terrace walks and flower beds formed.'[54] It appears that the earlier bare courts were starting to be replaced with more decorative garden areas similar to those at Ticehurst Place and Brislington House.

In 1866 a 'huge mound' was formed in the male paupers' court but as soon as it had been created it was considered 'so unsatisfactory that it has been determined to remove the mound at once'.[55] There is no indication as to why it was found to be unsatisfactory but it seems possible that it was for the same issues outlined above with regard to the female airing court in 1859. There appears to have been a difficult balance to be struck between patients being able to see out over the walls when in the airing courts and views being available from inside the asylum. Once the mound had been removed the court was planted and turfed, and laid out for croquet and bowls.[56] Similar issues concerning views out versus the height of walls seem to have been considered at the Brighton Workhouse, built in 1866. According to the *Brighton and Hove Herald*, the airing courts 'are encircled by a high walk which some say is unnecessarily high and blocks out the view of the surrounding countryside. Others contend that it is not sufficiently high to prevent ill-judged friends from passing in spirits or other things contrary to the regulations.'[57] In this case the permeability of the walls to the outside world is under question.

The planting and turfing of courts is something that appears to take place in the years following the Commissioners in Lunacy Report of 1854, recorded in the Visitors' Books. In this report they state that they 'think that the accommodation provided for the patients in the wards is not good. That the confined nature of the airing courts, and the absence of all the actual articles of furniture, and objects calculated to occupy and interest the patients tends to promote refractory, and disorderly habits.'[58] Here the Visitors are clearly linking the size of the airing courts, as well as the lack of homeliness, with the behaviour of the patients. As the ability of a patient to apply self-control to disorderly habits was seen as part of their recovery, they are, in turn, relating the inability to see the surrounding landscape and the overt feeling of confinement to a reduction in the possibility of a cure. Part of the solution to this problem seems to have been to allow the patients frequent opportunities to take exercise in the wider grounds. Later they also suggest further changes to the design of the airing courts.

The belief that order was important was reflected in the use of this term as a positive description of the patients and the gardens:

> The Patients, with one or two exceptions, are perfectly tranquil and orderly.[59]

> The airing courts and gardens are kept in the best order, and are most agreeable and cheerful.[60]

> The garden and grounds are in excellent order and well kept and evidently afford much enjoyment to the patients.[61]

This adds weight to the argument discussed above about order and its direct relationship with the landscape. The use of the term 'tranquil' also reflects Wordsworth's tranquillity through harmony with nature and was a term used until the late nineteenth century as a positive term for patient behaviour at the General Lunatic Asylum.

After describing the new male airing court as gravelled and tiled in 1858, the Commissioners go on to suggest 'that it should be laid out in walks and planted'.[62] They describe how the 'Male Airing Court No. 1 has been extended to nearly three times its size, by the addition of the Kitchen Garden to the North, and is about to be sown with grass seeds, and intersected with walks. We think that a portion of this ground might be beneficially appropriated as a Bowling Green.'[63] It appears that the Commissioners' suggestions were generally acted upon as they also suggest that there should be 'cheerful illustrations and publications, statuettes, flowering plants, singing birds, domestic animals etc'.[64] Two years later they record that their suggested improvements had been carried out: a bowling green had been formed and 'birds, animals, and gold and silver fish' had been introduced in the wards.[65]

Further ornamentation was provided at the General Lunatic Asylum by the introduction of seats, sunshades and fountains. From 1846, concerns were raised that there was no shelter for the patients: 'The airing courts on both sides of the House are sadly deficient in shelter against the excessive heat of the sun.'[66] The Commissioners reiterate this plea in 1860 when they recommend that the asylum provide 'Summer Houses, or sunshades, in the Airing Grounds which are urgently required.'[67] The suggestions of the Commissioners were eventually complied with. In 1862 six circular seats were constructed around the trees in the new male airing court, as was a 'shed with seats'.[68] Similarly for the women's large airing court in 1864, a 'shed, or covered promenade, 95 feet long and ten feet wide, with a roof of corrugated iron' was erected at a cost of £95. Fixed under this was a seat '95 feet long with elbows at intervals of eight feet'.[69] Other features created at this time in the large women's airing court include a fountain (1863) and an aviary (1864).[70] These elements reflected the design of country houses at the time as illustrated by a plan of Eleveden Hall, Suffolk from *The Builder* in 1871, which also included an aviary and a fountain, albeit at opposite ends of the house.[71]

The developments in the gardens throughout the first forty years of the asylum's existence meant that by the first Ordnance Survey Map of 1887, the grounds were considerably more ornamented than those shown on the 1847 map. It is not possible to ascertain if, when the asylum first opened, the gardens were considered to be appropriate in their unornamented state or whether there were simply not enough funds remaining for the landscape after the completion of the building. It seems likely that it was due to lack of funds as the gardens seem to be continually discussed and developed over the early period of the asylum. However, during the last decades of the nineteenth century, the gardens were not mentioned in either the Visitors' Books or the Annual Reports. Whether this omission was because the gardens had been completed to a satisfactory level, so there was no need for discussion, or because their significance had decreased it is impossible to establish.

On improvement of the airing courts attention started to shift to the wider landscape and the Visitors and the Commissioners began to discuss the enhancement of the landscape outside the airing courts. In 1872, the Visitors record that they 'have much satisfaction in observing that a broad walk is in course of construction which will afford the means of daily extended exercise along the boundary of the estate'.[72] In the same year, they stated that a 'wide gravel path around asylum grounds, with shrubs and lime trees planted beside it' was in formation.[73] There were also ornamental grounds within the estate as these were referred to in 1865 when the Visitors discussed developments in the grounds. After 1881 the area outside the immediate airing courts and ornamental grounds became predominantly parkland, as the agricultural production was moved to Moulton Park.

By the time that the General Lunatic Asylum appears to have completed the design of the airing courts and surrounding gardens to the satisfaction of the Visitors and the Commissioners, the new Northampton County Asylum was being built. The airing courts on the first Ordnance Survey Map of 1886, ten years after the asylum opened, appear to be less ornamented than those belonging to the General Lunatic Asylum at the same time. This could partly be because the rate payers were still paying for the new, expensive building.[74]

Designed by Robert Griffiths, County Surveyor of Staffordshire, the County Asylum was described by Burdett in 1891 as 'the finest specimen of the corridor-pavilion type and of the quadrangular arrangement of the blocks'.[75] In the twentieth century, Nikolaus Pevsner wrote that it was 'a large red-brick building with a prominent tower, vaguely Rhineland Romanesque in inspiration'.[76] Although (or perhaps because) the asylum displayed the best design layout of the day, it was not without its problems, specifically its high cost. In 1878, the *Northampton Herald* wrote:

> Of course the Commissioners in Lunacy were much gratified by their visit. They have not to pay . . . But now comes along the worst part of the story. You sir and I and other victims, would expect to obtain something for their money, a building that the country would be proud of . . . And what have we obtained? – a monstrously ugly structure whose chief architectural feature is a 'tall chimney'.[77]

The high cost of the building would have meant that there was little money left for the gardens on completion. There could also have been concerns over using even more of the rate payers' money, as its use for ornamenting the grounds could have led to further vitriolic attacks from those such as the *Northampton Herald* who felt that the asylum was already wasting money. However, the economic situation of the asylum improved once it opened as 'maintenance costs were covered by "out county" and private patients without the need for funding by the county' and by 1878 it was running at a profit.[78] This could explain why there were gradual improvements once the asylum was up and running and it does mirror the developments at the General Asylum, and earlier institutions such as the York Retreat.

According to Fred Golby, during the first year of the asylum's existence concern was raised that the airing courts had not yet been built and it was felt that 'no time should be lost in turfing them and planting them, and getting them generally in proper order'.[79] This suggests that the courts were created after the opening of the asylum and when finished would have been similar to those at the General Lunatic Asylum as they also had a combination of turf and planting. The planting was probably an amalgamation of shrubs and bedding but there is little written evidence to indicate what species of plants were used.

Gradual improvements were also implemented on the wider estate. Henrietta Ayres has stated that in 1877 a considerable number of trees and shrubs were planted throughout the estate but that little else was done initially, except for 'an extension of walks in the grounds to enable patients to take exercise beyond the airing courts'.[80] The records in the General Ledger suggest that expenditure on the grounds was ongoing. For example, in 1876 the asylum spent £19 2s on seeds, some of which were flower seeds, and in 1884 they purchased 'lawn grass and flower pots &c.' for £4 14s 6d, as well as shrubs, including lilacs and roses for £4 14s 2d.[81] The rose was a particular favourite of the Victorians and has been described by David Stuart as 'almost the Victorian flower' which suggests that fashion influenced even pauper asylum landscapes to some extent.[82] The asylum also purchased several rhododendrons, another Victorian favourite, between 1886 and 1894.[83] Although there is less evidence of structural ornamentation than at the General Lunatic Asylum, the County Asylum purchased materials for the construction of an eighty-foot long conservatory in 1881.[84]

Like the Governors of the General Lunatic Asylum, the County Asylum Governors continued to improve and enlarge the airing courts in the initial years following its opening. In December 1898 they resolved that the airing courts on the male and female side be enlarged and improved at an estimated cost of £1,739.[85] On the 1900 Ordnance Survey Map the courts were still depicted as the same size but there appear to be mounds in the south-east facing areas, presumably to improve the ability of the patients to view the surrounding landscape. The Ordnance Survey Map of 1926 provides the first evidence that new courts had been created to the south-east of the asylum. These additions appear to have been broken into quadrants by paths. A round circle in the central front court on the west side represents a band stand which was still present in the grounds in 2001.

The County Asylum had two distinct areas of landscape outside the airing courts; the woodland area to the north and the parkland/agricultural land to the south. Much of the woodland would have been inherited with the estate as the sales particulars describe the land as 'finely timbered with oaks of good growth and ornamental appearance'.[86] On the 1886 Ordnance Survey Map this woodland is shown as mixed deciduous and coniferous. The recent report by aboriculturalist Mark Hinsley on the site in 2000 commented on the lack of woodland ground flora which suggests that this area was managed as semi-parkland with mown grass between the trees.[87] The environmental statement also goes on to suggest that a 1911 photograph of a lady walking within the grounds adds further evidence for this method of management, although it is not clear in which part of the estate it was taken.

According to Hinsley, most of the trees on the estate are introduced exotics. Of particular interest are the *Thuja plicatas* (Western Red Cedar) which form a major feature of the landscape and the single *Sequoiadendron giganteum* (Giant Canadian Redwood). According to Hinsley's report, these species were only introduced into this country twenty years before the asylum was built, which proves that they were planted specifically as part of the landscape and implies that the Governors were interested in using novel species on the estate. The *Sequioadendron* was planted in an airing court to the east of the building, according to a map associated with the Environmental Statement. Although Hinsley has dated the planting of this tree at around 1880 it is not shown on any of the Ordnance Survey Maps after this time, although there is a deciduous tree symbol placed in the same location on the 1886 Ordnance Survey Map. This means that the symbols for coniferous and deciduous trees may not be entirely accurate and the fact that a tree of this level of interest and size is not featured on the Ordnance Survey Maps post-1886 indicates that there could have been a more detailed design within the airing courts than the maps suggest. This theory is supported by an engraving of a slightly earlier pauper asylum, Essex County Asylum, Brentwood (1857), which was printed in *The Builder*.[88] The airing court gardens portrayed appear to have areas of turf intersected by paths and Gardenesque style flowerbeds.[89]

Many of the early trees, including several *Thuja plicatas*, are planted either side of the main entrance drive. Rutherford has suggested that parkland planting in pauper asylums 'tended to be limited to the areas closest to the core of the site which were visible from the wards and, or, from the approaches' in comparison to more extensive ornamentation in the domestic landscape park.[90] She uses the Northampton County Asylum to illustrate this point, and the planting of the novel trees alongside the drive provides further evidence for her argument. This planting also implies that such ornamentation would have been for the benefit of the external world rather than the patients. Other trees in the landscape include a number of horse chestnuts, some of which may date from 1881 when the Marquis of Exeter, who was a member of the asylum's Visitors' Committee, donated eighty chestnut trees.[91] Further tree planting took place throughout the twentieth century, including the planting of *Pinus nigras* around 1905–10 to the west of the site, rows of poplars in 1920 and rows of limes in the 1940s. The last major tree planting was probably the poplars north of the laundry in the 1960s.[92]

Even with the additional planting the County Asylum seems to have remained less ornamented than the General Asylum. This might reflect general concerns about rate payers' money being used for ornamentation or even beliefs about differences in class. This is an area that Peter Bartlett has discussed at length and he argues that 'the Lunacy Commissioners were perceived as a check on extravagant construction, and to that end they emphazised the pauper clientele of the asylum. In their 1844 report, for example, they argue that no unnecessary cost ought to be spent on decoration "especially as these Asylums are erected for persons who, when in health, are accustomed to dwell in cottages".'[93] According to a mid-nineteenth-century report for the private Boston Lunatic Asylum in the United States:

> Paupers . . . or those in the lower walks of life, whose means are limited, are provided for by various City, County and State Institutions. It has seemed necessary to maintain here, a class of accommodations and a style of living more than simply comfortable, and even in a degree, luxurious, meeting the wants, artificial though they may be, of those in a higher social position, and possessed of a competency, who in a state of disease cannot be placed in the best condition for cure, or even present relief, unless surrounded by the comforts to which they have been accustomed.[94]

In the case of the Newcastle-upon-Tyne Borough Pauper Lunatic Asylum, economic considerations appear to have led to unornamented airing courts and resultant complaints from the Commissioners in Lunacy.

The 1871 *Annual Report* for the asylum stated that, 'The grounds are being gradually made to assume a neat and orderly appearance, but as the Committee are anxious that no expense should be incurred in the laying of them out, the labour is entirely contributed by patients, and the work is necessarily of slow progress.'[95] In 1875 the Commissioners complain that 'little has been done to put the airing courts into a proper state. They are still quite bare, and the paths are in a rough condition. The roads and shrubberies are in very good order, and there is no reason whatever why a matter of so much importance as the due planting and cultivation of the patients' airing courts should have been so long neglected.'[96] Then again in 1876 they report that, 'In the principal male airing court, some trees have been planted but it would be a great improvement if flower beds were laid out, both here and in the female courts, to which nothing has at present been done, and which are still in the same bare and unattractive condition.'[97] This suggests that the reports of the Commissioners had little weight in this matter and that, although the Commissioners considered well-laid-out gardens to be important, financial considerations could prevent such concerns being addressed in institutions catering for poorer inmates.

In contrast to this, Thomas Prichard, the proprietor of the Abington Abbey Retreat[98] which according to its promotional literature admitted 'invalids of respectability and education, but of limited incomes',[99] stated that

> In each county, but with few exceptions, will now be found an Asylum, well built and well appointed, cheerfully situate, and surrounded by extensive and well-planned grounds and gardens for the use and recreation of the inmates. The old, dreary, walled in airing courts, in which in former times the patients were accustomed for years to tramp to and fro like so many felons in a gaol, are now transformed into cheerful parterres, the flowers affording pleasing objects of contemplation.[100]

Again, Prichard seems to be suggesting that gardens filled with flowers helped achieve homely, in contrast to prison-like, environs. However, he was of course aiming at a group of patients, who although not wealthy, could afford to pay for their care. The use of the term 'cheerful parterres' probably also reflected the Victorian love of bright bedding plants, particularly those found in public parks of the period.[101] It should also be noted that he uses the terms 'cheerful' and 'tranquil', which provides further evidence for the significance of these terms throughout the nineteenth century.

Use of the landscape for recreation, exercise and work

In line with other superintendents, Prichard felt that the gardens had an important therapeutic role:

> the care of the gardens being, in many instances entrusted to patients, serves as a double purpose – of affording wholesome occupation, and of promoting a tranquil and cheerful tone of thought. The operations of husbandry are largely carried out upon the asylum farm, and many acres of ground are profitably cultivated, both in an economical point of view and as a remedial and curative process.[102]

However, as is common when researching the history of psychiatric care, it is hard to know what the patients themselves thought about the gardens and how much access they actually had to such spaces. The only other view of the gardens at Abington Abbey Retreat is found in a letter written by a patient in 1884. Addressed to the Visitors' Committee, Mrs Capron wrote:

> when I came here nearly three years ago, I was told I should find nice gardens and grounds to walk in. I have always been accustomed to these pleasures and amusements and appreciate them. For the first year and a half the Gardens were open and I enjoyed them; but, for the last few months the Gardens have been kept closely locked giving the surroundings a dismal and prison-like appearance; and very much interfering with the enjoyment of the peace.[103]

This is an unusual letter because it is from a patient discussing their access to the gardens. Sadly there is no mention of this letter or Mrs Capron's complaint in the Visitors' Books, which means there is no explanation as to why the gardens were locked or whether this situation was resolved. Her letter does imply that there were ornamental gardens and that she initially enjoyed these. However, of more interest, is that her concerns reflected the views of the medical profession at this time, which was that the landscape did much to relieve the sensation of confinement and prevented patients feeling that they were held within a prison. This suggests that some patients did appreciate the landscape and felt that it was of some therapeutic value to them. The sentiments expressed by Mrs Capron have also been echoed by some twentieth-century psychiatric patients, as discussed later on.

Mrs Capron's letter acts as a reminder that, just because superintendents and visiting committees stated that patients were actively using the grounds, this does not necessarily mean this was actually the case. There is, however, a substantial amount of documentary evidence that suggests that patients could spend a considerable amount of their time outdoors. One of many such examples is *The New Regulations of Wonford House Hospital for the Insane Near Exeter* (1880) which stated that 'the gardens and pleasure grounds into which the several galleries open, shall be accessible to the patients at all suitable times, and at least three hours in the morning, and two hours in the afternoon of everyday, when the weather is favourable'.[104] Similarly at the County Asylum in the 1880s:

> Those who were not able to work were still encouraged to occupy themselves in some way and all were taken outside into the 'airing courts' at about 10.30 a.m. and were not allowed to return until lunch at 12.30. Once outside, patients were goaded into 'walking around sufficiently', and in damp weather they were to be prevented from lying down on the gravel or grass while in hot weather they were ushered into the shade. All were to be 'carefully prevented from eating plants'.[105]

This regimented approach to the landscape has been related to the size of the asylum by Scull. He argues that 'large numbers from the outset required the development of a bureaucratic routine'.[106] This seems to have been the case at the County Asylum, which started with 510 patients in 1877 but expanded rapidly to have over 1,000 patients in 1913.[107] These large numbers would have placed pressure on the staff and the kind of one-to-one walk with conversation described by Tuke earlier would have been practically impossible.[108]

The practice of regimented time in the airing courts apparently continued into the twentieth century at the County Asylum. According to Ayres, in the early decades of the century, 'assuming the weather was reasonable the practice of turning patients out into the exercise yards for two hours in the morning and another two in the afternoon was still a part of daily life, and, as in previous years there was nothing for them to do but trudge round the walks within the walled courts'.[109] The last part of this sentence is subjective and, although it may be true, it should remembered that this history was written in 1976 when there was a strong anti-psychiatry movement and the hospital was trying to distance itself from its Victorian reputation.

Like the York Retreat and Brislington House, the various landscapes of the Northampton asylums were used by the patients for exercise, recreation and employment as part of the implementation of moral therapy. The importance of spending time within the landscape was a particularly strong notion at the General Lunatic Asylum. Infirm patients were even provided with the use of a carriage so that they could enjoy the landscape. In 1863 one of the members of the Visitors' Committee suggested 'the propriety of an invalid carriage to be drawn by hand so that Patients who are unable to walk have the advantages of fresh air on the grounds there are such carriages at the infirmary'.[110] By 1883 the Commissioners in Lunacy could record that 'carriages are used daily'.[111]

Exercise outdoors remained important throughout the century and all three of the Northampton asylums appear to have used this as part of the daily routine. In 1890 it was noted that at the General Lunatic Asylum, 'several of the patients have carriages, many walk daily in the grounds and about double their number walk weekly from the male side beyond the estate and about 47 women'.[112] At Abington Abbey, Thomas Prichard cites a number of cases where exercise outdoors had effected an alteration in the external behaviour of the patients. This again provides evidence for the idea that the patient's mental state was measured by their external behaviour.

> One case, a gentleman, had been a resident here for twenty years . . . he was for many years a harmless and incurable patient; was accustomed to walk in the grounds from day to day alone, never attempting to pass beyond the bounds of the park or to interfere with others taking exercise therein.[113]
>
> His was a case of dementia and he resided here for fifteen years . . . he was always quiet and contented, walked out at his pleasure, and seemed to enjoy existence.[114]

These cases probably tell us more about Thomas Prichard's beliefs than whether exercise taken outdoors was an effective treatment, particularly as he was writing about his private asylum, whose continued existence relied on giving the impression that it could help patients recover by pursuing moral therapy within an attractive environment. Annual reports would have been a powerful form of rhetoric and superintendents would hope that the descriptions of their therapeutic approaches and recovery rates would encourage relatives to send patients to their particular asylum. In Northampton the competition would have been fierce between the General Lunatic Asylum and the Abbey Retreat.

Recreational activities within the landscape remained important throughout the century. In 1883 the Commissioners in Lunacy recorded that patients at the General Lunatic Asylum were able to participate in 'tennis, bowls, archery, croquet'.[115] In fact the Visitors were concerned that outdoor activities were curtailed during the winter and one member of the Committee suggested that 'fives courts, asphalted Tennis courts,

Bowling and Skittle Alleys, or at least some of these would be desirable additions to the Hospital. A covered promenade for walking exercise in wet weather would also be very useful.'[116] By 1890 the variety of amusements appears to have increased so that they now included 'dances, and other concerts, theatrical entertainments, cricket matches, tennis, archery, football, billiard handicaps, fishing parties and excursions of various sorts. A few patients have joined hunts with hounds and beagles. There is a good band which plays frequently in the grounds.'[117]

The therapeutic effects associated with recreational activities meant that in the first year of the County Asylum's existence there was dancing and cricket as well as an ample supply of books. An American Bowling Alley was also built and a billiard table provided for the men's day room.[118] According to Ayres, it took until 1960 for a bowling alley to be opened in Northampton town for the general public, yet the pauper asylum acquired one in the nineteenth century. Later, football pitches and tennis courts were added, and a bandstand situated in the grounds was testament to outdoor concerts. However, there was no mention of hunting, which one can assume was reserved for patients of a higher class at the General Lunatic Asylum, as was the case at Brislington House and Ticehurst Place earlier in the century.

The other function of the landscape was to provide employment for the male patients. In Browne's description of how an asylum 'ought to be', his utopian vision conjured up 'a hive of industry' where 'you meet the gardener, the common agriculturalist, the mower, the weeder, all intent on their several occupations and loud in their merriment'.[119] In contrast, William Ellis, superintendent of Wakefield Asylum, was more overtly concerned with employment as a form of control as he felt that when pauper patients were left unemployed they behaved in a 'depraved and abandoned manner'.[120] Another argument for the importance placed on employment other than as part of the moral therapy regime was that it rehabilitated patients so that they could resume their place in industrialised society as productive and economically viable subjects.[121] There is no doubt some truth to this, particularly in relation to the publicly funded pauper asylums.

By the Victorian period the idea of idleness was seen as immoral and closely associated with dissipation. Prichard also held the view that:

> By the operation of the same wholesome discipline, the patient on quitting the Asylum is restored to his friends and family, endowed with those habits of industry which may secure him against being a burden to them, or, through the effects of idleness, relapsing into his recent malady.[122]

Prichard was superintendent of an asylum which took both paying and pauper patients but he suggests that the patient needs to be able to work so that they are not a burden on their family. This suggests that a central role of the asylum is to re-orientate the patient so that they can return and fulfil their allotted role within society. However, Prichard also suggests that idleness could cause the patient to relapse, so this demonstrates another layer in the relationship with immorality; in this case, idleness and insanity.

In relation to agricultural employment within the asylum, Philo rightly argues that 'at root it was still the moral identification of labouring in nature as vital to the cure of insanity that energised . . . the retreat of the asylum from the realm of the urban-industrial to that of the rural-agricultural'.[123] In terms of the location and size of the asylum the belief in the importance of agricultural work ensured a rural setting and the ownership of vast tracts of land. Philo goes on to say that in the nineteenth century a '*working* asylum called for yards, gardens, fields and other lands in quantity only available in rural districts'.[124] This, alongside other beliefs concerning physical and mental health, ensured the rural siting of the asylum.

It can be argued that the growth of industrialisation and urbanisation changed man's relationship with the natural world. Along with the popularity of representations of landscapes in both art and literature came fears that civilisation itself was causing both unhealthy bodies and minds as man moved further away from nature. As the ideas of mental health and morality are so closely intertwined during this period, it is, therefore, unsurprising that being close to nature could also be seen as conferring moral values. Landscape art in this period is suggestive of some level of rural morality. According to Rosemary Treble, 'one of the most powerful images of the Victorian countryside for the modern viewer and for the Victorians themselves, was provided by scenes of cottage life, featuring rustic simplicity, sometimes in picturesque poverty, sometimes in virtuous and provident, though rude, conduct'.[125] This suggests that there was a desire to portray the moral benefits of rural life.

Christiana Payne has argued that there are three myths associated with the countryside, which were portrayed in Victorian paintings of agricultural workers, and that these were as follows: 'that people are happier in the countryside, that country people are more virtuous, and that country people were more virtuous and happy in the past than they are now'.[126] She has also suggested that in the nineteenth century these myths were related to the contrast of the corrupt city and industrialised towns, 'with their horrific living and working conditions and their irreligious and riotous populations'[127] and that 'the countryside . . . is a place of moral and physical health free from the corruption of city and court'.[128] It is this moral element which is interesting in relation to idea of mental health and rural living. Payne has also suggested that, 'paintings helped establish the cultivated counties of the south as the setting of demonstrations of rural virtue; and already in the 1840s they were seen as symbolic of England as a whole'.[129] It is likely that this view of the countryside influenced the idea that a rural situation, and work within such a setting, could have a positive effect on the mind. Industriousness is seen as one of the virtues of the rural labourer, as well as a therapeutic element within the asylum. Therefore, the Romantic ideal of the cheerfully industrious agricultural labourer helped establish the concept that rural conditions were better for mental health.[130]

Jean-Jacques Rousseau had postulated in the mid-eighteenth century that as civilisation developed, men alienated themselves from nature and that primitive man was superior because he was closer to his natural state.[131] His idea of the 'noble savage' influenced later ideas, in particular those concerning mental illness. Scull has written that, 'the Rousseauist myth that the noble savage was somehow immune from the ravages of insanity was quite widely canvassed by Regency and early Victorian writers on the subject'.[132]

Examples of this belief can be found in the work of a number of writers on the subject, including Browne, who described in great detail how the development of civilised communities had increased the chance of individuals suffering from mental disturbance. From his point of view, it would not be surprising that a patient could develop a mental disorder from the excitement of visiting the Great Exhibition (a reason once given for the onset of madness) as it was the increased excitement created by civilisation that was the key problem:

> With luxury, indeed, insanity appears to keep equal pace. Nay, the opinion has been hazarded, that as we recede, step by step, from the simple, that is the savage manners of our ancestors, and advance in industry and knowledge and happiness, this malignant persecutor strides onward, signalising every era in the social progress by an increase, a new hecatomb of victims . . . The truth seems to be, that the barbarian escapes this scourge because he is exempt from many of the physical, and almost all the moral sources of mental excitement; and that the members of civilized communities are subjected to it, because the enjoyments and blessings of augmented power are abused; because the mind is roused to exertion without being disciplined,

> it is stimulated without being strengthened; because our selfish propensities are cultivated while our moral nature is left barren, our pleasures becoming poisonous; and because in the midst of a blaze of scientific light, and in the presence of a thousand temptations to multiply our immediate by a sacrifice of our ultimate gratifications, we remain in the darkest ignorance of our own mind, its true relations, its dangers and destiny.[133]

This belief that civilisation was an important factor in the causation of madness was confirmed by the recommendation that an asylum needed an airy and healthy situation and, according to Rutherford, 'indicated that, practically, a rural situation, rather than one within a cramped town centre was called for'.[134]

Similarly Klaus Doerner has argued that the rural asylum offered 'an escape from the anarchy of industrial society . . . Nature was to heal insanity like all other problems caused by chaotic social progress.'[135] This ideology of the aesthetic power of nature to tame the unruly industrial crowds has also been explored by Amy Woodson-Boulton in relation to nineteenth-century public art galleries where it was hoped that even artistic representations of landscapes would encourage moral reform.[136] She has argued that 'nineteenth-century aesthetic ideology developed as a reaction to the centrifugal forces of industrial capitalism, which unmoored traditional society, remade the natural landscape, and seemingly destroyed the bonds among man, nature and God. Nineteenth century art reformers hoped that art would heal those wounds.'[137]

It is worth exploring the role of pastoral landscape within the nineteenth century asylum in detail, beginning with the York Retreat (Figure 19). Edginton has suggested that, although the intention of the Retreat's design was to effect a cure, its relationship with nature was not as simple as it appeared: 'The Retreat did not place the lunatic closer to the calm influence of nature but closer to the influence of a constructed nature, and in "moral treatment" we find a discourse similar to the control of nature itself.'[138] Similarly Michel Foucault sees this ruralisation as the separation of the unreasonable mad person from the reasonable people of the town. Within moral therapy:

> Confinement, as the separation of reason and unreason, is not suppressed; but at the very heart of its intention, the space it occupies reveals natural powers, more constraining for madness, more likely to subjugate it in its essence, than the whole of the old limiting and repressive system. Madness must be liberated from that system so that, in the space of confinement, now endowed with a positive efficacy, it will be free to slough of its savage freedom, and to welcome the demands of nature.[139]

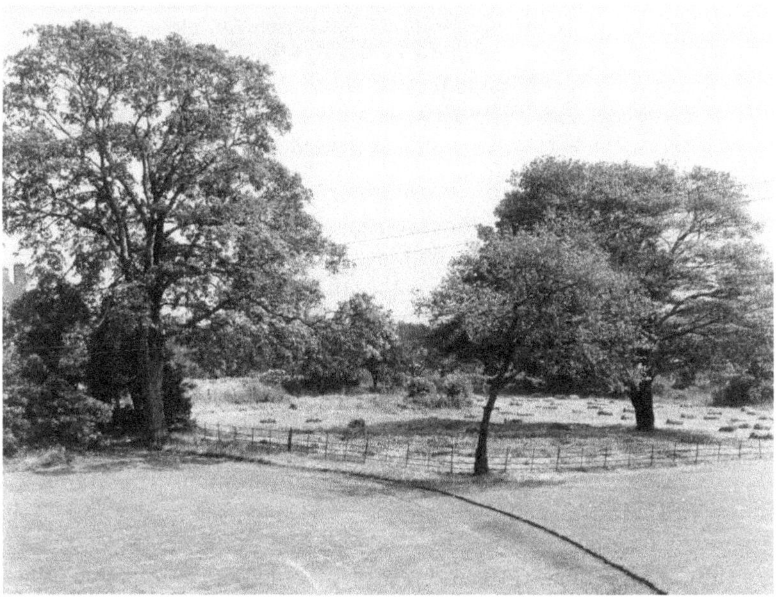

Figure 19 The ordered agricultural landscape at the York Retreat, presumably taken during hay-making (mid-twentieth century photograph).

Similar to pastoral ideas of landscape, this concept of nature is one that is 'mediatized by morality'.[140] Agricultural lands that are ordered and tamed by man are, therefore, considered to be more effective in restoring reason than wilderness, as nature untamed could act as a trigger for the expression of unsuitable, or immoral, passions. As Parr has summarised, 'Nature here was seen as a therapeutic space, the promise of health premised in part on the passive absorption of the inherently healthy and rational properties of moral and manicured asylum land.'[141]

According to Philo the moralised nature of the Retreat's landscape meant that it was 'composed as attractive scenes full of agricultural endeavour'.[142] In the case of the pauper asylums of nineteenth-century England, Rutherford suggests that beyond the immediate ornamental planting around the asylum, the land tended to be agricultural in character, which supports the idea that agricultural land formed a considerable part of the landscape that patients were exposed to.[143] As Parr has argued, 'to be a labourer among nature, for example, was to be (potentially) freed from the "artificial clutter" of society and to be subjected only to the "gentle constraints of nature", where living by the seasons and the demands of the land was to submit oneself to powers of "natural obligation" that might help to counter the confusion of the insane mind'.[144] That said, it is essential to emphasise that in the case of pauper asylums in particular, it was necessary to use the land for agricultural purposes to make the asylums economically viable.[145]

The Cambridgeshire Asylum provides an unusual example of the combination of aesthetics and agricultural use of the land. In front of the asylum huge petal-shaped beds were created (they are shown on the 1886 Ordnance Survey Map) surrounded by curved paths. In the aerial photograph taken around 1927 (Figure 20) the beds are shown planted with crops.[146] This reflects the original design as according to Benjamin Ward Richardson in 1864, 'the Asylum property includes about fifty eight acres of land, thirty two of which ore devoted to the cultivation of cereals and root crops, twenty are under spade husbandry as garden, and six

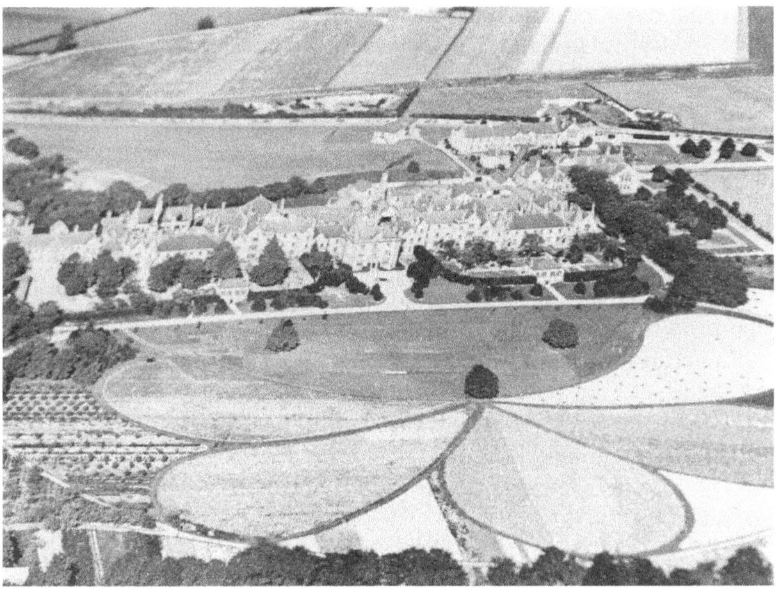

Figure 20 An aerial photograph taken around 1927 of the Fulbourn Hospital (previously Cambridgeshire Asylum) clearly showing the petal beds.

are occupied by buildings and airing-courts'.[147] Here the curving paths would have allowed patients close access to the ordered land. This use of agricultural land as part of the asylum landscape was also taken up in America. In 1854 Thomas Kirkbride, who at the time was the physician to the Pennsylvania Hospital for the Insane, wrote that:

> To enable the patients to have the greatest amount of benefit from their pleasure grounds, those of the males and females should be entirely distinct; and one of the best means of separating them will be found to be the appropriation of a strip of neutral ground, properly enclosed between them as a park for various animals, or to be otherwise handsomely cultivated.[148]

Another consequence of the discourse recommending that a close relationship with nature was the key to good mental health was that nineteenth-century doctors developed the idea that agricultural workers were less likely to develop insanity, as illustrated by these two examples:

> The cultivators of the earth are not so liable to derangement as the cultivators of the mind itself; but it is not because there is anything peculiar or injurious in the latter, but because, from accessory circumstances, it is more calculated to destroy that tranquillity and equilibrium of the powers which is favoured in the former.[149]

> We seldom meet with insanity among the savage tribes of men ... Among the slaves in the West Indies it very rarely occurs; and ... the contented peasantry of the Welsh Mountains, the Western Hebrides, and the wilds of Ireland are almost free from this complaint.[150]

The idea that people closer to the land did not develop insanity indicated that, from the very beginning of the nineteenth century, doctors viewed labour on the land as an effective part of moral therapy.[151]

Rutherford has shown that the size of asylum estates increased throughout the nineteenth century so that from the 1870s most estates covered more than 100 acres.[152] Size still appeared to be important at the end of the century even though medical treatments had taken over from moral ones in perceived importance. In 1891 Henry Burdett wrote that:

> Many of our English county asylums are placed on high, exposed situations, it being apparently forgotten that the building is to be used as a hospital and a residence for feeble invalids ... The two points which have hitherto determined the choice of a site have been cheapness of land and the view from it. Both of these admirable in their way, but both may have been purchased too dearly.[153]

However, given these reservations, he still viewed gardens as important features and suggested that the 'courts should be laid out as gardens, and orchards, and lawns'.[154]

The use of land for agricultural purposes is more obvious at the General Asylum and County Asylum because they were purpose-built. However, the estate of Abington Abbey did have a farm with associated agricultural land within its boundary. At the General Lunatic Asylum the growing need for agricultural land meant that the Governors had to purchase extra acreage throughout the nineteenth century. The Visitors' Books of the General and County asylums suggest that patients were employed on the land, even if the actual numbers were not as high as one would necessarily expect. At the General Lunatic Asylum in 1865 out of a possible 221 male patients, twenty-seven were employed on the farm and in the garden.[155] In 1887 the numbers of patients had grown so that out of 116 men, twenty were at Moulton Park (the farm estate) where they were employed in farm and garden work 'with great advantage to themselves'.[156] A further thirty-eight were working in the gardens surrounding the asylum and the remaining eighteen 'help in the workshop or domestic work'.[157] Both Scull and Rutherford have questioned the disparity between the amount of documentary evidence stressing the importance of employment, particularly outdoors, and the actual rates in practice, which appear to be very low.

It is clear that whatever work was carried out, it was intended to be of therapeutic benefit, as well as for economic reasons. In 1891, the Commissioners report that 'as many as 81 male patients are induced to employ themselves, of these 61 help on the farm or in the garden'.[158] They go on to say that 'Dr Bayley is quite convinced of the value of out-door employment in the proper treatment of many male patients and hopes to give this exercise to many more gentlemen upon the land newly acquired.'[159] This suggests that class was not necessarily a barrier, at least by this point in the century, as Bayley appears to have thought exercise upon the land was suitable for 'gentlemen'. Thomas Prichard was also keen on work as part of the therapy (see above) although research for this book has not ascertained whether this was practised at Abington Abbey.

As would be expected, work at the pauper County Asylum was economically essential as well as retaining some therapeutic value. These two factors are intertwined in the management of pauper asylums, as has been discussed in great depth by Rutherford.[160] In 1884, according to Golby, records from the County Asylum state that:

> The Asylum Farm has been carried on with great advantage to the Asylum. A certain quantity of land must be attached to every Asylum and outdoor exercise is beneficial to the patients. It may indeed be said that independently of the great service rendered by the Farm towards the management and treatment of the patients, the Asylum has to farm from necessity as well as choice.[161]

Ayres suggests that the rates of employment at the County Asylum were high. Within two years of the asylum opening, '60 percent of the men were employed and 50 percent of the women. For example, there were 75 men who worked as gardeners, six in the laundry, two as stokers, one as an engineer, seven as carpenters, 21 on domestic duties and a further 44 who undertook various jobs.'[162] It appears that outdoor employment was given to a greater number of the employable population than at the General Lunatic Asylum, but as Scull and Rutherford have suggested, one should be wary of such figures as they were sometimes manipulated for the benefit of the Commissioners in Lunacy.

There is some evidence that some sort of distinction was made in terms of how work was divided according to social class. In Browne's utopian asylum, labour is 'apportioned so that it may suit the powers and taste of each labourer'.[163] He goes on to describe the following as employment for patients of a higher class:

> You may visit rooms where there are ladies reading, or at the harp or the piano, or flowering muslin, or engaged in some of those thousand ornamental productions in which female taste and ingenuity are displayed . . . Another wing contains those gentlemen who can engage in intellectual pursuits, or in the amusements of the station to which they belong.[164]

This idea of suiting the employment to the station and skills of the patient explains in part why John Clare was employed in the kitchen garden at the General Lunatic Asylum even though he was a private patient.[165] He was registered as a gardener on admission to the asylum (although his occupation was later changed to 'poet' in his case notes) because he had previously been employed as a gardener. This included a brief period as a temporary kitchen garden apprentice at Burghley House, Stamford, Lincolnshire.[166] As he was a 'fifth class' or 'harmless' patient he was allowed considerable freedom and was allowed to walk into Northampton unaccompanied.[167] This provides additional evidence for the idea that employment on the land was mainly an activity for those who were seen as being in a state of recovery. This could be a factor in the explanation for why actual employment numbers were so low in relation to the widespread rhetoric.

The twentieth century

The general model of the rural asylum continued to be implemented into the twentieth century. This is in contrast to the general and specialist hospital where access to gardens and a view of the wider landscape was generally relinquished in favour of technological progress, as will be discussed in later chapters. When Severalls Hospital, Essex was opened in 1913 it was still based on the nineteenth-century model.[168] As late as 1911, The Board of Control were still suggesting that 'no estate less than 50 acres would be a suitable site'.[169] There were some changes to the architectural and landscape design in relation to idiot asylums, epileptic colonies, and mental deficiency colonies, but much of the landscape associated with mental asylums appears to remain the same, although often with lower walls around the airing courts.[170]

A few years after the Northampton County Asylum changed its name to St Crispin's Hospital, in 1947, the high walls that had enclosed the patients' exercise wards were demolished.[171] However, the parkland remained and, as discussed above, throughout the twentieth century the hospital still continued to add trees to the landscape. This implies that the landscape retained some level of importance until the hospital closed in the 1980s. In particular there are a number of *Metasequoia glyptostroboides* that, according to the 2000 aboriculturalist's report, could only have been planted post-1950 and, given their small size, were probably planted considerably more recently.[172] The landscape has been recognised as significant since the closure of the hospital and was made a conservation area in September 1996.

The landscapes of the asylums in Northampton still taking patients in the twentieth century (Abington Abbey Retreat was granted its last licence in 1891) were also still being used for therapeutic purposes. Part of the overarching philosophy of the moral therapy of the nineteenth century transformed itself into occupational therapy in the twentieth century. In 1915, Dr Daniel Rambaut, at the General Lunatic Asylum, 'introduced a scheme whereby patients were encouraged to hire small plots of land on the estate, grow their own produce and sell it to the Hospital; this proved a great success and was continued for many years'.[173] This was not based solely on economics as he also reported that 'employment in gardening has had a marked curative effect'.[174] Rambaut's successor, Dr Thomas

Tennent, also saw gardening as a valuable therapeutic tool and in 1938 he acknowledged the 'excellent progress already made by the Hospital, especially in gardening work, but was anxious to see even greater emphasis on this form of therapy'.[175]

At the same time, St Crispin's also introduced Occupational Therapy and in the 1958 review of the hospital's progress under the newly formed NHS they record that:

> One striking feature of out-door work organised by one Head Occupational Therapist is the now almost completed conversion of a former extensive rubbish tip, adjacent to one of the Centres, into a delightfully laid-out garden with lawns, flower beds and other features. The patients have carried out this work enthusiastically over the last six years and their efforts are much appreciated.[176]

This suggests that the landscape was still being used in a way that would have been recognisable to the Victorians even though new advances in treatments meant that medical intervention was at the forefront of psychiatric treatment.

One thing that has been missing in this discussion, as in most research concerning the history of psychiatric care, is the voice of the patient. Apart from Mrs Capron's letter from her time at Abington Abbey, Merivale's account of Ticehurst, and Perceval's diary of his time at both Brislington and Ticehurst, there is little evidence from non-fiction sources describing how nineteenth-century patients responded to the asylum landscapes. In the late twentieth century a small number of interviews were conducted with contemporary patients. The results of these suggest that these patients value the landscape in much the same way as the medical profession did in the nineteenth century.

In one interview conducted by Diana Gittins, a female patient was asked to compare Severalls Hospital with the new acute unit, The Lakes, attached to Colchester General Hospital. She said that, 'the grounds at Severalls, they were safe, they were – there were places where you might catch the odd glimpse of beauty. I mean, there was more than the odd glimpse then, but when you're in that state, you only see the odd glimpse. No, The Lakes is all wrong. Wrong.'[177] Similarly, in a study carried out for the King's Fund in 1977, Winifred Raphael found that 'most of the hospitals had lovely gardens and grounds and these were often a source of great pleasure; indeed they were frequently given in answer to the question, "what do you like best about the hospital?"'[178] She goes on to say that 'it was abundantly clear that wandering or sitting in spacious grounds served as a welcome antidote to the crowded wards and departments'.[179] It seems that the landscape was one of the few elements of the old asylum regime that was still viewed with affection by the patients. It also appears that in 1977 one of the patients was still responding to the grounds in the way the nineteenth-century medical profession had intended: 'The grounds have a soothing effect.'[180]

Similarly, Philo interviewed ex-patients of the old Inverness District Asylum and found they also had a positive response to the grounds. Comments that he recorded included the following: 'It is the grounds that make this place'; 'The Craig itself was quite helpful, quiet grounds to be in'; 'Well, that's what everyone misses, the grounds. I used to love walking up to the duck pond and over . . . The grounds were brilliant, used to wander around.'[181] This is just a snapshot, but it does suggest that the grounds were significant for at least some patients. In the case of Inverness, some of the users indicated to Philo that they still went up to the grounds even though it was theoretically inaccessible and the hospital had closed down. One interviewee articulated his worries over the site being developed by a private owner stating that, 'I'm wondering what's going to happen. Robertsons want to develop it, and what not, and when that happens, there's going to be nowhere for people to go. I think it's quite important. Most people are looking for peace and quiet when they are in hospital, so must have somewhere to walk.'[182]

The patients interviewed appear to have responded in a more positive manner to the gardens than the building itself. It could be argued that this was in part because it represented an area of greater freedom. One of the results of the development of moral therapy was the increased surveillance of patients. Some asylums, such as the one at Bodmin in Cornwall, were developed on a radial plan, which reflected the Benthamite principles of surveillance found in his Panoptican plan for prisons. According to Foucault, the benefit of this plan was that it was 'not necessary to use force to restrain the convict to good behaviour, the madman to calm, the worker to work, the schoolboy to application, the patient to observation of the regulations'.[183]

Although moral therapy has been replaced by newer therapies there can still be a strong element of surveillance within secure psychiatric units. In an institution where one of the modes of treatment is surveillance it could be argued that the gardens represent a less closely observed space. In Jennifer Dawson's 1961 novel, *The Ha-Ha*, the garden provides a place where two patients, who become lovers while confined, can meet away from prying eyes.[184] However, as Kerry Davies has written, 'while accounts from participants may not be as explicit or dramatic as that of Dawson . . . there is a significant emphasis on grounds as places of escape, rest and reflection'.[185] Here the garden represents a place that allows more freedom, perhaps even a more 'normal' life, within the institution and it is perhaps this notion that explains the more positive response to the external space. The garden also represents a marginal area between the enclosed space within and the open world outside. The role of the garden as a contested border area between the internal organisation of the psychiatric institution and the external world would be an interesting subject for further research.

The second half of the twentieth century saw a dramatic decline in the use of asylums and the closure of the majority of institutions. The decline began in relation to the effectiveness of newly developed drugs and an increase in the social unwillingness to place people in asylums. Gittins has described the replacement of asylums with drugs as a change in the use of space from outside to that within the patient themselves: 'Some of the history of a changing use of space in mental hospitals in recent years can be related to the increasing use of pharmacological means as a primary source of restraint and control . . . The space of control as a result has increasingly gone into the patient's body itself, instead of the body being restrained by outside forces.'[186] It can be argued that following Enoch Powell's speech as the new Minister of Health in 1961, the public asylum was doomed.[187] Alongside the government policy of care in the community, criticism of the ruralisation of these institutions, which had been so key to nineteenth-century treatment, was voiced by the mental health charity MIND. In 1975 they stated that:

> many of the institutions are totally unsuitable for anyone to live their lives in; too often they are large, isolated, old, built as self-contained 'colonies' outside the main centres of population, segregated from the rest of the community to protect it from the supposedly contaminating and corrupting influence of the 'mentally disordered'.[188]

The Victorian rural vision had become a twentieth-century curse. MIND went on to say that hospital care was now unnecessary and inappropriate for many.

In response to this changing philosophy, St Crispin's finally closed its doors to patients in 1995 and the estate, like many ex-institutional sites, is now being developed as housing. The Northampton General Lunatic Asylum, now known as St Andrew's, however, bucked this trend, mainly because it remained outside the public sector. When the NHS was formed, St Andrew's was one of only four hospitals to be disclaimed and consequently has been run on a charitable basis throughout the twentieth century and is still going strong at the beginning of the twenty-first. The landscape still performs an important function at the hospital and its upkeep is paid for by subscriptions to a private members' golf club which is located within the parkland to the south of the hospital. The current website describes the hospital as follows: 'St Andrew's largest range of services is located at its main site in Northampton. Situated across 120 acres of parkland and with excellent therapeutic and recreational facilities.'[189] The rhetorical language used in this quote would have been familiar to a nineteenth-century audience. Here, at least, the landscape is still perceived as performing a therapeutic role today.

The ruralisation and increasing size of landscapes surrounding the nineteenth- and early twentieth-century asylums reflected cultural perceptions of the health benefits of the countryside as well as the concept that recreation and work outdoors was part of the therapeutic regime. The effect of gardens and contact with nature seems to have been connected to the desired outcomes of tranquillity and cheerfulness. This research also demonstrates that although economic considerations and concerns over class influenced the design and use of the gardens, the theoretical underpinning remained the same. Although enforced time outdoors was not always enjoyable or even particularly beneficial for patients, accounts and interviews suggest that the gardens and landscape could represent a positive element of the institutional experience.

Notes

1 Browne, *What Asylums Are*, p. 229.

2 He later became Medical Superintendent at the Royal Crichton Institute, Dumfries (1839–57), before becoming Senior Medical Inspector in Lunacy for Scotland (1857–70) until an accident forced him to retire.

3 For more on the changes in legislation see Kathleen Jones, *Asylums and After: A Revised History of the Mental Health Services from the Early Eighteenth Century to the 1990s* (London: Athlone Press, 1993) and Scull, *The Most Solitary of Afflictions*, 1993.

4 Philo, *A Geographical History*, p. 535. For a history of the parliamentary enquiries and other factors that led to this see Scull, *The Most Solitary of Afflictions*, 1993, and Porter, *Mind Forg'd Manactes*, 1987.

5 Rutherford suggests that county asylums based on the designs of Brislington and the York Retreat were later Victorian developments and that the first

three public asylums to be built in the nineteenth century (Nottingham 1810–12, Bedford 1810–12 and Norwich 1811–14) owed more to earlier charitable institutions such as St Luke's and Bethlem. Therefore, on the whole they did not use the model of an asylum which included an extensive landscape to be used for therapeutic purposes. However the Nottingham asylum was more of a hybrid between the older model and the newer country estate asylum. Rutherford, *The Landscapes*, i, pp. 136–7.

6 Philo, *A Geographical History*, p. 572.

7 Deborah Kirklin and Ruth Richardson, eds, *The Healing Environment: Without and Within* (London: Royal College of Physicians, 2003), p. 28.

8 Philo, *A Geographical History*, p. 572. See also Cherry and Munting, 'Exercise is the Thing', in which they discuss the ruralisation of the asylum in relation to recreation, particularly cricket.

9 Showalter, *The Female Malady*, p. 35.

10 *Ibid.*

11 Philo, *A Geographical History*, p. 596.

12 For a discussion of the lay influence within the Lunacy Commission and its effect on the psychiatric profession see N. Hervey, 'A slavish bowing down: The Lunacy Commission and the psychiatric profession 1845–60', in Bynum et al., *The Anatomy of Madness*, ii, 98–131.

13 W.J. Keith, 'The land in Victorian literature', in Mingay, *The Victorian Countryside*, i, 136–49, p. 138.

14 *Ibid.*

15 Northampton County Asylum (hereafter NCA) was also known locally by the name of Berrywood Asylum after the name of the estate on which it was built.

16 Rutherford, *The Landscapes.*

17 In 1845, T.O. Prichard left his post as the first superintendent of the Northampton General Lunatic Asylum to run his own private asylum. He took on the rental of Abington Abbey, a country house whose estate as Manor of Abington had been recorded in the Domesday Book.

18 Quoted in Henrietta Ayres, *A Changing Community: The Brief History of St Crispin Hospital, Duston, Northampton, 1876–1976* (Northampton: Northamptonshire Area Health Authority, 1976), p. 8.

19 Jonathan Reinarz, 'Receiving the rich, rejecting the poor: towards a history of hospital visiting in nineteenth-century provincial England', in Graman Mooney and Jonathan Reinarz, eds, *Permeable Walls: Historical Perspectives on Hospital and Asylum Visiting* (New York: Rodopi, 2009), 31–54, p. 32.

20 Northampton General Lunatic Asylum (hereafter NGLA), Visitors' Books, 16 June 1846. All NGLA Visitors' Books and Annual Reports are held at St Andrew's Healthcare Archives, Northampton.

21 See also Showalter, *The Female Malady.*

22 Ayres, *A Changing Community*, p. 12.

23 Merivale, *My Experiences*, p. 78.
24 Arthur Foss and Kerith Trick, *St Andrew's Hospital, Northampton: The First One Hundred and Fifty Years, 1839–1988* (Cambridge: Granta Editions, 1989), p. 7.
25 Taken from Ayres, *A Changing Community*, p. 7.
26 See Porter, *Mind Forg'd Manacles*, 1987, pp. 184–7.
27 Foss and Trick, *St Andrew's Hospital*, p. 15.
28 Philo, *A Geographical History*, p. 583 (original emphasis).
29 For more on the changes from town-based facilities to more rural ones see Philo, *A Geographical History*.
30 NGLA, Visitors' Books, 8 October 1850 and 20 December 1853.
31 St Andrew's Hospital, *150 years of Progress, Saint Andrew's Hospital* (Northampton: St Andrew's Hospital, 1988).
32 NGLA, Visitors' Books, 12 October 1889.
33 For more on mineral water and sea bathing hospitals see Richardson, *English Hospitals*, pp. 124–7. Also for the history of the seaside and its role in health see Fred Gray, *Designing the Seaside: Architecture, Nature and Health* (London: Reaktion Books, 2006) and John Hassan, *The Seaside, Health and Environment in England and Wales Since 1800* (Aldershot: Ashgate, 2003).
34 Quoted in Pinon, *L'Hospice de Charenton*, p. 49.
35 *The Northampton Herald*, 10 March 1878, quoted in Scull, *The Most Solitary of Afflictions*, p. 314.
36 Scull, *The Most Solitary of Afflictions*, p. 314.
37 Ayres, *A Changing Community*, p. 22.
38 Quoted in Philo, *A Geographical History*, p. 440.
39 Conolly quoted in Philo, *A Geographical History*, p. 581.
40 *Ibid.*
41 William Wordsworth, 'Lines composed a few miles above Tintern Abbey, on revisiting the banks of the Wye during a tour', 13 July 1798, in Wordsworth, *Complete Poetical Works*, ed. Thomas Hutchinson, revised by Ernest de Selincourt (Oxford: Oxford University Press, 1973), p. 164, lines 22–30.
42 Showalter, *The Female Malady*, p. 36.
43 For more on the relationship between women and the psychiatric profession see Showalter, *The Female Malady*.
44 Foss and Trick, *St Andrew's Hospital*, p. 180.
45 NGLA, Visitors' Books, 28 April 1858.
46 NGLA, *Thomas Octavius Prichard's Second Annual Report* (Northampton: Freeman, printer and bookseller, 1840), p. 35 (Northampton Local Studies Library-hereafter NLSL).
47 There are various entries regarding Perkins in the *General Ledger* for the County Lunatic Asylum (July 1876 to May 1897) between 1881 and 1894.

For example, in 1881 the asylum bought trees and shrubs, including Austrian pines, from Perkins for £25 18s (Northampton Record Office – hereafter NRO).

48 Rutherford, *The Landscapes*, i, p. 241. See also Rutherford, 'Landscapers for the mind: English asylum designers, 1845–1914', *Garden History*, 33:1 (2005), 61–86.

49 NGLA, Visitors' Books, Commissioners in Lunacy report, 5 May 1860.

50 NGLA, Visitors' Books, 26 January 1846.

51 See Chapter 2.

52 NGLA, Visitors' Books, 18 February 1859.

53 Giraudy, Assistant Doctor at the Charenton Hospital, 1803, quoted in Pinon, *L'Hospice de Charenton*, p. 72.

54 NGLA, *The Report of the Northampton General Lunatic Asylum*.

55 NGLA, Visitors' Books, 21 February 1866.

56 *Ibid.*, 20 August 1867.

57 Quoted in Janet Gooch, *A History of Brighton General Hospital* (London and Chichester: Phillimore Books, 1980), p. 5.

58 NGLA, Visitors' Books, 6 July 1854.

59 *Ibid.*, 1 December 1869.

60 *Ibid.*, 6 October 1871.

61 *Ibid.*, 14 August 1879.

62 *Ibid.*, 28 April 1858.

63 *Ibid.*

64 *Ibid.*

65 *Ibid.*, 5 May 1860.

66 *Ibid.*, 16 June 1846.

67 *Ibid.*, 5 May 1860.

68 NGLA, *Annual Report*, 1862, p. 48.

69 *Ibid.*, 1864, p. 31.

70 *Ibid.*, 1863, p. 64 and 1864, p. 31.

71 *The Builder*, 18 November 1871, pp. 906–7.

72 NGLA, Visitors' Books, 17 May 1872.

73 *Ibid.*, 25 February 1876.

74 Scull, *The Most Solitary of Afflictions*, 1993, pp. 313–14.

75 Henry Burdett, *Hospitals and Asylums of the World; Their Origin, History, Construction, Administration, Management and Legislation*, 4 vols (London: Churchill, 1893), ii, p. 111.

76 Nikolaus Pevsner, *The Buildings of England: Northamptonshire*, second edition revised by Bridget Cherry (Harmondsworth: Penguin, 1973), p. 358.

77 The *Northampton Herald*, 10 March 1878, quoted in Scull, *The Most Solitary of Afflictions*, 1993, p. 314.

78 John Thompson and Partners, 'Cultural heritage study', in *A Proposal for a New Community: St Crispin, Northampton, Environmental Statement,*

Appendix 2, Architectural Appraisal (held at Northampton Council Planning Office: N/2000/404) p. 4 and Scull, *The Most Solitary of Afflictions*, 1993, p. 314.

79 Fred Golby, *A History of Upton and Berrywood* (Warwick: Warwick Printing Company Limited, 1994), p. 70.

80 Ayres, *A Changing Community*, pp. 10–3.

81 NCLA, *General Ledger* (NRO).

82 David Stuart, *The Garden Triumphant: A Victorian Legacy* (London: Viking, 1988), p. 174.

83 NCLA, *General Ledger.*

84 *Ibid.*

85 *Northampton County Asylum, Berrywood; How it was Established and a Sketch of its History from its Opening to March, 1913* (Northampton: Jos. Tebbutt, 1913), p. 26.

86 Quoted in Ayres, *A Changing Community*, p. 8.

87 Mark Hinsley, 'The survey', as reported in Thompson and Partners, 'Cultural heritage study', p. 15.

88 *The Builder*, 16 May 1857.

89 For more on Gardenesque planting see Chapter 2.

90 Rutherford, *The Landscapes*, i, p. 224.

91 NCA, Visitors' Books, 17 March 1881 (NRO).

92 Mark Hinsley, 'Appendix 3: Tree survey', in FPD Savills incorporating Shaw Crammond, *A Proposal for a New Community, Environmental Statement.*

93 Peter Bartlett, *The Poor Law of Lunacy: The Administration of Pauper Lunatics in Mid-Nineteenth Century England* (London: Leicester University Press, 1999), p. 206.

94 Quoted in Alex Beam, *Gracefully Insane: The Rise and Fall of America's Premier Mental Hospital* (Cambridge, Mass.: PublicAffairs, 2001), p. 23.

95 *Annual Report*, 1871 (Tyne and Wear Archives, HO. SN/34).

96 *Ibid.*, 1875.

97 *Ibid.*, 1876.

98 The Retreat was opened in 1845 as a private institution by Thomas Octavius Prichard, who left his post as the first superintendent of the General Lunatic Asylum under a cloud of accusations concerning his drinking habits. It was later run by his son, also called Thomas. The quote from the 1860s is from him. For a time he was the medical superintendent of Glasgow Royal Lunatic Asylum, according to Parry-Jones, *The Trade in Lunacy*, p. 79.

99 Quoted in Foss and Trick, *St Andrew's Hospital*, p. 60.

100 Thomas Prichard, *Report of Cases of Insanity Treated at Abington Abbey, Northampton from Jan 1 1862 to Dec 31, 1867*, No VI (Northampton: Cordeux and Sons, 1868), p. 54 (NLSL). This Thomas Prichard was the son of the first superintendent, Thomas Octavius Prichard.

101 For more on Victorian planting see Brent Elliott and Stuart (*The Garden Triumphant*).
102 Prichard, *Report of Cases*, p. 54 (NLSL).
103 Letter to the Visitors of Abington Abbey Retreat from Mrs Capron, 1884 (NRO: Bundle of correspondence with the Visitors covering the years 1876–85, x3323 C).
104 *The New Regulations of Wonford House Hospital for the Insane Near Exeter, Adopted at a General Court of Governors Held on the 11 February 1880* (Exeter: William Pollard Printer, 1880).
105 Ayres, *A Changing Community*, p. 13.
106 Scull, The Most Solitary of Afflictions, p. 169.
107 Figures from Ayres, *A Changing Community*, pp. 9 and 21.
108 Tuke, *Description of the Retreat*, p. 155.
109 *Ibid.*, p. 23.
110 NGLA, Visitors' Books, 24 October 1865.
111 NGLA, Visitors' Books, Commissioners in Lunacy Report, 24 May 1883.
112 *Ibid.*, 16 July 1890.
113 Prichard, *Report of Cases*, pp. 28–9.
114 *Ibid.*, p. 29.
115 NGLA, Visitors' Books, Commissioners in Lunacy Report, 24 May 1883.
116 NGLA, Visitors' Books, 12 November 1891.
117 NGLA, Visitors' Books, Commissioners in Lunacy Report, 16 July 1890.
118 Ayres, *A Changing Community*, p. 13.
119 Browne, *What Asylums Are*, p. 229.
120 Rutherford, *The Landscapes*, i, p. 156.
121 See Rutherford, *The Landscapes*, i, Scull, *The Most Solitary of Afflictions* and Michel Foucault, *Madness and Civilization: A History of Madness in the Age of Reason* (1961), translated by Richard Howard (Cambridge: Routledge, 1995).
122 Quoted in Foss and Trick, *St Andrew's Hospital*, p. 34.
123 Philo, *A Geographical History*, pp. 601–2.
124 *Ibid.*, p. 597 (original emphasis).
125 Rosemary Treble, 'The Victorian picture of the country', in G.E. Mingay, ed., *The Victorian Countryside*, 2 vols (London: Routledge and Kegan Paul, 1981), i, 166–75, p. 169.
126 Christiana Payne, *Toil and Plenty: Images of the Agricultural Landscape in England 1780–1890* (New Haven and London: Yale University Press, 1993), p. 24.
127 *Ibid.*
128 *Ibid.*, p. 25.
129 *Ibid.*, p. 41.
130 There are obviously tensions surrounding the portrayal of the countryside and agricultural workers, which have great economic and social class

significance. For more on this see John Barrell, *The Dark Side of the Landscape: The Rural Poor in English Paintings, 1730–1840* (Cambridge: Cambridge University Press, 1980), Michael Rosenthal, *British Landscape Painting* (Oxford: Phaidon, 1982) and Payne, *Toil and Plenty*.

131 Jeremy Black and Roy Porter, eds, *A Dictionary of Eighteenth-Century History* (Bath: Penguin Books, 2001), pp. 650–2 and pp. 597–8.

132 Andrew Scull's introduction to Browne, *What Asylums Are*, p. xxxi.

133 Browne, *What Asylums Are*, pp. 52–3.

134 Rutherford, *The Landscapes*, i, pp. 95–6.

135 Doerner, *Madmen and the Bourgeoisie*, p. 80.

136 Amy Woodson-Boulton, 'A window onto nature: visual language, aesthetic ideology and the nature of social transformation', in Minsoo Kang and Amy Woodson-Boulton, eds, *Visions of the Industrial Age, 1830–1914: Modernity and the Anxiety of Representation in Europe* (Hampshire: Ashgate, 2008), 139–62.

137 *Ibid.*, p. 144.

138 Edginton, 'Moral architectore', p. 98.

139 Foucault, *Madness and Civilization*, pp. 195–6.

140 *Ibid.*, p. 196.

141 Parr, *Mental Health*, p. 83.

142 Philo, *A Geographical History*, p. 593.

143 Rutherford, *The Landscapes*, i, p. 224.

144 Parr, *Mental Health*, p. 83.

145 For more on economic uses of pauper asylum landscapes see Rutherford, *The Landscapes*.

146 Skene, 'The development of the gardens', pp. 33–4.

147 Benjamin Ward Richardson, 'The medical history of Cambridge', *Medical Times and Gazette*, 2 (1864), p. 658.

148 Thomas Kirkbride, *On the Construction, Organization and General Arrangements of Hospitals for the Insane* (Philadelphia: Lindsay and Blakiston, 1854), pp. 7–8.

149 Browne, *What Asylums Are*, p. 57.

150 Dr Andrew Halliday quoted in Showalter, *The Female Malady*, p. 24.

151 This has already been discussed in relation to Fox at Brislington House, which, although a private asylum, still viewed outdoor work as important.

152 Rutherford, *The Landscapes*, i, p. 221.

153 Burdett, *Hospitals and Asylums*, ii, p. 2.

154 *Ibid.*, p. 13.

155 NGLA, Visitors' Books, Commissioners in Lunacy Report, 9 May 1865.

156 NGLA, Visitors' Books, 6 May 1887.

157 *Ibid.*

158 *Ibid.*, 16 February 1891.

159 *Ibid.*

160 See Rutherford, *The Landscapes*.
161 Golby, *History of Upton*, p. 73.
162 Ayres, *A Changing Community*, p. 12.
163 Browne, *What Asylums Are*, p. 229.
164 *Ibid.*, p. 230.
165 Jonathan Bate, *John Clare: A Biography* (London: Picador, 2003), p. 71.
166 *Ibid.*
167 *Ibid.*, p. 469.
168 For more on Severalls see Diana Gittins, *Madness in its Place: Narratives of Severalls Hospital, 1913–1997* (London: Routledge, 1998).
169 Board of Control, *Annual Report of the Board of Control* (London: HMSO, 1911), p. 12.
170 This does not seem to have had much of an impact on the Northampton asylums. For more on this see Rutherford, *The Landscapes* and Richardson, *English Hospitals*.
171 Thompson and Partners, 'Cultural heritage study', p. 5.
172 Hinsley, 'Tree survey', p. 58.
173 Foss and Trick, *St Andrew's Hospital*, p. 215.
174 Quoted in Foss and Trick, *St Andrew's Hospital*, p. 215.
175 Foss and Trick, *St Andrew's Hospital*, p. 247.
176 St Crispin Hospital Management Committee, *Review of the Hospital During the First Ten Years of the National Health Service* (Northampton: St Crispin Hospital, 1958).
177 Gittins, *Madness in its Place*, p. 11.
178 Winifred Raphael, *Psychiatric Hospitals Viewed by their Patients*, second edition (London: King Edward's Hospital Fund for London, 1977), p. 14.
179 *Ibid.*, p. 28.
180 *Ibid.*
181 Chris Philo, 'Scaling the asylum: three geographies of the Inverness District Lunatic Asylum (Craig Dunain)', in Topp et al., *Madness*, 107–31, p. 115.
182 *Ibid.*, p. 116.
183 Michel Foucault, *Discipline and Punish: The Birth of the Prison* (1975), translated by Alan Sheridan (New York: Random House, 1979), p. 202.
184 Jennifer Dawson, *The Ha-Ha* (London: Virago, 1961).
185 Davies, 'A small corner', p. 315.
186 Gittins, *Madness in its Place*, p. 27.
187 For more on these developments see Jones, *Asylums and After*.
188 MIND, *Hospital Land: A Resource for the Future* (MIND, July 1975).
189 St Andrew's Group of Hospitals, *About St Andrew's*, www.stah.org/about-us/about-us.aspx (accessed 7 August 2011).

4

Pavilions and palaces of health: the gardens of the Victorian general hospital

> There is no escape from a sick ward, when sunlight, trees, plants, grass, and the external air, would do more for patients than all the medicine and doctors in the world. Thousands of lives might be saved annually if sick men could be turned out so as to look upon Nature, feel the sunshine, and breathe pure air.
>
> *The Builder*, 1856[1]

In the 1860s two doctors, John Syer Bristowe and Timothy Holmes, travelled around Britain visiting hospitals and making notes on their design and how they were run. These findings were published in a report for the Medical Officer of the Privy Council in 1863 and included descriptions of a number of hospital gardens.[2] Of the sixty-seven hospitals Holmes and Bristowe visited in England, forty-six were described as having some kind of external grounds: this figure includes any mention of acreage of land around hospitals, as well as more detailed descriptions of garden grounds, so it gives us a snapshot of the state of hospital gardens in the mid-nineteenth century.

The forty-six gardens mentioned could be an underestimate of the actual number. On their visit to Leeds General Hospital, for example, where there was definitely a garden in existence[3] the doctors do not comment on it. So a lack of a description does not necessarily indicate that gardens did not exist. The men actually only positively state that three London-based hospitals did not have gardens: Kings College Hospital, Westminster Hospital and Charing Cross Hospital. In the case of Charing Cross they wrote that it 'has no airing grounds whatever attached to it, so the patients needing exercise have to take it in the streets'.[4] This suggests that they were inclined to make a note of hospitals where space was severely limited, so where gardens were omitted it could be because they thought it was more important to list other factors in the design or management of the hospital. In the case of Leeds they seemed more concerned with the problems created by the existing hospital building and the fact that a replacement was about to be built. Taking all these factors into account it does suggest that some form of external space was common to a great proportion of hospitals by the middle of the nineteenth century.

Bristowe and Holmes divided their report into three sections: London hospitals, provincial hospitals and rural hospitals. As would be expected there were fewer gardens mentioned in relation to hospitals located in London. They commented that the London Hospital was 'distinguished as being almost the only one in London which stands in a large piece of garden ground'.[5] However, even at St George's Hospital, which apparently had no 'exercising grounds', there was still a 'small gravelled courtyard, in which males and females are allowed to walk at different times in the day'.[6] Provincial and rural hospitals were often described in the report as having some form of airing court or garden for the use of patients, and they recorded that Birmingham Queen's Hospital even had a bowling green.[7]

Most of these hospitals could be classed as general hospitals. In 1858 the role of the general hospital was defined by Bristowe, who was a physician at St Thomas's Hospital, London, as 'that, which has for its object the effecting of the greatest possible amount of good, to the greatest possible number of sick persons. In short, a Hospital is, and ought to be, and is acknowledged to be, specially a place for the care and cure of the emergencies of disease and accident'.[8] This description, which can still be applied to general hospitals today, was used by him to differentiate the general hospital from both its historical roots and the other newly emerging forms of medical institution.

At the start of the century in which Bristowe and Holmes found themselves acting as official hospital auditors, there were only about thirty general hospitals in England.[9] These hospitals were traditionally places that provided limited treatment, food, shelter and opportunities for convalescence rather than the intensive medical care we expect today. They were also highly selective about who they admitted. According to Porter, although 'by 1800, London's hospitals alone were handling over 20,000 patients a year . . . they restricted themselves to fairly minor complaints likely to respond to treatment, and they excluded infectious cases'.[10] Their function was to provide medical care for the poor, but not paupers, who were excluded from general hospitals. After the passing of the Poor Law Amendment Act in 1834, most paupers were treated in workhouse infirmaries, which had developed out of necessity and practicality.[11] On the other hand, people who were better off and could afford to pay for medical treatment were still treated in their own homes.

All the general hospitals founded pre-1800, and almost of all of those established in the nineteenth century, were funded by voluntary subscriptions, which added an extra layer of patient selection. Apart from patients requiring immediate hospital treatment for accidents (acute injuries), anyone requiring medical treatment at a hospital needed to obtain an admission letter from one of the hospital's subscribers before a doctor could see them. This meant that the subscribers rather than the medical staff made decisions about who should be treated. This began to change at the start of the nineteenth century with the formation of hospitals such as the London General Institution for Gratuitous Care of Malignant Diseases (better known as the Royal Free Hospital) founded by Dr William Marsden in 1828. This was the first hospital to provide treatment for the poor without letters of recommendation. However, many hospitals such as Bristol General Hospital retained the system of admission based on subscribers' letters into the twentieth century.

The influence of lay people in the form of subscribers began to decline during the nineteenth century as medicine took a more central role within the hospital, particularly as the teaching of medical students within the hospital setting came to be seen as an essential part of the physician's education. Again, according to Porter, with 'the development, around 1800, of the new medical science typified by physical examination, pathological anatomy, and statistics, the hospital gradually ceased to be primarily a site of charity, care and convalescence; it turned into the medical powerhouse it has been ever since'.[12]

In response to this medicalisation, many voluntary hospitals that had previously used converted houses began to build their own purpose-built establishments. Christine Stevenson has suggested that these were often in the style of Palladian villas, which reflected the prevailing architectural idiom of the time.[13] For example, the 1810 Derbyshire General Infirmary was described by one of the consultants in 1890 as 'rather according to the then prevailing idea of what the proper arrangement for an ordinary dwelling-house should be, than for ... [the] best arrangement for a hospital'.[14]

The gardens might similarly have reflected domestic designs of the period. Interrogating the map of Derbyshire General Infirmary, surveyed by the Board of Ordnance for the local Board of Health in 1852, and two photographs, the Derbyshire General hospital appears to have been set in parkland with a garden laid out with paths and Gardenesque-style plantings to the rear of the building, which is what one might expect for a domestic garden of this period.[15] Similarly, the 1847 garden at Leeds General Infirmary depicted on the Ordnance Survey map of that date also appears to be Gardenesque in style (Figure 21). Comparisons can perhaps be made with some of the domestic examples in Loudon's *The Suburban Gardener and Villa Companion*. In particular Loudon's

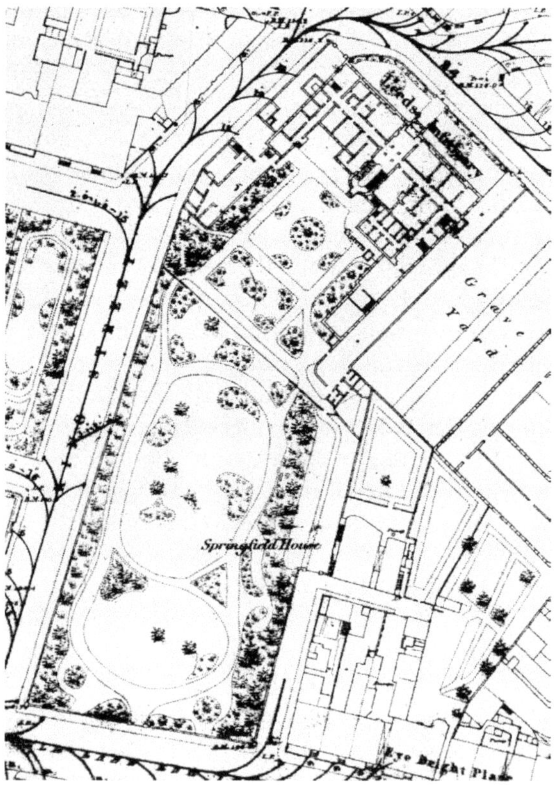

Figure 21 Old Leeds General Infirmary as depicted on the Ordnance Survey map of Leeds, surveyed in 1847 and published in 1850. This shows the extent of the garden at this time. It also suggests that there were distinct Gardenesque-style clumps of planting and winding paths, as well as a more formal area directly behind the hospital building.

description of a garden that was about to be laid out 'with winding walks of different breadths, and with clumps and scattered trees, in the manner of modern pleasure-grounds' could just as easily relate to the garden at Leeds.[16] This suggests that they were laid out in the style of the day and were similar to domestic gardens.

A number of texts were written towards the end of the eighteenth century in relation to hospital design which denote a shift to gardens with specific elements identified for institutional use. One of these was written by Edward Foster as a dissertation while he was at Edinburgh University in 1768. In this text, described by Stevenson as 'a new way of writing about hospitals in the English-speaking world', he discussed the role gardens should play in association with hospital design.[17] As an Irish physician he was interested in the design of hospitals in relation to the recent Parliamentary Act to build county hospitals in Ireland. His section entitled *The Recovery of the Sick in Relation to Construction and Appurtenances of Hospitals* begins with a suggestion that the 'external appurtenances requisite to a hospital are a rivulet and garden'.[18] Foster described the role of the rivulet as primarily a sanitary one. However, he suggested that the garden had four functions: to provide fresh air; to give patients a place where they could exercise; to be used as a kitchen garden; and as a place where the apothecary could grow the plants needed for medicaments:

> That a garden is very requisite, no one can deny, who knows, how necessary exercise is, to the cure of most chronic diseases, or who considers how salutary a pure, fresh air must prove to people confined, for any time, in a bad one. To say nothing of the number of vegetables necessary for nourishment, as well as for medicinal uses of various kinds. I would, therefore, have an Acre of ground at least, about every hospital, laid out in a garden, with proper walks, some straight, some winding, some level, and some ascending, to answer the various uses of the patients[19]

The role of the garden in relation to therapy seems to have predominantly been its ability to provide fresh air and to allow opportunities for exercise. This notion appears to have been generally accepted at the time, which may explain why, although many early hospitals have gardens, little is written to justify why they were constructed.

It is possible to confirm that the gardens in existence were intended to be used by the patients, although whether this intention was realised in practice is harder to establish and is outside the parameters of this study. Northampton General Infirmary, for example, was described by

Bristowe and Holmes as standing 'in a large open space not less than sixteen acres of land around belonging to the hospital . . . The patients have a garden of more than three acres for exercise.'[20] Like the examples of the Derbyshire and Leeds hospitals, there are also suggestions that the gardens were often laid out in the style of the day. For example, the Ipswich and East Suffolk Hospital had 'large and pleasant grounds around, which are partly laid out as plantations, partly as kitchen garden, and partly as flower garden'.[21]

However, in some cases the use of the gardens by patients was limited in some manner. In John Penfold's biography of the Essex County Hospital, Colchester (opened in 1820), the land to the rear of the hospital was initially laid out with an area containing a plantation of fir trees and shrubs, but the rest of the land, apart from the courtyard, was rented out, possibly for sheep grazing. Later in 1838–39, the shrubbery and fir plantation were removed and the land turned into a vegetable garden for the hospital's benefit. It seems that it was not until 1869 that 'part of the grounds were laid as recreation areas . . . for the patients, the males and females having separate "wired off" parts. In 1876, due to vandalism, notice boards were fixed in the men's part cautioning them to keep to the paths and not to do further injury to the shrubs.'[22] This suggests there was a change of emphasis over time regarding the amount of land needed for recreation by the patients, and some of the attendant problems in terms of vandalism. Sometimes the amount of land available was also restricted: in the case of the Radcliffe Infirmary, Oxford, 'such patients as could walk were forced to take their exercise in the back court, which until 1845 had posts and lines for drying clothes'.[23]

At the Ipswich and East Suffolk Hospital patients only had access to the grounds at certain times. Taunton and Somerset Hospital and the Nottingham Hospital also only allowed patients to use the airing grounds at defined hours. The Salisbury Infirmary had limitations too but they appear to reflect concerns about allowing both sexes of convalescing patients to mix in the gardens. As Foster stated, the concern was that 'as the desires of nature are apt to return with health, a division betwixt the men's and women's walks, may be necessary to prevent any indecent, or immodest behaviour'.[24] Their restrictions meant that male and female patients were only allowed access to the airing grounds at different times.[25] The idea of gender separation was taken further at the Chester Infirmary where they had two gardens, one at the front for the male patients and one at the rear for the female patients.[26] This was of continual concern, particularly when patients were convalescing or resident for any period of time. As well as in psychiatric institutions, patients in twentieth-century tuberculosis sanatoria were also separated by gender.

A more detailed idea of the importance attached to gardens for these provincial hospitals can be gained by looking at the example of the old Leeds General Infirmary. According to S.T. Anning's history of the hospital, the 1771 hospital had a garden to the south of the building which was 'from the first an important feature, and more so from 1817 when the Trustees acquired a large area of open land to the south of the property'.[27] The fact that the Trustees extended the garden suggests that, by the start of the nineteenth century, the garden was growing in importance. This garden fulfilled several of the functions recommended by Foster. From 1805 the apothecary used part of the garden and 'benches with backs were provided for the use of patients', presumably for them to sit and take the air as well as exercising.[28] The main reason for the extension of the garden appears to have been for patient use. According to Anning, 'the enlarged garden was soon in danger of being lost for the use of patients on account of the expense of laying it out. In 1819 it was decided to let it as a kitchen garden but the Board changed this decision a few weeks later and resolved to lay it out as an "ornamental pleasure ground"'.[29] The levelling, planting and laying of gravel paths was completed by April 1821 and, to cover the costs of the garden, the Trustees charged an annual sum for the privilege of walking round the grounds. The grounds were also used from 1849 by the Leeds Horticultural and Floral Society (founded 1837) for their annual grand horticultural and floral exhibition.[30] This continued until 1861 when the Trustees decided to start the process of building a replacement hospital.[31]

From the evidence above, the map of 1847, a photograph from 1867 and the following description in John Mayhall's *The Annals of Yorkshire, Leeds*, in 1861, it appears that great care was taken in designing the garden. Mayhall wrote that, 'the land is carefully laid out as a garden and pleasure ground, and is enclosed by a substantial wall, surmounted with iron palisades, and forms an ornament to the western part of the town'.[32] Its primary function, like many other hospital gardens, does appear to have been as a place for the patients to exercise and take the air. It would also appear that it was important enough for the Trustees to spend money that they could ill afford to create this garden.

The development of large gardens associated with provincial hospitals seems to have continued well into the nineteenth century. In 1849, *The Builder* reported that the Cheltenham General Hospital and Dispensary, 'lately erected in Sandford-fields, Cheltenham, by Mr Darby, builder, from plans prepared by Mr D.J. Humphris, architect . . . Around the building is an area of two acres in garden ground.'[33] Popular belief, as voiced by *The Builder* and reproduced at the start of this chapter, still appeared to have held on to the idea that nature had more power than the doctors.[34]

One other function of the general hospital garden may have been as a purely rhetorical device. As the hospitals were paid for by local subscription the gardens might have been intended to both display the extent to which money had already been spent on the institution and to encourage new subscribers. Harriet Richardson has suggested that this was the case in relation to the architecture, 'as voluntary and paid for by local community the buildings were seen as visible expressions of pride in their foundation as well as an encouragement to potential subscribers'.[35] This may correspond to gardens such as the small, planted area at the front of the Leeds General Infirmary (Figure 22) and the gardens shown in an illustration of the Radclife Infirmary, Oxford (Figure 23).

As towns expanded through the success of Victorian industry, these gardens can be seen to reflect the movement that made a general hospital or infirmary 'a source of civic pride along with the town hall, public library, literary society, and notable ancient building or monument'.[36] By 1911, *The Hospital* journal was lamenting that hospital guidebooks were

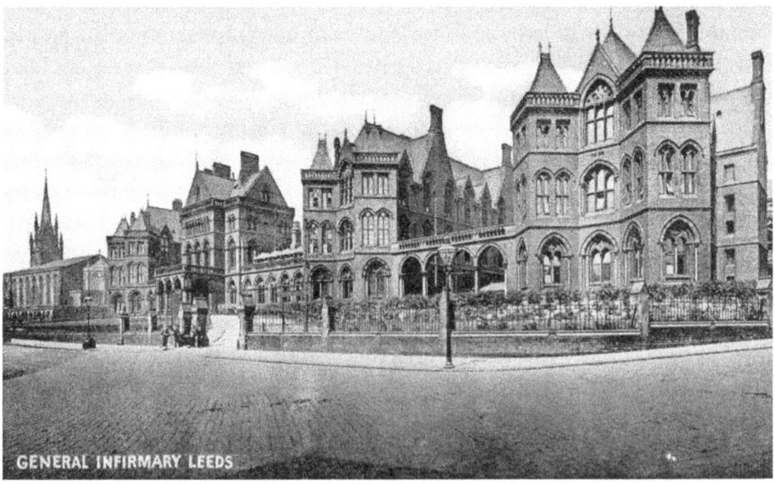

Figure 22 The small, formal gardens at the front of Leeds General Infirmary, date unknown.

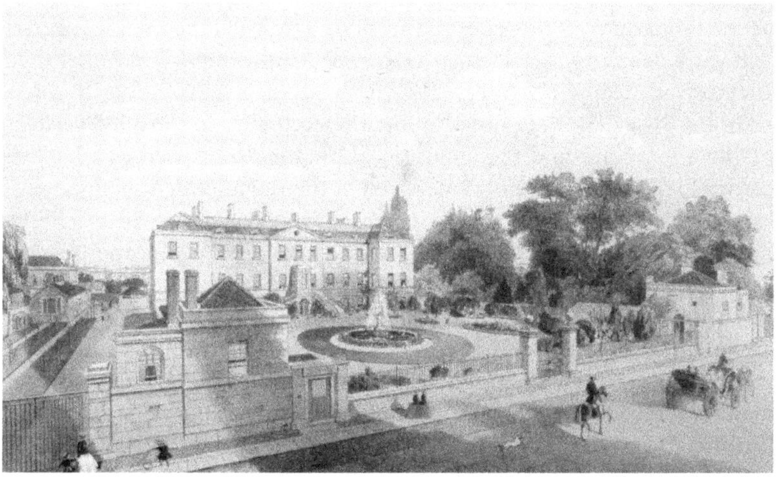

Figure 23 The front gardens of the Radcliffe Infirmary with fountain and colourful parterres. These were evidently designed to be seen by those passing by.

needed to overcome the 'dour and depressing' hospital exteriors.[37] They argued that 'till the day comes when hospital architects are able to meet reasonable aesthetic demands on the exterior of their buildings, illustrated hospital Guides will remain the best way of overcoming ignorant prejudice against them, and of attracting public sympathy and interest'.[38] One can extrapolate from this that gardens at the front of hospitals were also used to encourage these benevolent and potentially charitable feelings towards the institution.

However, in many cases, gardens used by the patients were to the rear of the hospital, such as the garden at Leeds General Infirmary, and, as such, not on general display. The rhetorical role is complicated by a tension between a display of wealth and the need for charity to be seen to be serving those in need, rather than flattering its benefactors.[39] This suggests that these gardens could only play a limited rhetorical role and that they would have needed some utilitarian function. If they were of no benefit to the patients they might have been seen as a waste of charitable funds. This type of wastage was often discussed in journals, such as *The Builder*, and appears to have been a preoccupation of the Victorians. This could have been a considerable problem for hospital gardens, as many of them extended over several acres, according to

Bristowe and Holmes, and could, therefore, have been seen as an unnecessary luxury. As this does not seem to have been the case, it suggests that gardens were generally seen as therapeutically important rather than an extravagance.

In his dissertation, Foster also mentioned the use of hospital gardens by the apothecary and the inclusion of an area to be used as a kitchen garden. This book is mainly interested in the therapeutic use of gardens by patients but the other roles of the hospital garden will briefly be discussed in order to complete the picture. Firstly, the apothecary's garden will be described. In the eighteenth century, much of the apothecaries' *materia medica* consisted of herbal remedies that were mainly designed to act as either emetics or laxatives. It is, therefore, unsurprising that Foster, in 1768, mentions the importance of growing plants for medicinal uses within the hospital. In the case of the Radcliffe Infirmary, Oxford, the ground at the back of the hospital in the 1770s was at first intended to be used 'as a vegetable and wort garden for culinary and pharmaceutical purposes under the direction of the apothecary'.[40] However, by 1788 the garden was being offered on a contract to anyone who would maintain it and provide the hospital with whatever it needed. By the nineteenth century it seems that the garden for medicinal uses has become less worthy of mention. For example, there do not appear to be any references to this use of the garden in relation to new hospital plans published within *The Builder* in the nineteenth century. This may be because new drugs were developed in the nineteenth century, as people became skilled in refining the therapeutic agent from various substances. This new chemistry altered therapeutics, as doctors had access to 'potent medicaments which included morphine, codeine, quinine, cocaine, colchine, ephedrine, atropine, reserpine and digitoxin'.[41] This chemical armoury would have played a part in the decline of the apothecary's garden. From the centre stage they had maintained in the eighteenth century, herbal remedies became relegated to the status of alternative and folk medicine.

The use of an area of the garden as a kitchen garden to produce food for the patients is also something which is not generally discussed in the literature. However, there are illustrations of a large vegetable garden attached to Gloucester Infirmary in an engraving of 1764[42] and there appears to have been a walled garden on the 1852 Local Board of Health Survey Map of Derbyshire General Infirmary.[43] Bristowe and Holmes also mention the existence of kitchen gardens at some of the hospitals they visited. In the case of the London Fever Hospital, patients were apparently given access to visit the kitchen garden, which took up a large part of the three acres of ground surrounding the hospital.[44] Again, this reflects the general model of the domestic house of the time, which would not have been complete without a kitchen garden.

Gardens and the new pavilion plan

By the Victorian period, medicine was, according to Joan Lane, 'a recognised and respected profession, with registration, professional journals and a career structure in both private practice and institutional appointments'.[45] Unsurprisingly, therefore, the medical profession became more involved in the design of hospitals. This was particularly the case by the middle of the nineteenth century, when hospitals came to be seen as being at the centre of medical research, the development of new medical techniques and the education of the next generation of medical practitioners.

The idea that hospitals themselves could cause disease was promoted by Sir John Pringle in his *Observations on Diseases of the Army* published in 1752.[46] He suggested that sick people gave off poisons (known as miasmas) and that in sufficient concentration the resulting tainted atmosphere, when inhaled, caused fevers such as typhus which was known as the 'hospital' or 'jail' fever.[47]

During the nineteenth century, the idea of hospitals as dangerous places full of miasmata became of crucial importance to the medical profession, so much so that they invented a specific term for it. The Scottish surgeon, Sir James Simpson, coined the term 'hospitalism' in 1863 to describe this phenomenon. He defined it as 'the hygienic evils, which the system of huge and colossal hospital edifices has hitherto been made to involve'.[48] Simpson's phrase was the result of a debate that began in earnest in the 1850s when the difficulties of hospital design began to be widely addressed in Britain and brought to the attention of the general public. The bulk of eighteenth- and early nineteenth-century medical texts appear to have had nothing to say about hospital construction. However, this had changed radically by the middle of the nineteenth century. Much of the miasmatic view was promoted within the pages of the influential journal *The Builder*, by the editor George Godwin, and through the works of Florence Nightingale, who is now better known for her reform of the nursing profession in England.

The idea of the hospital as a dangerous place was obviously prevalent when Nightingale began her *Notes on Hospitals* with the phrase: 'The very first requirement in a Hospital is that it should do the sick no harm.'[49] She went on to describe the high mortality rates in hospitals that she felt were directly related to the institution itself. The miasmatists, of whom she was one, felt that there were two solutions to the problem. As the poisonous miasmas built up within the hospitals over time, 'the obvious solution was to tear down old hospitals on a regular basis and build new, smaller ones, preferably in the countryside'.[50] The alternative was to increase the ventilation through the building as much as possible to dilute the miasmas with fresh air.

Ventilation was an older idea which had often been perceived to be the key to reducing the mortality rates in hospitals. According to Joan Lane, 'at Manchester there was an awareness that death rates could be affected by poor ventilation, and in 1799 The Medical Register, having described the room layout in detail, noted that, in the rented house first used as a hospital there, of 403 patients, admitted in three years, twenty-two had died, a death rate of 1:18, while in the new infirmary it was reduced to 1:24.5'.[51] Statistics such as these were appropriated by reformers, and the size of the wards and the number of windows came to be seen as crucial.

An early reformer who was much concerned with ventilation was John Howard, whose influential work, first published in 1789, *An Account of the Principal Lazarettos in Europe*, also included descriptions of both existing European hospitals and his guidance for new designs. In relation to Lazarettos, which were places used to quarantine the sick, he wrote that they should have 'a spacious and pleasant garden' as it would be 'convenient as well as salutary'.[52] This concern with gardens continued as he recorded 'the wards round the garden of the Hospital of San Maria Nova being very properly contrived for promoting the health and spirits of the patients, especially convalescents'.[53] In this description he echoed earlier ideas about the benefits of gardens to both physical and mental health. The significance of outdoor space, particularly for convalescents, was still recognised in the mid-twentieth century.

Howard included a plan of the gardens with a fountain in the centre of a courtyard broken into quadrants, presumably of turf, stating that this is 'the usual form of hospitals in many Roman-Catholic countries'.[54] The gardens he described were designed to be visually appealing as well as functional. The Hospital at Pisa is described as having 'an elegant botanic garden, which, through the iron-grates, affords a pleasant view'.[55] They were also productive spaces. He stated that at Scio Hospital for Lepers, the patients are 'accommodated with little gardens, which supply them with almonds, pot-herbs, and delicious figs and grapes'.[56] Therefore, it is unsurprising that in his recommendation for the construction of hospitals in Britain, Howard argued that 'a piazza and spacious walk to induce patients to take the air and exercise' should be included.[57]

Howard was also concerned with the need for 'windows lofty and opposite' and argues that 'one of the windows should open from the ceiling to the floor' to admit air.

The miasmatists took these earlier concerns with ventilation and developed a particular method of hospital design which appeared new to the Victorians. The favoured way of increasing fresh air was to build hospitals where the individual wards were in separate pavilions and where each of these pavilions was cross-ventilated by opposing windows.

Colonnades were often included as features within the pavilion design and they were described in *The Builder* as being for the use of patients:

> The colonnades not only form a feature in the design, but afford ambulatories for the patients to take out-door exercise in showery weather. One is appropriated to males, the other to females; and both these and the garden command an uninterrupted view of the busy scenes occurring at every tide, from the arrival and departure of the passengers, &c. by the Welsh steam-boats and the large no. of coasting vessels always entering and leaving the basin.[58]

A description of Bristol's General Hospital (described in more detail below) stated that there were colonnades for each sex and that these were designed so that the patients had a view to look at while they were walking. This also has parallels in domestic architectural design. Loudon describes the design of a house which has been 'calculated for invalids, and, therefore, furnished with verandas extending nearly round the whole building, for taking exercise during inclement weather'.[59] This again suggests that the use of outdoor space and external hospital architecture reflected widely held beliefs about the role of the physical environment in the recovery from illness.

Ensuring the patients had a view also appears to have been considered important when the wards were designed at Bristol General Hospital:

> Two large and cheerful day-rooms are provided in the tower for the male and female convalescents, each room being octagonal, and having five windows commanding fine views, and overlooking the river, harbour, and basin.[60]

The notion of octagonal day rooms can be seen as a precursor to the design of circular wards at later hospitals. However, this later development appears to have been influenced less by the need to provide views but was instead predominantly a response to the desire to provide patients with the optimum amount of light and air.[61]

Although there was some opposition to the ideas of the miasmatists there was a general perception of the importance of ventilation, and those promoting the pavilion design, in particular Nightingale, had both popular public support and the ear of those with influence in government. One other reason for Nightingale's active support for the pavilion design, alongside its sanitary benefits, may have been that it was also more convenient for the practice of nursing.[62]

The idea of the pavilion design for hospitals was promoted in *The Builder* in the context of the general call for sanitary reform. This was championed by its editor, George Godwin, within the pages of his journal. An editorial written by him personally in 1856, along with four other articles published in *The Builder* in 1858, laid out the basis of the pavilion design.[63] These were based on the work of John Roberton, a Manchester surgeon, and Godwin put this work into the wider context of the sanitary movement:

> The sanitary history of hospitals may be summed up in very few words. There are hospitals on very bad sites: there are hospitals on comparatively good sites; but there is hardly an instance, in this country at least, of both hospital and site fully embodying those sanitary principles which are essentially necessary for a rapid recovery of the sick and maimed. The one paramount sanitary condition, which ought to be observed in all hospitals, is that of having pure and dry air both within and without the walls of buildings.[64]

The principles of sanitation were held in near-veneration in the second half of the nineteenth century. In fact the importance of air and light became such that there was a brief vogue for circular pavilions, which provided the optimum amount of light and air for patients.[65]

Like the domestic model of hospital design, the pavilion design also lent itself to the inclusion of gardens. In one of the 1856 editorials in *The Builder* which laid down the rules of pavilion design, John Roberton described the Bordeaux Hospital, France. Roberton wrote that it was the 'most attractive altogether, that I have examined' and that:

> Passing into the hospital by the centre gateway, the visitor beholds a beautiful court, for the most part planted with evergreens and flowering shrubs; and on the two sides thereof, facing each other, a succession of pavilions or tiers of building, standing parallel, and having the ends towards the square. The tiers of building are separated from each other by a flower

> garden, and in these tiers are the sick-wards, each ward isolated from the rest . . . and in every ward when you look out of a window it is into a garden, there being, as before mentioned, a garden between each pair of tiers of building.[66]

His only criticism was that, 'it would be better if the open gardens between the wards at Bordeaux were wider, so as to ensure a visit from the rays of the sun'.[67] Again light and air are the key things here and, in a later editorial, *The Builder* suggested that, 'the square within the hospital, and the spaces between the pavilions, should be laid out as garden grounds with well-drained and rolled walks, and shaded seats for convalescents'.[68]

Both the above editorials are quoted within Nightingale's *Notes on Hospitals*, which no doubt increased their audience and gave them extra weight. Nightingale herself went further and suggested that views, as well as colour, also had therapeutic benefits:

> Among kindred effects of light I may mention, from experience, as quite perceptible in promoting recovery, the being able to see out of a window; instead of looking against a dead wall; the bright colours of flowers; the being able to read in bed by the light of a window close to the bed-head. It is generally said that the effect is upon the mind. Perhaps so; but it is no less so upon the body on that account.[69]

This may not have been a widely held view at the time, but it does suggest that Nightingale, at least, considered the environment to be an element affecting the patient's well-being.

Similarly, the public parks movement of the nineteenth century can be seen to reflect views concerning disease-causing miasma and the consequent need for fresh air. In the *First Annual Report of the Registrar-General* in 1839, Dr William Farr wrote that 'in other terms, the mortality of cities in England and Wales is high, but it may be immeasurably reduced. A good, general system of sewers; the intersection of the dense, crowded districts of the metropolis by a few spacious streets; and a park in the east end of London would probably diminish the annual deaths by several thousands, prevent many years of sickness, and add several years to the lives of the entire population.' He then went on to state that this would be of advantage because 'the poorer classes would be benefited by these measures, and the poor-rates would be reduced; but all classes of the community are directly interested in their adoption, for the epidemics, whether influenza, typhus, or cholera, – small-pox, scarlatina, or measles, which arise in the east end of the town, do not stay there; they travel to the west end, and prove fatal in wide streets and squares'. One of the outcomes of this report was indeed the creation in the 1840s of Victoria Park in the east end of London.

This interest in health and urban space was also echoed by philanthropists and active societies.[70] One example of these was the Kyrle Society which was established in 1875 by Miranda and Octavia Hill. In 1894 they described their goal as '"bringing beauty home to the people" in the widest and most catholic sense. Indeed it may be said that all that tends to brighten, better, and beautify the lives of the poorer members of the community has the full sympathy of the Society.'[71] One example of such enterprise is the art work the Birmingham branch donated to the Isolation ward of the Queen's Hospital, Birmingham.[72] As well as encouraging the appreciation of art and music, the Kyrle Society were also involved in the preservation and creation of open spaces and had a specialist branch to campaign on this basis. The central aims of the Open Spaces Branch were:

> To secure and assist in securing any open spaces in or near the metropolis . . . To provide gymnasia and playgrounds for the use of the poorer classes and to assist other bodies, both public and private, in such provision. To distribute cut flowers, plants, ferns, and bulbs to hospitals, workhouses and other institutions, and amongst the homes of the poor.[73]

The Metropolitan Public Gardens Association, which was founded in conjunction with National Health Society, also argued that the preservation of health was one of its central motives: 'To endeavour to secure, for purposes of health and recreation, available vacant plots of grounds, large or small, within the Metropolitan area; to obtain the right of laying out, and planting, and seating, all Disused Burial Grounds, waste places and enclosed squares.'[74]

In this way a direct connection can be made between the wider movement to create green spaces in cities in order to encourage health and the inclusion of gardens within hospital designs. This wider movement was also often encouraged by miasmatists and those involved in the temperance movement. The National Health Society, founded in 1871 by Elizabeth Blackwell for the promotion of health to all classes, could count such influential sanitarian reformers amongst its members as Edwin Chadwick, Edwin Hart, George Godwin and William Farr.

St Thomas's Hospital

The largest and most prominent example of the pavilion hospital design to be built in the late 1860s was the new St Thomas's Hospital (Figure 24).

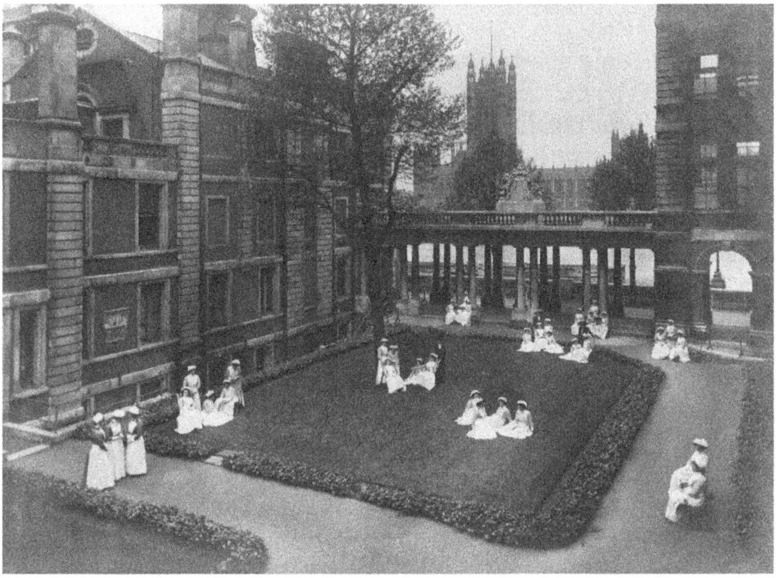

Figure 24 This photograph was taken of the nurses in Nightingale Square at St Thomas's Hospital, London, in the early twentieth century (1910–20). It gives an idea of what the gardens may have looked like in the late nineteenth century with views of the Thames between the colonnades.

It was built in the Italianate style by Henry Currey in 1868–71, on a prominent site on the Embankment, opposite the Houses of Parliament, and it was seen to represent a limited triumph by the miasmatists.[75] The desire for fresh air became such that miasmatists such as Nightingale called for hospitals to be moved out of cities altogether and rebuilt in the countryside. In the 1860s, when the Governors of St Thomas's tried to decide on the site the new hospital should occupy, after it was forced to move to make way for a new railway station, Nightingale was one of those who suggested that it should be rebuilt in leafy Surrey. A similar idea was also advocated in *The Builder*: 'One can quite understand that if St Thomas's Hospital for instance, were moved along the South-Eastern line to some breezy upland down in Kent or Sussex, that it would be a very great sanitary advantage'.[76] The gardens associated with hospitals of this time reflect this desire for fresh air. Although the new St Thomas's was eventually built in the city rather than the countryside, it was built as a pavilion hospital. In fact some doctors began to suggest that the hospital's location by the river could in fact be beneficial. Dr Albert Bernays suggested in a letter to the Governors of the hospital that there might be 'healing effects produced on the minds of the Patients and convalescents by the very calm of a river's ebb and flow'.[77]

When the new building was completed *The Lancet* hailed St Thomas's as 'one of the finest hospitals in the world, as well as an architectural beauty worthy of the metropolis'.[78] The size of the hospital and its prominent location suggests that hospitals were 'becoming almost as important as institutions like churches and their Victorian replicas, railway stations'.[79] The cost of the construction, its location and the fact that its design was hotly debated in publications such as *The Builder* and *The Lancet* before it was built, means that St Thomas's can also be seen as the embodiment of the medical ideas of the time in relation to hospital construction.

As Nightingale strongly influenced its design, it is not surprising that the hospital appears to have courtyard gardens similar to those at the Lariboisière Hospital, Paris, and the Bordeaux Hospital. Lariboisière's design was recommended by her in the first edition of *Notes on Hospitals* and she also reprinted *The Builder* editorial describing Bordeaux in the appendix. A plan reproduced in *The Lancet* of the Menilmontant Hospital, near Paris, suggests that such courtyard gardens were still popular in France later in the century (Figure 25).

The gardens at St Thomas's appear to have been incredibly expensive. Apparently the cost of laying out the grounds and planting came to £2,820 14s.[80] There are no references to the gardens within the *Contract for Building a New Hospital at Stangate*, 1867, which described the proposed fabric and method of construction of the hospital in minute detail.[81] However, there were references to some external construction, which suggest that the exterior appearance of the hospital was of some rhetorical importance. The description of the forecourt enclosure next to Palace New Road stated that 'the ornamental case ironwork is to be of the best description metal, and the castings perfectly sound and clean'.[82] It is, therefore, hard to ascertain how the gardens were laid out. A lithograph of St Thomas's Hospital published in 1883 depicts gardens between the pavilions although it is not possible to discern the detail of the design.

There are also later photographs that give an indication of the nineteenth-century design of the gardens. Here they appear to have areas of lawn as well as flowerbeds and some trees. These may reflect the original planting as a lithograph of the St Marylebone Infirmary, London, for the sick poor (opened in 1881) depicts similar gardens between the

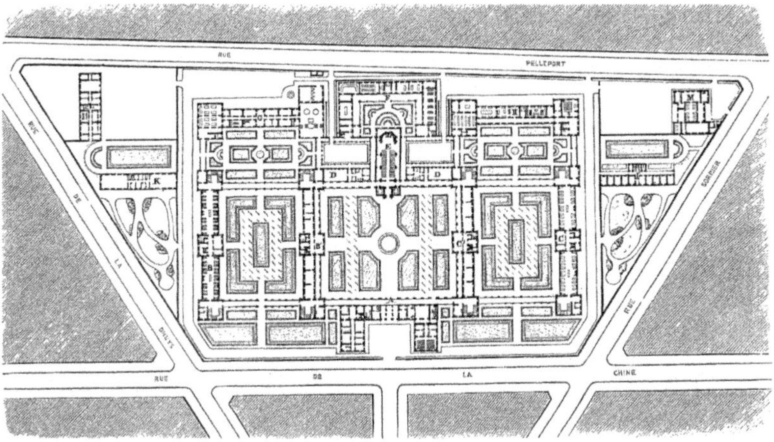

Figure 25 A plan of Menilmontant Hospital, near Paris, published in *The Lancet*, 2 July 1881 as part of series of essays 'On Hospitals' by Frederic Mouat, in which it is depicted with a series of geometric gardens between the pavilions. The article described it as 'a very fine hospital and much in advance of what was, at one time, considered a model for imitation, the unhealthy Lariboisière'.

pavilions, with predominantly grass plots, a few trees and some flower-beds. The photographs also show that views of the River Thames could be obtained through the colonnades from within the gardens. Colonnades were particularly important in pavilion hospitals as they were used to connect the separate buildings as well as to provide walks for the patients.

It is possible, given the location of the hospital opposite Parliament and its representation as the epitome of pavilion design, that the gardens had a rhetorical function as well as a therapeutic one. The whole building, as well as its gardens, could be said to have raised the profile of hospitals and with it the importance of the medical profession. According to Grace Goldin, 'a fair American visitor taking tea upon the terrace of the Houses of Parliament, and looking across the river to the sevenfold splendours opposite, is said to have inquired, "Are those the mansions of your aristocracy?"'[83] This suggests that the external image portrayed by St Thomas's was one of regal splendour.

However, within two weeks of its opening, the hospital was advertising for funds to pay for the new building and at one time there were no patients in thirteen of the twenty-one wards.[84] In order to raise funds the hospital decided to take in paying patients in the 1880s and a new layer to the perceived role of the gardens was added in consequence. Two private wards were opened as St Thomas's Home in 1881. In the regulations published in Frederick J. Mouat and H. Saxon Snell's book in 1883 they were advertised as being 'situated in a large garden facing the river Thames and the Albert Embankment, and . . . in close contiguity to Lambeth Palace' and therefore 'the occupants of the Home have the advantage of these open spaces'.[85] The gardens and other open spaces can, therefore, be seen as part of the rhetoric to encourage paying patients at this time.

There is also another aspect to the role of the gardens as described by a writer in *The Lancet* in 1862. Describing the size of the gardens at the re-opened St Thomas's Hospital, the writer discusses the use of them by medical students as well as patients: 'The student will here, in modern academic groves pursue his duties in a little oasis of quiet and beauty . . . The patients themselves will enjoy the advantages of free air, repose pleasant prospects and exercise, to an extent unknown in other London hospitals.'[86]

The design and utilisation of the gardens by staff, and in particular nurses, becomes a common feature towards the end of the nineteenth and beginning of the twentieth century. In 1899, *The Hospital* reported that, 'one of the most impressive points connected with our present-day hospital construction and management is the superior way in which the nurses are cared for in the matters of accommodation, board, leave of absence and amusement'.[87] This is reflected in the increase in provision of purpose-built accommodation and associated garden or recreational spaces, even using spaces that previously had a separate purpose:

> This charming garden was at first more or less opened . . . to the parish, but lately it has been put to the most suitable use of giving a quiet place for rest and recreation to the nurses of the London Hospital . . . A high brick wall encloses this oasis, and the nurses and some privileged people have keys to the door, which opens, from a side street close to the noise of the Mile End Road, suddenly into a peaceful, picturesque garden. The idea in the formation was a willow-pattern plate, and the little bridge over a miniature stream is reproduced. Plane trees in a formal array are kept trimmed to give a dense shade, and the hammocks hung from them in summer provide the most ideal resting-places for the worn-out nurses.[88]

In 1946, Carl A. Erikson wrote of the importance of providing places of recreation for nurses. He stated that, '"refreshment of strength and spirits after toil" needs to be ever in mind when nurses' recreational areas are being planned'.[89] He was discussing accommodation for nurses in America but it is reasonable to assume that similar concerns were also present in England. He went on to state that 'open-air activity – tennis, shuffleboard, skating on flooded grounds, and similar activities should be considered. If there isn't space enough around the nurses' home for such facilities, then it is almost safe to say that there isn't room enough for the building . . . Such grounds will be large enough for attractive landscaping and thus become an inviting part of the social facilities of the school.'[90] This active use of the hospital landscape was certainly present in England and tennis courts for the use of nurses were built at places such as the Homeopathic Hospital, Bristol.

Technology and design

As well as the development of the pavilion plan, the Victorian period also saw the creation of hospital gardens that utilised new and exciting technologies, such as the winter garden at Leeds General Infirmary and the roof-top garden at Bristol General Hospital. As with many other hospitals, by the mid-nineteenth century the old Leeds hospital was no longer able to cater for the city's rapidly increasing population. To solve this problem George Gilbert Scott was appointed as the architect for a new hospital in 1862. After taking up this post he appears to have taken a trip around Europe accompanied by one of the hospital's doctors and one of the governors. The Minutes of the Building and Finance Committee recorded that it was 'resolved that Dr Chadwick and Mr Lipton be earnestly requested to accompany Mr Scott to the Continent for the purposes for which Mr Scott had been invited to go by the Committee'.[91] It is also known that the Building Committee corresponded with Nightingale.[92] The combination of these two factors led to the hospital being one of the first to be based on the pavilion principle and, like St Thomas's, one that was also modelled on 'Florence Nightingale's original *beau ideal* of a pavilion layout, the Lariboisière Hospital, Paris' (Figure 26).[93] As this suggests, the Governors at Leeds wanted their new building to be 'in accordance with the present state of science as regards Hospital Hygiene'.[94] This demonstrates great respect for contemporary medical thinking, and therefore one could expect that any garden associated with the building would similarly relate to current trends.

In 1864, plans and an etching of Gilbert Scott's designs were published in *The Builder*. There was no mention of a garden on any of these although an open central courtyard was depicted. However, when the

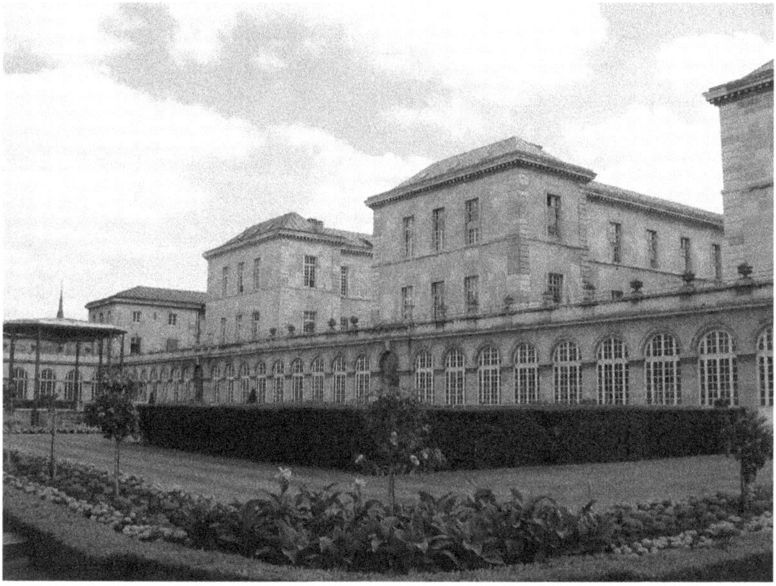

Figure 26 The original model for pavilion hospitals, Lariboisière in Paris, which still has manicured gardens and a bandstand.

building was completed the central courtyard was covered in a glass roof and was referred to as a 'winter garden' in an article in *The Builder* in 1868 (Figure 27). It appears that the roof was requested by the organisers of the 'National Exhibition of Works of Art', which was holding its exhibition in the new building to help raise funds for the hospital. According to the Building Committee's Minutes, 'the Exhibition Committee having represented to this Committee . . . for the purposes of the exhibition it will be necessary to cover with a glass roof the large Central Court'.[95] However, given their interest in ensuring that the building followed the most recent ideas concerning hospital hygiene the Committee reported that they asked for advice from the hospital's medical staff. They received assurance and recorded that, 'on the recommendation of Mr Scott and with the approbation of the Medical Officers of the Infirmary, it appears desirable that the Central Court should be permanently covered in'.[96] The cost of this roof was financed by both the Building and Exhibition Committees, and it can be seen on one of Gilbert Scott's architectural drawings.

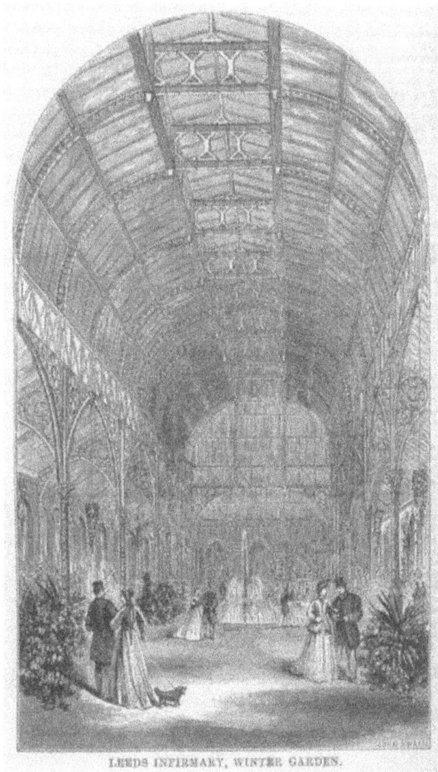

Figure 27 Engraving of the Leeds General Infirmary winter garden originally used in a trade book published by Messrs Handyside. This was published in *The Builder* on 26 June 1868, which corresponds to the time when the garden was being used for a fundraising art exhibition.

Although the roof appears to have been created as a direct result of the Exhibition Committee's request, the use of a glass-covered area by patients had already been suggested in an editorial concerned with pavilion hospital design in *The Builder* in 1858:

> The square within the hospital, and the spaces between the pavilions, should be laid out as garden grounds with well-drained and rolled walks, and shaded seats for convalescents. It is of great importance to provide places of exercise under shelter, for patients, to be appropriated to that purpose alone. Such recreation and winter-airing grounds may be comparatively large, and yet of cheap construction, if roofed on the Crystal Palace Plan.[97]

The idea of covering a whole area can be seen as an extension of the idea of using colonnades as sheltered walks. This was still popular in the 1890s as a means of providing a covered area for exercise within a domestic setting. *The Beeton Book of Garden Management* suggested that 'the conservatory may appropriately be termed a winter garden, for such is its most useful purpose; it is really an essentially necessary adjunct to a well-ordered country house of any pretensions, affording means of exercise to the ladies and visitors in inclement weather'.[98] The concept of a whole garden covered in glass, can, like the Bristol General Hospital roof garden, also be seen as a direct result of developments in technology.[99]

Conservatories and glasshouses became both fashionable and affordable during the nineteenth century. The combination of these elements was famously demonstrated by Joseph Paxton in his building to house the 1851 Great Exhibition of the Works of Industry of all Nations, which became known as the Crystal Palace. Paxton also drew up plans for a glass house to be used as a sanatorium by the City of London Hospital for Diseases of the Chest in 1851 (Figure 28) and argued that it would

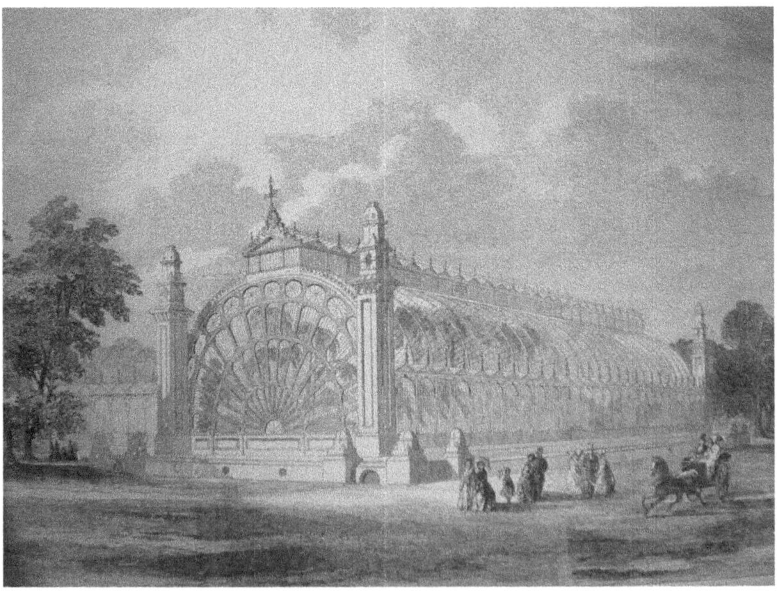

Figure 28 Joseph Paxton's unbuilt design for a sanatorium in the style of a winter garden for the City of London Hospital for Diseases of the Chest. The *Illustrated London News*, 5 July 1851.

ensure 'a healthy climate, and sufficient space for exercise to their inmates, without exposure to the open air'.[100] This was never constructed but the publication of the design in the *Illustrated London News* is likely to have influenced Scott and others. Intriguingly, in the same article Paxton suggested that 'some of the squares of London might, by being covered with glass, form the most delightful and interesting places of resort at all seasons'.[101]

The doctor Benjamin Ward Richardson also hypothesised the use of glass to cover gardens to create 'Palaces of Health'. He proposed that city squares could be covered in glass so that the internal air could be kept at a constant temperature similar to the south of France. This was based on his idea that man can, 'if he will, compete with Nature in the matter of climate, and in the matter of steadiness of climate can beat her'.[102]

Ward Richardson used the city of Bath as an example of where the palaces could be built and argued that 'if a large winter palace was constructed and heated with water from warm springs it would become one of the grandest resorts in the kingdom, perhaps in the world, for sufferers from various affections of the chest'.[103] He went on to say that 'in these gardens flowers and subtropical plants could be cultivated in all their beauty, and with all their health-giving properties; and that in such grounds, leading directly out of the residences, the sick could find every amusement, mental and physical, that was best adapted to their condition, treatment, and possible cure'.[104] To reinforce that this is perhaps a scientific solution to the fact patients are travelling to the Continent in search of cures, he also states that:

> In a palace of health of this kind there need be no monotony nor one whit less of good exercise than is obtainable at foreign resorts, while the immense advantage would be secured of entire freedom from treacherous winds and the other accidents of atmospheric variability which the best climate within easy reach of Great Britain fails altogether to secure.[105]

Brent Elliott suggests that 'public winter gardens began to appear in many towns and cities in the 1860s, and the process continued into the 1890s'.[106] Other contemporary examples of winter gardens include those at Edinburgh, Bournemouth and Folkestone. The concept was also taken up later by the New York Hospital, where the top storey of the building was in effect a winter garden filled with 'rare plants, aquaria, and means for occupying and amusing the patients'.[107] According to Mouat, describing the garden in 1881, 'it would be difficult to over-estimate [its] value, in accelerating the recovery of the sick and injured'.[108] In another associated article in *The Lancet* he reproduced a plan by Mr Booth which also included a top storey winter garden. Winter gardens and conservatories were to become common features attached to the convalescent homes and sanatoria of the twentieth century. An early example of convalescent home in Cheadle, Cheshire, already had 'a summer and winter garden, elegant in design, 100 by 61 feet in extent, and with a gallery on the first floor', according to Mouat in 1881.[109]

In 1868 the new Leeds General Infirmary was completed and the National Exhibition of Works of Art was held in the winter garden the same year. An illustration of this, taken from a trade catalogue advertising glass and iron constructions, appeared in *The Builder* in 1868. This illustration shows the winter garden with a fountain, plants hanging from the pillars and what appear to be containers full of plants. Although this engraving was made a year before the hospital finally opened to patients in 1869 it is possible that it was intended to be the type of conservatory garden popular at the time and one that could be used by the patients. An illustration from the same catalogue, also reproduced in *The Builder*, shows an unnamed, but presumably domestic iron conservatory, which contains a fountain and similar planting.

The popularity of the winter garden at Leeds Infirmary was short lived. Criticisms about the stagnation of air caused by the roof over the courtyard were being voiced as early as 1869 in the *British Medical Journal*, as one writer suggested that the roof should be taken down.[110] This demonstrates a tension between providing constant climatic conditions and all-weather areas for patients, and the desire for natural ventilation. When Henry Burdett visited in 1893 the area was being used as a carpenter's shop and he too suggested that the roof should be taken down.[111] Finally, in 1911, the roof was removed, and a hard tennis court was laid in 1914. Today the area has once again been converted into a garden for the use of patients, staff and relatives, albeit without a roof.

Like the new Leeds Infirmary, Bristol General Hospital was also the result of an increased need for medical support. It was founded in 1831, in response to the 'well-known fact that the Bristol Infirmary has for some time past (owing to the increase of its funds not having kept pace with that of the population of this City) been incompetent fully to answer the demands made upon the charity by those for whose benefit it was instituted'.[112] The General Hospital saw a rapid increase in patients after 1850, which was 'in part due to the fact that in that year the rule excluding patients from outside Bristol was abolished'.[113] The increase in patients coincided with a period of widespread Victorian prosperity and the hospital's finances appear to have been in a more affluent state.[114] In 1850 the Governors started an appeal for a new hospital building and in 1852 they bought the Bathurst Iron Works and three houses in Guinea Street.[115] Work was completed on the new building in the autumn of 1857 in accordance with the Italianate designs of the architect William Bruce Gingell. Plans and an engraving of the hospital appeared in *The Builder* in 1858. The plans make no mention of a garden but there is evidence of planting on a roof-top area above the warehouses to the right of the hospital on the engraving (Figure 29).

There was also a description of the garden published in *The Builder* when the hospital opened:

> The warehouses under and about the hospital, are all fire-proof . . . and over those to the southward, there is a spacious airing ground, laid out as a garden, the walks and beds being formed in Pilkington's asphalte [*sic*], with upwards of 250 tons of mould deposited upon it . . .[116]

The creation of this garden appears to have relied upon the invention of asphalt. A new substance, asphalt was introduced from France in the

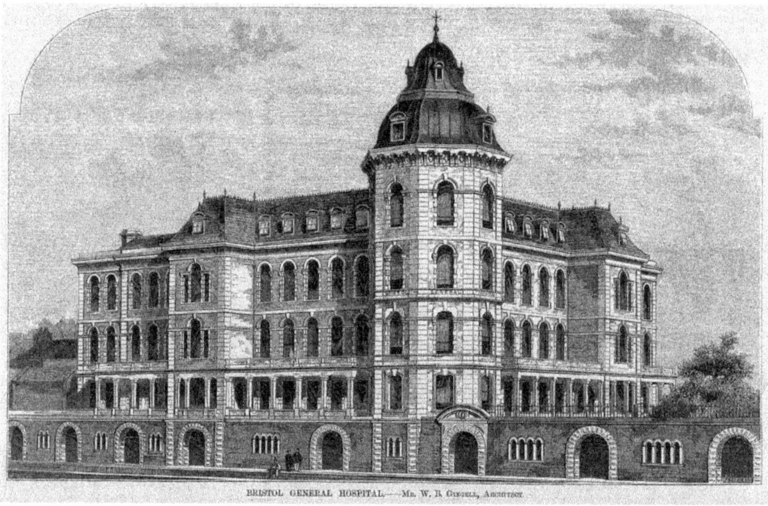

Figure 29 Engraving of William Bruce Gingell's Italianate design for the Bristol General Hospital as published in *The Builder* on 17 April 1858. The colonnades can be seen clearly running around the building on the first floor level and the roof garden is the area to the right of the engraving above the warehouses.

late 1830s. Originally it was used as a surface material for roads and cemetery catacombs and only later did it begin to be used for garden paths.[117] However, in Bristol they took this one stage further to create a roof garden and solve the problems concerning the lack of space. People walking in the garden can be seen in an engraving reproduced in *A Short History of the Bristol General Hospital* by J. Odery Symes.

There does not appear to be any description or engraving showing the garden at Bristol General Hospital in any detail, so it is hard to know what form the design took. However, it is known that beds were created from the asphalt, as this was described in *The Builder* article quoted above. Later discussions relating to problems with the garden also suggest that trees were once planted in it. According to Symes, 'the garden was a frequent source of trouble, and in 1873 Messrs. H. Pritchard & Company wrote complaining of the bad state of repair of No. 2 Warehouse situated beneath the garden. The Committee adjourned to the garden and directed the Secretary to have all the large trees removed and asphalt laid down to prevent further leakage.'[118] The trees appear to have been removed by the time a photograph was taken of the hospital in 1875. One can only speculate, but, given the creation of asphalt beds, it is quite likely that the roof garden took the traditional form of a Victorian garden with walks between the flowerbeds.

Similarly the Italian Hospital in London was reported in 1900 as having 'a flat roof which will make a pleasant retreat in fine weather, being provided with sheltered seats'.[119] These examples may have been relatively rare cases though. In 1899, *The Hospital*, reported that 'it is a wonder hospital architects do not oftener make use of roofs for providing places of recreation'.[120] However, the concept, if not the reality, of roof gardens as places that could engender health was not only limited to hospital settings. According to Richardson, the houses described in his utopian city of health, Hygeia, would have roofs that were

> but slightly arched, and are indeed all but flat. They are covered either with asphalte [*sic*], which experience, out of our supposed city, has proved to last long and to be easily repaired, or with flat tile. The roofs, barricaded round with iron palisades, tastefully painted, make excellent outdoor grounds for every house. In some instances flowers are cultivated on them.[121]

This idea was echoed in 1907 by Dr James Dunbar Brunton. *The Lancet* reported that he had postulated that flat roofs of the poorer houses could be 'used as playgrounds and might be beautified with trees and flowers in tubs and pots'.[122] He went on to state that 'the public health authorities would appoint a medical officer whose duty would be daily inspection of all roof gardens'.[123] This suggests that the concept that roof gardens could provide healthy spaces had a wider reach outside hospital design, and could impact upon wider urban design concepts. Again there is a two-way dialogue between the design of domestic and institutional spaces.

From convalescence to cure

The role of general hospitals changed during the nineteenth century, as can be seen in the example of Bristol General Hospital. Towards the end of the period the types of case admitted became more acute and the patients' length of stay was shorter. This was also related to an increase in the use of convalescent homes for patients in need of longer-term care. At Bristol the roof-top garden itself was built on in 1930. According to Symes, 'it was decided that the new Children's Ward should be built on the old "deck" side by side with a new Men's accident or emergency ward . . . these were opened and occupied at the end of December, 1930'.[124] The need for the creation of new hospital departments has often put pressure on hospital gardens and in many cases led to their loss.

In response to this wider change in the role of hospitals the perception of the importance of hospital gardens in therapeutic terms also altered. The subject of the hospital's external environment was hotly debated during the last half of the century. There were some who believed that general hospitals in small rural buildings with gardens were the ideal therapeutic environment. For example, in response to *An Address on the General Principles which should be Observed in the Construction of Hospitals* delivered to the British Medical Association at Leeds on 29 July 1869 by Douglas Galton, Dr George H.B. MacLeod from Glasgow said that:

> He hoped a time would come when small buildings placed among fields and gardens, and having all the aids to recovery which amusements, flowers and music could contribute, would be the type of our hospitals, and not the present huge piles of courts and towers crowded into the heart of our great manufacturing centres.[125]

This view was, however, not without some opposition. For a brief period of time (1862–71) St Thomas's was based in the Surrey Gardens, London, while a site was found for the new pavilion hospital. While there,

Bristowe gave an address to the Medical School entitled *The Future of St Thomas's*. During this address he commended the decision to place the hospital within the gardens:

> The site, which they have selected, is certainly the best which could, under the circumstances of the case, have been chosen. It may have some drawbacks; but it has, on the other hand, many and great advantages of position, advantages of space, and advantages of beauty, both natural and acquired. The latter especially are striking, and must approve themselves to everyone who feels any interest in the well-being of the establishment.[126]

However he went on to criticise those who felt that hospitals should be set in vast areas of land:

> Next, as regards the space of ground which a Hospital should occupy. On this head, I have no hesitation of course in admitting that, for many reasons, the more space one can obtain the better. But, I am far from thinking that a very large surface is absolutely necessary for the welfare of the patients. What is space wanted for? Eventually, I presume, for the erection of Hospital-buildings, and for the recreation and exercise of patients . . . as regards airing courts for patients; there is no doubt that these are desirable, but they are far more important for a sanatorium, or a convalescent institution, than for a general Hospital; because, for the most part, in the case of these latter, it generally happens, that when that stage has been reached, at which out-of-door exercise or air is desirable, the patients have to be discharged to make room for more pressing cases of disease.[127]

This illustrates a change in the perceived role of the general hospital and in consequence a modification of the status of the gardens associated with them in terms of their therapeutic value. It appears from MacLeod's speech and the editorials in *The Builder*, as discussed above, that many saw gardens as fulfilling the same therapeutic role in general hospitals as that described by Foster almost a century before: mainly fresh air and exercise. However, Bristowe's argument suggests that the role of general hospitals was beginning to change and, consequently, so was that of the gardens. The main difference appears to have been that patients were no longer staying in general hospitals to convalesce, as there were now special institutions for this purpose. With the rise of surgery and scientific medicine, general hospitals began to focus solely on acute medicine. From Bristowe's argument it appears that the main function of the garden in terms of therapy was to help patients during convalescence. In turn, this meant that if convalescent patients were being sent elsewhere, gardens no longer had a therapeutic function.

However, it is interesting to note that in 1862 Bristowe still felt that airing courts were important, and, as late as 1883, Mouat and Snell were still recommending that general hospitals needed gardens:

> The interspaces, which should be found in all hospitals in town or country, should not be paved or concreted yards shut in by buildings, but open cultivated gardens, accessible to the convalescent, with shelter from the weather, so as to enable them to be as much in the open air as possible, whenever it is prudent or proper for them to be out of doors.[128]

In 1893, Burdett also wrote that, 'the site of the London Hospital is self-contained . . . It is entirely surrounded by streets; it has ample grass and garden space within its area . . . The garden and grass plots are essential to the well-being of a hospital in a large town'.[129] However, the focus was perhaps shifting away from the patients and towards the staff as he goes on to say that the London Hospital's gardens are important, 'because they not only secure to the patients the requisite light and air, but they enable the resident staff to have an amount of exercise which is essential to their health and consequently to the well-being of the whole establishment'.[130] As indicated above, one of the reasons for this change might have been that more of the staff were living on the hospital site and, therefore, required a share of the external space.

The change in the function of the general hospital, with the focus increasingly on medical treatment rather than convalescence, may be one of the main explanations for the decline of general hospital gardens. Other factors include the pressure on external space as hospitals continued to expand, and the arrival of the car, which necessitated the construction of car parks. This is illustrated by the following description of the courtyard at St Bartholomew's Hospital, London, in 1992:

> The Square has been a centre of Hospital life ever since it was built. In the summer months beds are brought out into the Square so that patients can enjoy the sunshine – a custom of many years' standing which still continues. Since the 1960s, however, an increasing demand for car parking space has led to the Square being full of parked vehicles for much of the time.[131]

Of the main examples of hospital gardens discussed, only the courtyard at Leeds currently functions as a garden but its survival has more to do with its location in the heart of the hospital than its role as a therapeutic place. Although it has been reinstated as a garden and is used by patients, relatives and staff, for much of its life it was used as a staff tennis court and even its location has not saved it from being encroached on at one end by twentieth-century developments in the form of extensions to the hospital buildings.

As this chapter has demonstrated, gardens were seen as an important part of the physical environment of the nineteenth-century general hospital and they performed a variety of functions; from spaces for the recreation of patients to embellishments of civic splendour. They have been built in a range of sizes: from large acreage around provincial rural hospitals which often incorporated vegetable gardens, to small flat roofs where space was at a premium in urban centres. In the case of winter gardens, hospitals have also utilised cutting-edge technologies to provide spaces that could be used all year round. However, what is clear is that gardens were viewed as most therapeutic in relation to convalescence or where there was necessarily a longer hospital stay. The result of this is that by the twentieth century they were no longer seen as an essential element of general hospital design, but remained crucial for psychiatric institutions, convalescent homes and specialist institutions.

Notes

1 *The Builder*, 4 October 1856, p. 544.
2 Bristowe and Holmes, 'Report on the hospitals'.
3 This garden will be discussed in detail later in the chapter.
4 Bristowe and Holmes, 'Report on the hospitals', p. 573.
5 *Ibid.*, p. 583.
6 *Ibid.*, p. 575.
7 *Ibid.*, p. 601.
8 John Syer Bristowe, *An Introductory Address on the Future of St Thomas's Hospital Delivered at the Hospital in the Surrey Gardens on the Occasion of the Opening of the Session of its Medical and Surgical* College, 1 October 1862 (London: J.W. Roche, 1862), p. 8. At this time Bristowe was lecturing on *Materia Medica* at St Thomas's Hospital.
9 Richardson, *English Hospitals*, p. 16.
10 Roy Porter, ed., *The Cambridge Illustrated History of Medicine* (Cambridge: Cambridge University Press, 1996), p. 213.
11 Richardson, *English Hospitals*, p. 54.
12 Porter, *Cambridge Illustrated History*, p. 224.
13 Christine Stevenson, 'Medicine and architecture', in W.F. Bynum and Roy Porter, eds, *The Companion Encyclopedia of the History of Medicine*, 2 vols (London and New York: Routledge, 1993), ii, 1495–1519, p. 1500.
14 Quoted in Taylor, *Hospital and Asylum Architecture*, pp. 5–6.

15 For a definition of Gardenesque style see Chapter 2, pages 52–3. All are reproduced in V.M. Leveaux, *The History of the Derbyshire General Infirmary, 1810–1894* (Cromford: Scarthin Books, 1999).
16 Loudon, *The Suburban Gardener*, p. 302.
17 Stevenson, *Medicine and Magnificence*, p. 125.
18 Foster, *An Essay on Hospitals*, p. 23.
19 *Ibid.*, pp. 24–5.
20 Bristowe and Holmes, 'Report on the hospitals', p. 657.
21 *Ibid.*, p. 650.
22 John Penfold, *The History of The Essex County Hospital, Colchester, 1820–1948* (Essex: John Penfold, 1984), pp. 128–9.
23 Alexander George Gibson, *The Radcliffe Infirmary* (Oxford: Oxford University Press, 1926), p. 60.
24 Foster, *An Essay on Hospitals*, p. 23.
25 Bristowe and Holmes, 'Report on the hospitals', p. 669.
26 *Ibid.*, p. 636.
27 Anning, *The General Infirmary*, i, pp. 19–20.
28 *Ibid.*, p. 20.
29 *Ibid.*
30 *Ibid.*
31 *Ibid.*
32 Quoted in Anning, *The General Infirmary*.
33 *The Builder*, 19 May 1849, p. 235.
34 *Ibid.*, 4 October 1856, p. 544.
35 Richardson, *English Hospitals*, p. 3.
36 W.F. Bynum, *Science and the Practice of Medicine in the Nineteenth Century* (Cambridge: Cambridge University Press, 1994), p. 185.
37 'Hospital guide-books', *The Hospital*, 28 January 1911, p. 539.
38 *Ibid.*
39 Stevenson has discussed this issue in relation to hospital architecture in great detail in *Medicine and Magnificence*.
40 Gibson, *The Radcliffe Infirmary*, p. 59.
41 Roy Porter, *The Greatest Benefit to Mankind: A Medical History of Humanity from Antiquity to the Present* (London: Fontana Press, 1997), p. 334.
42 1764 engraving of Gloucester Infirmary, which shows a vast kitchen garden to the rear of the hospital. The engraver also appears to have emphasised the rural location of the hospital. This is reproduced in Richardson, *English Hospitals*, p. 24.
43 Reproduced in Leveaux, *History of the Derbyshire Royal Infirmary*.
44 Bristowe and Holmes, 'Report on the Hospitals', p. 772.
45 Lane, *A Social History of Medicine*, p. 11.
46 John Bart Pringle, *Observations on the Diseases of the Army in Camp and Garrison . . . With an Appendix, Containing Some Papers of Experiments, Read at Several Meetings of the Royal Society* (London: 1752).

47 Stevenson, 'Medicine and architecture', p. 1500.
48 Quoted in Bill Bynum, 'Discarded diagnoses: hospitalism', *The Lancet*, 357:9265 (2001), 1372, p. 1372.
49 Florence Nightingale, *Notes on Hospitals, Third Edition: Enlarged and For the Most Part Re-written* (London: Longman, Green, Longman, Roberts and Green, 1863), p. iii.
50 Bynum, 'Discarded diagnoses', p. 1372.
51 Lane, *A Social History of Medicine*, p. 85.
52 John Howard, *An Account of the Principal Lazarettos in Europe: With Various Papers Relative to the Plague: Together with Further Observations on some Foreign Prisons and Hospitals; and Additional Remarks on the Present State of Those in Great Britain and Ireland*, second edition (London: Printed for J. Johnson, C. Dilly, and T. Cadell, 1791), p. 23.
53 *Ibid.*, p. 57.
54 *Ibid.*, p. 58.
55 *Ibid.*, p. 57.
56 *Ibid.*, p. 65.
57 *Ibid.*, p. 142.
58 *The Builder*, 17 April 1858, p. 261.
59 Loudon, *The Suburban Gardener*, p. 325.
60 *The Builder*, 17 April 1858, p. 265.
61 For more on circular wards see Jeremy Taylor, *The Architect and the Pavilion Hospital: Dialogue and Design Creativity in England 1850–1914* (London and New York: Leicester University Press, 1997), pp. 134–67.
62 G.C. Cook, 'Henry Currey FRIBA (1820–1900): leading Victorian hospital architect, and early exponent of the "pavilion principle"', *Postgraduate Medical Journal*, 78:920 (2002), 352–9, p. 352.
63 There is some debate over who wrote these articles, as they are anonymous. Grace Goldin in 'Building a hospital of air', *Bulletin of the History of Medicine*, 49 (1975), 512–35 has suggested that Nightingale wrote them but it is more likely that they are the work of Roberton and edited by Godwin as suggested by Antony King, 'Hospital planning: revised thoughts on the origin of the pavilion principle in England', *Medical History*, 10:4 (1966), 360–73.
64 *The Builder*, 28 August 1858, p. 577. Jeremy Taylor has written extensively on the subject of the history of the pavilion design. See in particular *The Architect and the Pavilion*.
65 See Taylor, *The Architect and the Pavilion*, pp. 134–67.
66 *The Builder*, 20 September 1856, p. 509.
67 *Ibid.*
68 *Ibid.*, 11 September 1858, p. 610.
69 Nightingale, *Notes, Third Edition*, p. 19.
70 For more on this see in particular Hazel Conway, *People's Parks: The Design and Development of Victorian Parks in Britain* (Cambridge: Cambridge

University Press, 1991), Peter Thorsheim, *Inventing Pollution: Coal, Smoke and Culture in Britain Since 1800* (Ohio: Ohio University Press, 2006), Felix Driver, 'Moral geographies: social science and the urban environment in mid-nineteenth century England', *Transactions of the Institute of British Geographers*, 13:3 (1998), 275–87 and H.L. Malchow, 'Public gardens and social action in late Victorian London', *Victorian Studies*, 29:1 (1985), 97–124.

71 Mary Logan, Guide to the Pictures at Hampton Court with Studies of the Artists (London: Kyrle Society Pamphlet, 1894), p. 48.

72 'The Queen's Hospital, Birmingham', *The Hospital*, 9 November 1889, 94–5, p. 95.

73 Mary Logan, *The Guide to the Italian Pictures at Hampton Court*, Kyrle Pamphlets No. 2 (London: Innes & Co., 1894). The aims of the society are listed on the back cover.

74 *Fifth Annual Report of the Metropolitan Public Gardens Association* (in connection with the National Health Society), 1887, p. 40.

75 For more on Henry Currey and the design of St Thomas's Hospital see Cook, 'Henry Currey'.

76 *The Builder*, 11 February 1860, p. 90.

77 Quoted in Lindsay Granshaw, *St Thomas' Hospital, London, 1850–1900*, PhD Thesis (Bryn Mawr: Bryn Mawr College, 1981), p. 163.

78 *The Lancet*, 28 January 1871, quoted in Goldin, 'Building a hospital of air', p. 534.

79 Granshaw, *St Thomas' Hospital*, p. 187.

80 E.M. McInnes, *St Thomas' Hospital* (London: George Allen and Unwin Ltd, 1963) p. 138.

81 *St Thomas's Hospital Contract for Building New Hospital at Stangate*. Printed copy of the agreement 1867 – unsigned – between John Perry, Charles Edward Alfort, Joseph Brindley and Francis Hicks, Treasurer of the Hospital . . . 1867 (held in Kings College London Archives, TH/FR1/2 oversized).

82 *Ibid.*, p. 59.

83 Goldin, 'Building a hospital of air', p. 525.

84 *Ibid.*, p. 534.

85 Frederick J. Mouat and Saxon H. Snell, *Hospital: Construction and Management* (London: J. & A. Churchill and Co., 1883), p. 24.

86 'The reopening of St Thomas's Hospital', *The Lancet*, 27 September 1862, p. 335.

87 'Nurses' home at the Wandsworth and Clapham Union Infirmary', *The Hospital*, 7 October 1899, p. 18.

88 Alicia Amherst, *London Parks and Gardens* (New York: E. P. Dutton & Co., 1907), p. 295.

89 Carl A. Erikson, 'Planning space for recreation', *American Journal of Nursing*, 46:10 (1946), 696–700, p. 696.

90 *Ibid.*

91 Leeds General Infirmary, *Building Committee Minutes*, 7 May 1862 (West Yorkshire Archive Service: LGI/13/3–4).
92 Taylor, *The Architect and the Pavilion*, p. 13.
93 *Ibid.*, p. 18.
94 Quoted in Taylor, *The Architect and the Pavilion*, p. 41.
95 Leeds General Infirmary, *Building Committee Minutes*, 28 November 1866.
96 *Ibid.*
97 *The Builder*, Editorial, 11 September 1858. Also printed as part of an appendix in Nightingale, *Notes, Third Edition.*
98 Samuel Orchart Beeton, *The Beeton Book of Garden Management* (originally published as *Beeton's Illustrated Book of the Garden* in 1889–91) (facsimile reprinted Hertfordshire: Omega Books, 1985), p. 356.
99 For more on the wider context of the increased use of glass in the Victorian period see Chris Otter, *The Victorian Eye: A Political History of Light and Vision in Britain, 1800–1910* (Chicago and London: University of Chicago Press, 2008).
100 Joseph Paxton, 'Sanitariums for exercise of invalids and others in all weathers', in *The Illustrated London News*, 5 July 1851, p. 11. With thanks to Imogen Magnus for this reference.
101 *Ibid.*
102 Benjamin Ward Richardson, 'On winter palaces of health and camps of health at home. A practicable ideal', *The Asclepiad*, 4 (1884), 120–31, p. 122.
103 *Ibid.*, p. 123.
104 *Ibid.*, p. 124.
105 *Ibid.*, p. 125.
106 *Ibid.*
107 Frederic J. Mouat, 'On hospitals', *The Lancet*, 30 July 1881, p. 166.
108 *Ibid.*
109 Mouat, 'On hospitals', *The Lancet*, 1 October 1881, p. 580.
110 'Account of Leeds Infirmary', *British Medical Journal*, 31 July 1869.
111 Burdett, *Hospitals and Asylums*, iv, p. 129.
112 Taken from their first report, quoted in J. Odery Symes, *A Short History of the Bristol General Hospital* (Bristol: John Wright and Sons Ltd, 1932), p. 1.
113 *Ibid.*, p. 31.
114 *Ibid.*, p. 30.
115 *Ibid.*, p. 42.
116 *The Builder*, 17 April 1858, p. 261.
117 Brent Elliott, *Victorian Gardens* (London: Batsford, 1986), p. 17.
118 Symes, *Bristol General Hospital*, p. 46.
119 'The new Italian Hospital, Queen Square', *The Hospital*, 31 March 1900, p. 438.
120 'Nottingham General Hospital-Jubilee Wing', *The Hospital*, 28 October 1899, 67–8, p. 67.

121 Benjamin Ward Richardson, *Hygeia* (1876) (reprinted USA: Dodo Press, 2008), p. 24.
122 'Urban roof gardens and roof hospitals', *The Lancet*, 9 February 1907, p. 372.
123 *Ibid.*
124 Symes, *Bristol General Hospital*, pp. 94–5.
125 Douglas Galton, *An Address on the General Principles Which Should be Observed in the Construction of Hospitals*, delivered to the British Medical Association at Leeds, 29 July 1869 (London: Macmillan and Co., 1869), p. 79.
126 Bristowe, *An Introductory Address* (1862), p. 5.
127 *Ibid.*, p. 13.
128 Mouat and Snell, *Hospital*, p. 23.
129 Burdett, *Hospitals and Asylums*, iv, p. xi.
130 *Ibid.*
131 Geoffrey Yeo, *Images of Bart's: An Illustrated History of St Bartholomew's Hospital in the City of London* (London: Historical Publications Ltd. in association with the Archives Department St Bartholomew's Hospital, 1992) p. 30.

5

Fresh air and sunshine: the open-air institutions of the twentieth century

Give him air, he'll straight be well
Motto for Edward VII Sanatorium design competition, 1902[1]

In 1862 John Syer Bristowe argued that 'as regards airing courts for patients; there is no doubt that these are desirable, but they are far more important for a sanatorium, or a convalescent institution, than for a general Hospital'.[2] This reflected a change in the perceived role of the general hospital and a move towards the introduction of specialist institutions for chronic diseases and homes in which patients could convalesce.[3] It also marked a decline in the importance of gardens associated with general hospitals and a rise in gardens associated with specialist institutions, particularly those practising open-air therapies.

Open-air therapy was practised in many of the new specialist and convalescent institutions. This therapeutic approach ensured that patients spent as much time as possible in the fresh air and sunshine, as both were considered to have curative properties. On the surface this appears to be a direct continuation of the theories concerning the role of light and air in disease causation and recovery that were held by eminent Victorians such as Florence Nightingale. However, these therapies had a new medical basis, as developments in the understanding of disease causation meant that the role 'air' played in health and disease had changed. As Roger Cooter has argued, while bacteriology theories still permitted air to be thought of as a reservoir of harmful agents, they also allowed more emphasis to be placed on air as curative or constitutionally restorative in and of itself.[4]

The idea that there was a paradigm shift towards the end of the nineteenth century can be illustrated by comparing the reception of George

Bodington's essay on his use of open-air therapy at his sanatorium near Sutton Coldfield, in the West Midlands, in 1840 and in 1901. When first published in 1840 it received a hostile reception from the medical profession but when the Sydenham Society republished it in 1901 it had 'hosannas raised to it'.[5] According to Cooter this comparison implies that 'in the eyes of the medical establishment, while it was quite acceptable for Bodington's generation to recommend fresh air, it was clearly unacceptable for them to advocate open air as the major part of an exclusive medical regimen'.[6] This demonstrates that the early twentieth-century emphasis on open-air therapies was based on new medical theories, albeit ones that, initially, appear to be an extension of older ideas concerning the role of light and air in relation to disease.

A wide range of institutions embraced the idea of open-air therapies. In this chapter, four specialist hospitals and a convalescent home have been chosen for discussion. These are: the Winford Orthopaedic Hospital, Bristol; the Edward VII Sanatorium, Sussex; Hailey Open-Air Sanatorium, Oxfordshire; Bristol Homeopathic Hospital; and Blackwell Convalescent Home, Birmingham. These will enable a detailed analysis of individual institutions across an array of different medical concerns.

Open-air therapy

The notion of hospitals and schools based on the open-air regime is generally accepted to have originated Germany. It seems to have begun as a treatment for tuberculosis and then developed to become a therapeutic approach for other diseases. F.B. Smith suggests that the vogue for sanatoria began in Germany around 1860, 'inspired by a mixture of traditional cure-taking at spas, nature worship, and a new physiology of lung weakness'.[7] However, after Robert Koch discovered the tuberculosis bacillus in 1882, the concept that disease was caused by germs gradually became the standard theory of causation. While men like Koch tried to develop specific serum therapies for infectious diseases in the 1890s, other doctors developed therapeutic regimes which they believed would enhance natural immunity. According to research conducted by Paul Weindling:

> Critics of Koch like the public health experts Gottstein and the bacteriologist Hueppe argued for the importance of studying resistance to diseases. They emphasised the importance of strengthening the body's natural resistance to disease rather than promoting 'artificial immunity' through mass immunisation with injections of sera.[8]

Therefore, it can be argued that the use of open-air therapy in the specialist institutions and convalescent homes of the early twentieth century was in response to the belief that it would strengthen the body's natural immunity.

This theory was also expressed in a paper published in *The Medical Officer* in 1909 which suggests that open-air therapies were gaining popularity in Britain:

> In fact the 'fresh air cure' has become almost a household word. And many people seem to look upon fresh air as a kind of specific or panacea for phthisis in the same sense, as we look on opium as a specific for pain. To my mind, this is quite an erroneous view; what the fresh air does is to increase metabolism and thus increase the resisting power of the individual to the tubercle bacillus.[9]

Those who promoted open-air therapies appear to have viewed them as the most progressive form of health care and they do seem to have been represented as a popular method of treating a variety of diseases at the turn of the century. T.N. Kelynack, the editor of the first edition of *The Year Book of Open-air Schools and Children's Sanatoria* (1915) wrote that:

> With the rapid development of the movement for the open-air education and treatment of tuberculosis, tuberculously disposed and other diseased and delicate children, it has become clear that if the subject is to be adequately dealt with, a special volume must be devoted to it. The open-air sanatorium and school stand as embodiments of new principles and more rational practices in regard to Preventive Medicine and the science and art of the hygiene of education.[10]

Open-air therapies were often described as a natural cure and many conventional doctors appear to have been interested in the idea of giving the body the correct natural conditions to help it heal itself. In 1910, C. Muthu argued that open-air therapy was a 'natural treatment' and then suggested that:

> the secret of its widespread interest in Europe is due to the discovery – if discovery it may be called – that fresh air, hitherto regarded as an enemy to be shut out and barred, is really a friend, and one of Nature's best gifts to man, without which life slowly fades and disease lengthens its stay.[11]

Like many writers, he related the concept of open-air therapies to a time before industrialisation and urbanisation, and he stated:

> that man, by building towns and manufacturing dirt and disease, is undoing Nature's work, and that to put himself right again he must go back to Nature, and lead an open-life in the green fields and meadow, and breathe the sweet fresh air.[12]

As this suggests, there were wider social implications related to the rationale behind open-air therapies. It appears, as always, that the dirty air of the town was seen as part of the problem so that the clean air of the countryside became the obvious solution.

The medical ideas concerning the value of fresh air and sunshine also influenced wider movements, including the development of the Garden City ideal and modernist architecture. Throughout the nineteenth century there had been a growing concern regarding the lack of open spaces in urban areas. This led to the creation of parks, gardens, recreation grounds and playgrounds.[13]

An early example of the combination of such considerations can be found in Ward Richardson's description of his utopian city, *Hygeia*. Within this vision, which he argues is based on the latest scientific principles, gardens and open spaces were given a fundamentally important role:

> The acreage of our model city allows room for three wide main streets or boulevards . . . They are planted on each side of the pathways with trees, and in many places with shrubs and evergreens. All the interspaces between the backs of houses are gardens . . . other public buildings, as well as some private buildings such as warehouses and stables, stand alone . . . They are surrounded with garden space, and add not only to the beauty but to the healthiness of the city.[14]

Ebenezer Howard, the visionary behind the Garden City movement, was heavily influenced by Ward Richardson and argued that although the country 'is the source of all health, all wealth and all knowledge' it needed to be combined with society as symbolised by the town (Figure 30).[15] The solution to the problems caused by urbanisation was to bring the countryside into the towns in the form of gardens – the 'rus en urbe' ideal.

Some of the medical profession also appear to have viewed the garden city as a potential weapon in the war against the degeneration of the population. In 1919 a writer in *The Medical Officer* argued that garden cities could help create a more vigorous and happy nation:

> It was open air and exercise, good feeding and well-regulated rest which had converted weedy citizens into robust soldiers, which restored the weakly in open-air schools, and the consumptive in sanatoria. Preventable sickness

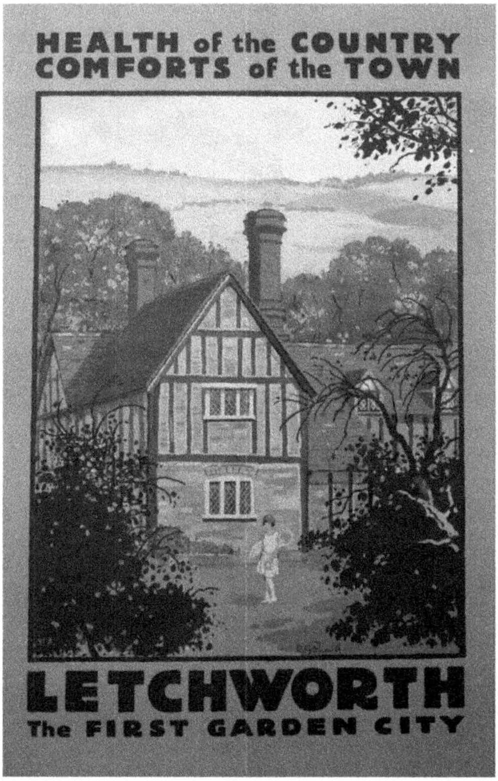
HEALTH of the COUNTRY
COMFORTS of the TOWN
LETCHWORTH
The FIRST GARDEN CITY

Figure 30 A poster issued by the First Garden City Ltd, c.1925, demonstrating the importance of combining the town and the country through the use of gardens.

was maiming and killing as many and causing economic loss as much as the late war. If for that reason alone, Dr Hill, urged that garden cities should be built and big towns not added to . . . An immediate and pressing demand should be made for garden cities and the bringing up of the young in the discipline of taking pride in and keeping perfect bodily health.[16]

As well as the creation of garden cities, Muthu thought a solution could be found if the Poor Law was abolished and the poor were given free access to the land. Again the rural life is seen as the healthiest and the idea of men becoming noble yeomen relates to the Romantic view of an idealised England that existed before industrialisation and urbanisation. According to him these measures would mean:

> more employment in the country, more honourable work done under health-giving conditions . . . It would mean pure and wholesome occupation to thousands of citizens living in the open air and pleasant sunshine, and engaged in the congenial task of tilling the fields and gathering in the harvest . . . It would mean that in many a cottage home the family altar would be set up, and a 'race of pure heart, iron sinew, splendid frame, and constant faith', would keep alive the bygone traditions of its yeoman fathers.[17]

Again this reflects the fear that the race is degenerating in terms of physical and moral health and suggests that there was an English golden age of health before the development of the towns, when people were employed on the land. This concept argued that, to stem this degeneration of the population, people needed to return to an earlier rural way of life. There is also of course a less savoury side to this, as similar ideas concerning the need for a pure, healthy race are those which were promoted in Nazi Germany a few decades later.

On a lighter note, Muthu's call for a return to rural living is a product of both earlier Romantic ideas and those of the Arts and Crafts movement. One writer who imagined a post-industrial paradise based on these notions was William Morris, whose utopian *News from Nowhere* (1890) was set in the future and described a socialist society in which everyone lived in the countryside. There are constant references to similarities between this utopian dream and the medieval period, for example, the houses 'were so like mediaeval houses . . . that I felt as if I were alive in the fourteenth century'.[18] There are also echoes of the open-air philosophy with open-air work being recommended as a method 'to clear the cobwebs' from the brain and children are described as playing in forests and sleeping in tents.[19] One of the characters inhabiting this utopian land explains to the protagonist that:

> these children do not all come from the near houses, the woodland houses, but from the countryside generally. They often make up parties, and come to play in the woods for weeks together in summer-time living in tents, as you see. We rather encourage them to do it . . . the less they stew inside houses the better for them.[20]

Similarly, the protagonist often comments on how healthy and young the people look in comparison to those of the industrialised society he has left. For example, the children in the forest are described as being 'especially fine specimens of their race'[21] and 'as to the women themselves, it was pleasant indeed to see them, they were so kind and happy-looking in expression of face, so shapely and well-knit of body, and thoroughly healthy looking and strong'.[22] Throughout the novel Morris argues that a life of physical labour in a rural setting with as much open air as possible was the reason for the health, youth and beauty of the fictional population. This is related to both the fear of ill-health caused by urbanisation and industrialisation and the myth that the predominantly rural medieval way of life had resulted in a stronger, healthier population.

Another sign of an increased interest in the rural way of life, as associated with the concept of Englishness in the Edwardian period, is reflected in the emergence of *Country Life*. First published by Edward Hudson in 1897, Anne Helmreich has suggested that its creation reflected the 'growing identification of the wealthy middle classes not with the city, the typical source of their money but with the countryside. Although they lacked the landed gentry's traditional hereditary ties to agriculture, these persons nonetheless (or perhaps because of this) worked to bind themselves to the land and to the English past.'[23] The English garden can be seen as a representation of this Edwardian move back towards the countryside and it was to be an integral part of the design of places such as sanatoria. As will be discussed later, Gertrude Jekyll, the designer probably most associated with the country garden style, was even brought in to design the gardens surrounding a sanatorium, thereby bringing the English garden style to a therapeutic space.

Design of open-air institutions

In around 1900, Burton-Fanning wrote that 'elaborate buildings are not necessary for the treatment of pulmonary tuberculosis . . . Granted free access of fresh air, the accommodation may be planned on the simplest lines.'[24] This meant that many early open-air institutions, like many nineteenth-century hospitals, shared design features with domestic houses. In fact country houses were often used with minimal adaptations as open-air institutions. David Lambert and Stewart Harding have suggested that from the 1880s 'country seats and parkland became available at knock-down prices as the aristocracy and squirearchy adjusted to leaner times'.[25] They go on to describe the 'Colony' system of national institutions for the mentally handicapped, instigated by Reverend Harold Burden, which 'were established from 1908 in a string of country houses purchased after they failed to reach their reserve prices at auction'.[26] It is also worth mentioning that during the First and Second World Wars country houses were often used as convalescent hospitals for service men.[27]

Hospital architecture, primarily with regard to sanatoria, developed specific design features in relation to open-air therapy, so that by the 1950s the National Association for the Prevention of Consumption and Other Forms of Tuberculosis (NAPT) suggested that it was unthinkable that anything other than a new building would be suitable for a sanatorium:

> Sometimes it happens that large mansions are presented for hospital purposes, and there is an understandable temptation to think that it is cheaper to convert such a building into a sanatorium rather than face the experience of new construction. This impulse should be firmly resisted. Modern hospital architecture is so specialised that it is nearly impossible to adapt an existing building for the purpose.[28]

The specialised designs for sanatoria included methods that would maximise the view available to patients and increase the accessibility of sunshine and fresh air. Taylor has argued that:

> Following the King Edward VII Prize Essay Competition (1902) to identify the best architectural and medical solution, and influenced by continental regimes such as Nordrach and Falkenstein, a distinctive new building form emerged . . . With its glass walls, balconies and distinctive 'butterfly' plan, it represented a suitable combination of new medical thinking with an innovative design response.[29]

The Homeopathic Hospital in Bristol was one such hospital built on the butterfly plan,[30] a design whereby the wings of a building are located at an angle to its core in order to maximise the sunlight reaching the interior of the building. The butterfly plan was also popular with Arts and Crafts architects and, according to Jane Brown, was used by E.S. Prior, M.H. Baillie Scott, Edward Lutyens and Charles Edward Mallows along with Edward Brantwood Maufe at Kelling Hall, Norfolk, in 1912.[31] Another example of innovative architecture designed to maximise the amount of sunshine and fresh air available to patients was Sully Hospital, Cardiff, built between 1932 and 1936. Designed by William Pite, Son and Fairweather on a 'double-v plan', with the wings of the building forming v-shapes, the wards were south facing and had views of the sea, and the idea of the v-shapes was that they would provide shelter from the south-westerly winds.[32] Orthopaedic hospitals were also often designed specifically in relation to open-air therapy. In this case they generally took the form of a single-storey building with large windows or doors that could be opened to allow beds to be wheeled outside.

The Sully Hospital design had been influenced by other modernist designs such as the Paimio Sanatorium, Finland, designed by Alvar Aalto in 1929–33. According to Jonathan Glancey, at Paimio the 'patient's rooms are awash with daylight for as much of the year as possible'.[33] Similarly the Birmingham Hospital Saturday Fund Convalescent Home for Women built at Kewstoke, near Weston-Super-Mare, and opened in 1933, exemplifies these ideals and also seems to have had a quite remarkable modernist garden (Figure 31). However, although NAPT argued that modern hospital architecture was a specific specialism, the styles used had much in common with domestic modern architecture.[34] For example, Glancey describes Paimio as having 'ship-like balconies projecting out into the forest landscape' and this seems to reflect the modernist movement in architecture as much as specific hospital design.[35] In 1939, Leslie Abercrombie wrote that:

> It used to be the aim of ship designers to make their interiors look as like as possible to long-shore buildings, with dummy fireplaces to preserve the illusion of stability: it now appears, *per contra*, to be the desire of some architects to make their houses look like ships, perhaps to create the feeling of rushing air and sunny decks. Streamlinism is a modern movement reflected equally in clothes and locomotives, and in an indefinite way connected with the cult of fitness.[36]

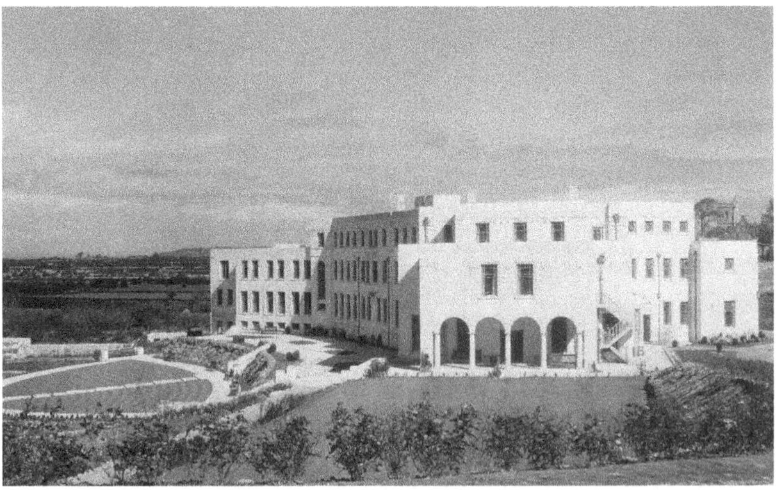

Figure 31 The modernist architecture and gardens of the Birmingham Hospital Saturday Fund Convalescent Home for Women, Kewstoke near Weston-Super-Mare, c.1930s.

This suggests that the interest in open-air lifestyles was reflected in both domestic and hospital architecture.

Pyrs Gruffudd has argued that the modern movement was concerned with 'hygienic design, utilization of sunlight and fresh air, and the value of propaganda in health education'.[37] This implies that concerns about sunlight and fresh air were as much about being healthy as curing disease, which is why they were relevant to architects designing houses as well as those working on institutions. Le Corbusier's Villa Savoye, designed in 1928–29, illustrates this relationship between health and modernist architecture. The villa was designed with horizontal windows to increase the amount of light inside the building and Dennis Doordan has argued that 'the rooftop solarium and the horizontal windows are clear responses to the emphasis on sunlight and fresh air that figured prominently in early-twentieth century descriptions of modern environments'.[38]

Although modernism was one form of architecture embraced by hospital designers, the Arts and Crafts movement was also influential. An unexecuted design by the architect Robert Schultz, for a new Male Infirmary at Holloway Sanatorium, Virginia Water, published in *The Builder* on 26 September 1906, demonstrates the strong influence of these concepts. According to David Ottewill, Schultz attached great importance to the relationship between house and garden and built up a strong reputation for garden design.[39] In this capacity he has been linked with the small garden rooms designed at Cottesbrooke Hall, Northamptonshire, in the 1910s which epitomise this Arts and Crafts garden style.[40]

Both modernism and the Arts and Crafts movement were concerned with the health of the nation, even if their resultant forms were very different, and, as Gruffudd has suggested, 'to an extent, the medical and even moral condition of urbanities was thought to be potentially improvable through the management and design of space'.[41] Clifford Holliday voiced this idea in 1939 when he wrote that 'ordered housing development creates a true philosophy of living capable of harmonising health, work and leisure'.[42] As Mark Wigley suggests, in the case of modernism even the whiteness of the architecture was important as this meant that it 'joins the doctor's white coat, the white tiles of the bathroom, the white walls of the hospital, and so on'.[43]

Winford Orthopaedic Hospital

One institution using the open-air approach was the Winford Orthopaedic Hospital, Bristol (Figure 32). In 1925 a sixty-acre site was purchased on

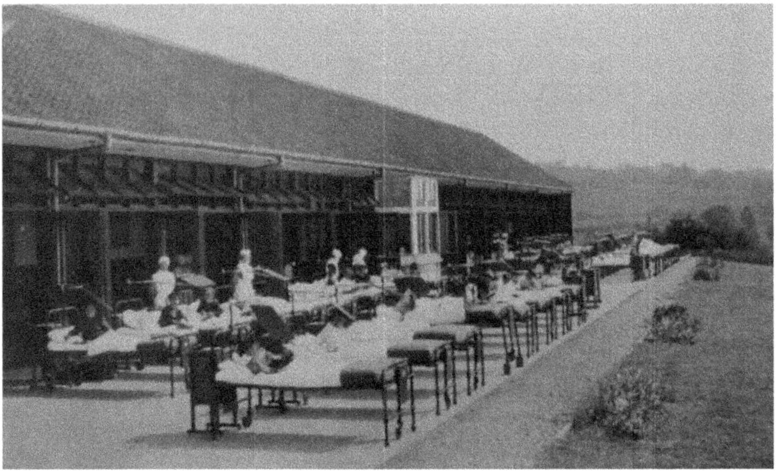

Figure 32 Photograph showing the children in beds that have been pushed outside at Winford Orthopaedic Hospital, Bristol, from the 1936 *Annual Report.*

the outskirts of Bristol and Sir George Oatley (also the architect of the Bristol Homeopathic Hospital) acted as honorary architect.[44] Robert Jones stated a number of factors of importance in making decisions about the site of an orthopaedic hospital:

- in the first place you want ample acreage
- the air should be pure and free from contamination of cities
- the site should be dry, and not subject to mist
- it should be on a hill, preferably several hundred feet above sea level
- the wards should open to south or south west and lie on a sloping surface[45]

He went on to say that, 'you can see that the great object is to obtain the maximum of sunshine and dry fresh air, and if in addition, breezes should come from over the sea, it would be an advantage'.[46] Therefore, like other open-air institutions of this type, Winford Orthopaedic Hospital was built on a rural site. This was described in the 1928 programme as, 'a beautiful site . . . facing south and at an elevation of over 400 feet above sea-level. Here open pavilions will be erected where the little patients can get every bit of sunlight available.'[47]

As Richardson has pointed out, the similarity of orthopaedic and tuberculosis treatment was due to the belief that orthopaedic conditions, like tuberculosis, were linked with 'poverty, poor diet and overcrowding, so the emphasis on sunshine, good food and fresh air continued to dominate their treatment'.[48] Although orthopaedics is generally seen solely as a surgical discipline, there were a number of surgeons in the nineteenth and early twentieth century who took a more holistic approach.[49] Cooter has argued that:

> Based on the principle of sacrificing as little of the body as possible to the surgeon's scalpel, the interest of curing rather than cutting, conservative surgery emerged in the eighteenth century out of the teachings of John Hunter. Linked to it was the belief in the healing power of nature (*vis medicatrix naturae*) which included appreciation of the curative value of fresh air, rest, the immobilization of injured limbs, and the notions of the use of minimal doses of physic.[50]

Influential in this movement were the London surgeons Sir William Fergusson (1808–77), Frederick Howard Marsh (1839–1915) and George Callender (1830–79). Cooter has suggested that the principles and practices indicated by these leading physicians:

> contributed to an appreciation of the value of good diet, clean environment, rest and gentleness on health, and to a respect for non-heroic surgery and physic. Holistic in their orientation, and inclined to prevention as much as to cure, these principles and practices owed something to popular 'alternative' medical cults and practices, but only as reworked *within* orthodox medicine according to ideas of the body's own natural restorative capacities.[51]

As in the other institutions discussed in this chapter, there was an emphasis on nature as a restorative power. This emphasis was apparent in the 1928 programme:

> Crippling diseases of children, e.g., infantile paralysis, advanced rickets, heart disease and tubercular bone disease, nearly always require prolonged treatment, often extending over one or two years. In addition to skilled medical and surgical treatment three conditions are needed to give the best chance of a permanent cure:
>
> - Continuous treatment
> - Pure clean air and all the sunlight possible over a long period
> - Pleasant surroundings with as much occupation for mind and hands as the patient's strength allows.[52]

Gardens were important in relation to two of these listed conditions, as they could encourage patients to spend time outside by providing pleasant surroundings as well as occupation in the form of gardening. One writer in 1909 noted that 'all sanatoria for children should be provided with gardens in which health-giving employment can be found for both mind and body'.[53] This language reflects the medico-moral discourse of the nineteenth century asylum with its use of gardens and gardening. According to G.R. Girdlestone, the children should spend most of the day outside: 'If it is not too bad a day, most of the cases will be having sun baths, or, if there is no direct sunlight, exposure to sky and air. This raises their vitality, gives them a good colour and well-developed muscles though they are in bed, and helps them in their fight against disease.'[54]

As the hospital was described as an 'Open-Air Hospital School' in the 1928 programme it was evidently used as both an orthopaedic hospital and a school. Until the outbreak of war in 1939 the hospital was used solely by children.[55] In a photograph from the *Annual Report* of 1938 the children are shown to be working outside (Figure 33). The schoolroom itself had folding shutters so that it could either be fully open or offer some protection from the wind. According to the 'School Report' of Miss S.A. Thomas (Headmistress) in 1936, 'the children who can get up

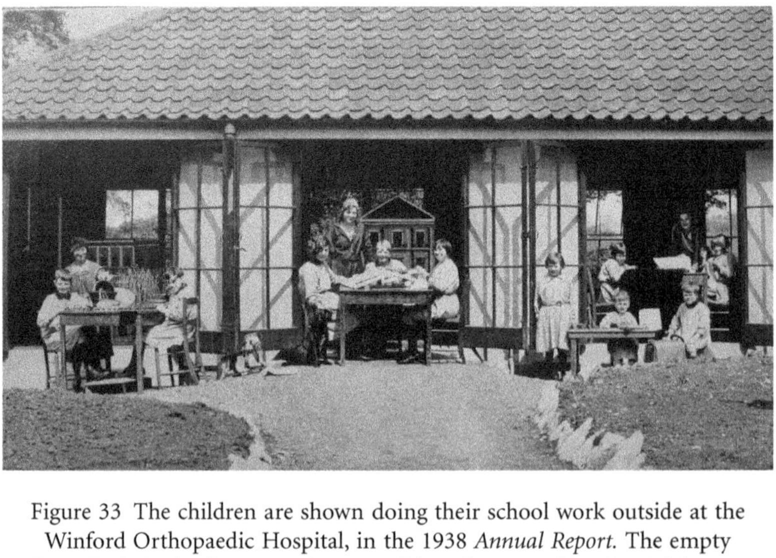

Figure 33 The children are shown doing their school work outside at the Winford Orthopaedic Hospital, in the 1938 *Annual Report*. The empty flowerbeds in the foreground may well have been used by the children as part of the educational programme.

are encouraged to take an interest in the garden and to look after their own little plots out of school hours'.[56] Gardening was seen to have both moral and physical benefits and was an important part of the open-air school regime.

The importance of clean air as a method of promoting health, particularly for children, led to the establishment of a number of charities that existed solely to send children from urban areas on country holidays. In the 1890 *Charities Register and Digest* four charities are listed which had this specific aim.[57] Similarly, the role played by the countryside in terms of good health is demonstrated by a cure for tonsilitis recommended in *The Medical Officer* in 1908. The cure was to 'give them cod liver oil and steel wine, and send them to the country, and they will get well quicker than if they remain in the towns'.[58]

An extension of this was the belief that some children could benefit from attending schools designed along the same lines as open-air hospitals. The movement in favour of open-air schools, originally known as open-air recovery schools or forest schools, began in Germany like the open-air hospitals. The London County Council opened the first open-air school in England at Plumstead in 1907. According to Smith this was based on the Charlottenberg Open-Air Recovery School of 1904, which was intended to 'instruct and cure simultaneously'.[59] One contemporary commentator described the value of the schools as:

> both curative and educational, curative to this extent, that the children are placed in the best possible hygienic surroundings, in order that they may build up their strength that they become resistant to any harmful tendency to which they are predisposed by heredity, on the one hand, or on the other, that they may so completely recover as to be fit to return to the normal school . . . What, then are the hygienic requirements of these debilitated children? I think you will agree with me that they require an abundance of fresh air, for the majority of these children come from homes that are dark, badly ventilated and over crowded.[60]

Again it is suggested that natural immunity needed to be strengthened in order to overcome predisposing factors to illness. In this case heredity is stated as the predisposing element but, according to Michael Worboys, poverty, overcrowding, poor sanitation, ignorance, fatigue and alcoholism were also invoked as ancillary causes of disease.[61]

Children with a variety of physical conditions were sent to the schools. The majority, according to Smith, had rickets, and the next largest group were consumptive or joint cases.[62] The children also often had learning difficulties and therefore the work was generally practical in nature and often took place outside, using the natural world as an instructive tool:

> The chief points about school work associated with the garden are the facts that children are brought into touch with actualities; they work and breathe the fresh air amidst surroundings they themselves largely help to shape . . . As to the garden itself for the open-air school, I would have it to embrace not only land for vegetable culture, but also borders for flowers and shrubs, a rock garden, fruit, Nature study, and geographical plots, and if by any means possible a nice sweep of lawn.[63]

In this way the outdoor landscape played a variety of roles in relation to the open-air school and was seen as having both moral and physical benefits.[64]

As in nineteenth-century psychiatric institutions, there was a focus on outdoor manual work, such as gardening and farming. This was considered by some to be a method of teaching the individual skills that would enable the children to play a role in helping to maintain the nation's efficiency. This relates to the Edwardian concern that the nation needed robust men and women, and one function of the open-air schools was intended to be the creation of strong, healthy adults from weak children:

> Education should not end, however with the teaching of ordinary school subjects, but be continued by such practical training as will eventually fit the child to take his or her place in the nation's life and activities; and the scheme must therefore include accessory buildings, together with garden land and small fields, in and upon which the children shall be taught a variety of fresh air or outdoor occupations.[65]

Some writers seem to have believed that the schools were just the start of a life spent outside:

> If the supply of workers was found in the future to be in excess of the needs of England, the students should at an early age emigrate to Canada or California. Trained as practical agriculturalists, and accustomed to plain living and hard working, they would be eminently suitable for a colonial career.[66]

During the summer months, open-air lessons were also held in urban parks, partly because there were only limited full-time places in schools practising open-air techniques. Although the open-air school movement was generally aimed at children from impoverished backgrounds, parents occasionally paid to send their children to summer schools. Mrs Joseph Cunning argued that open-air schools were valuable for children from the upper and middle classes.[67] She also stated that they were suitable for children who had not yet developed any physical illnesses. This emphasises the focus on an open-air lifestyle as a preventative measure as well as a method of curing disease. However, summer schools held in parks were, like the open-air schools, generally aimed at children from urban slum areas. Smith has suggested that there were a variety of social reasons for these summer schools and that free boots and tonsillectomies were used as bribes to ensure that children attended and that while the children were at the school their homes were sometimes visited and cleaned.

There was also a moral element attached to education in the open air. As well as advocating farming as part of the curriculum in open-air schools, Campbell also noted that in his work at reformatory schools for boys he had found that 'the boy benefits morally by work in his garden, and his physical improvement is decidedly apparent'.[68] The restorative powers of the garden on both the mind and the body are also literary themes in the Edwardian period.[69] The Edwardians appear to have been preoccupied with hard work and this influenced both the regime within the hospitals and schools, to try to strengthen the population and help make the nation more efficient, and the importance that health issues assumed.

The most famous example of the therapeutic powers of a garden in a literary work aimed at children is Frances Hodgson Burnett's highly didactic *The Secret Garden* published in 1911. Again it is the moral power of being outside in the garden that is therapeutic:

> So long as Colin shut himself up in his room and thought only of his fears and weaknesses and his detestation of people who looked at him and reflected hourly on humps and early death, he was a hysterical, half-crazy little hypochondriac who knew nothing of the sunshine and the spring.[70]

This also echoes nineteenth-century ideas about the moral power of landscape and its importance in the design of psychiatric institutions.

Hodgson Burnett appears to have believed in the importance of fresh air for health. One of the first factors in the hypochondriac Colin's recovery is the opening of the windows so that he can breathe in the fresh air. The heroine, Mary, also describes how Dickon, her friend who spends all his time outdoors and is close to nature, feels about fresh air:

> 'That's fresh air,' she said. 'Lie on your back and draw in long breaths of it. That's what Dickon does when he's lying on the moor. He says he feels it in his veins and it makes him strong and he feels as if he could live for ever and ever.'[71]

The strong message is that fresh air and being outdoors in a garden is good both mentally and physically, which reflects the ideology of open-air schools of this time and is strongly related to the practice of open-air therapies in medical institutions.

Tuberculosis sanatoria – Hailey and the Edward VII Sanatoria

Similar therapeutic approaches were taken in the battle against tuberculosis. As tuberculosis was responsible for approximately one death in every eight in Britain in the first decade of the twentieth century its eradication became a major national concern.[72] From 1898, when NAPT was founded, it was a significant organisation, with its first meeting attended by leading physicians as well as Lord Salisbury, the Prime Minister, and the Prince of Wales, later King Edward VII.[73] After the First World War the anti-tuberculosis campaign became part of local authority services and there was a distinct anti-urban emphasis.[74] For example, a series of lantern slides used in their exhibition was captioned as follows:

> The anaemic work girls of our towns.
> Look at the fisher-lass and see the contrast.
> See the pasty-white faces of the city children.
> See how different they look after they have been in the country.
> The poor fishermen hardly ever contract consumption.
> Live as much as possible in the open air.[75]

NAPT can be seen from this to have been in favour of a retreat to the countryside in line with other commentators and writers of the period such as Muthu and Morris.

In 1889, the first specialist institution to practise open-air therapies in the treatment of tuberculosis was opened – the Royal Victoria Hospital for Consumption, Edinburgh established by Sir Robert Philip. By 1907 there were ninety-six institutions providing open-air treatment in England and Wales,[76] once again influenced by work carried out in Germany. Hermann Brehmer popularised this form of treatment at his institution for tuberculosis established in 1859 at Goebersdorf, Silesia. According to Bryder he believed that 'fresh air and exercise, as a result of their beneficial effect on the heart and lungs, could cure tuberculosis'.[77] Other institutions influenced by Brehmer's work included one established by a former patient of Brehmer's, Peter Dettweiler, at Flakenstein in the Taurus Mountains in 1876, and one that was founded by Otto Walther at Nordrach-in-Baden in the Black Forest in 1888.

In the case of Nordrach, in an account of the sanatorium recorded in the *St Thomas's Hospital Gazette* in May 1900, it was stated that 'compared to . . . most of the other Continental sanatoria this life is extremely peaceful and monotonous'.[78] The article is written by an anonymous person who spent six months at the sanatorium. They record that the activities of patients, apart from a vast amount of eating, included walking twice a day, from a few yards to five or six miles, occasional tobogganing for the healthier patients, and resting, sometimes by lying in hammocks in the woods. There is a rather wonderful description of the patients as 'sitting solitary or in groups on their Moseses [oil-cloths], spread on wet seats or decaying tree trunks or mossy stones, looking like enormous fungi growing amongst the pine-trees: the best patients – those, who have profited most by the diet – may even present the appearance of ripe puff balls'.[79] The main complaints of the author are 'the indigestible and disgusting nature of some of the food and the absence of proper nursing for patients who are seriously ill'.[80]

Another insight into life in the sanatorium comes from Thomas Mann in his novel *The Magic Mountain* which is set in a sanatorium in the resort of Davos Platz, Switzerland. Mann's novel is particularly evocative as it is based on a three-week visit he himself made while his wife was being treated at Davos in 1912. His main concern about sanatorium life, according to his own notes, were the attendant dangers it held for the mainly young population. He writes of it as a 'substitute existence, and it can, in a relatively short time wean a young person from actual and active life'.[81] Within this fairytale world of the institution the protagonist, Hans Castorp, describes the folding of rugs to try and keep warm on the balconies in winter, the regular patterns of exercise and the daily routine. There are also glimpses of the sanatorium gardens: 'Among the dewy grass of the sloping terrace, short-stemmed, star-shaped gentians stood out. Part of the level ground had been enclosed for a garden, with flower-beds, gravel paths, and an artificial grotto under a stately silver fir.'[82] He also describes the mountains, meadows, waterfalls, views framed by the loggia windows and pine trees. In this way the natural setting of the sanatorium is described in detail.

Sanatoriums such as those at Davos and Nordrach were, without doubt, influential in relation to British sanatoria. For example, in the 1899 *Report on the 'Open-air' Treatment of Consumption at the North London Hospital for Consumption* the hospital stated that 'we have followed in the main the line of treatment which has proved most successful in many of the Continental Sanatoria and which appears to give as good results in some of English Sanatoria'.[83] An advertisement for the Vale of Clwyd Sanatorium also emphasised its relationship with Continental sanatoria:

> This sanatorium is established for the treatment of Pulmonary and other forms of Tuberculosis as carried out by Dr. Otto Walther of Nordrach . . . The physicians are fully conversant with Dr Walther's Treatment, having themselves been patients at Nordrach.[84]

This form of rhetoric would only be successful if the patients were aware of the success associated with Continental sanatoria. Presumably the English sanatoria were competing for the same middle- and upper-class clientele, and it would, therefore, be essential that they suggested that English sanatoria could offer therapies that would be as effective as those practised on the Continent.

C. Briane Hartnell in an undated pamphlet (c.1900) argued that 'we have in England many places where sanatoria might be built, and there is no reason why our results should be in any way inferior to those obtained in Germany'.[85] This suggests that this was a competitive area and that people needed to be persuaded that England could provide conditions that would be just as good. He goes on to list the advantages for patients if they were to remain in England:

> 1. They would avoid a long and tedious journey.
> 2. They would be surrounded by people of their own nationality.
> 3. They would not have to put up with foreign food, and foreign ways of cooking it.[86]

Given the account of the patient at Nordrach above, it perhaps seems more realistic than we would now expect that foreign food was classed as one of the problems.

One of the early proponents of open-air therapy for tuberculosis patients was Dr F.W. Burton-Fanning, and he is said to have designed the main Mundesley Sanatorium building in Norfolk, which with 'weather boarding, mock half-timbering, and broad gables . . . echoes a chalet Suisse' according to Richardson.[87] She goes on to suggest that this design was perhaps a 'deliberate ploy to recreate the atmosphere of the Continental sanatoria and woo a high-class clientele'.[88] There does seem to be a desire to mimic aspects of the Continental institutions. For example, many of the English sanatoria are named after Dr Otto Walther's Nordrach Institution, for example, Nordrach, Wales; Nordrach-on-Dee and Nordrach-on-Mendip.[89] However, a photograph of Kelling Sanatorium,

Norfolk, suggests that this style could also be utilised for plain wooden buildings with basic landscaping designed for the lower classes.[90] This particular sanatorium was described as a model for inexpensive sanatoria design for the use of working-class patients by its resident medical officer W.J. Burton-Fanning. It is starkly different from the examples of Hailey and the Edward VII Sanatorium discussed below.

As well as trying to establish that England was as suitable as Germany for the treatment of tuberculosis, doctors also had to establish that the climatic conditions could rival those of the Swiss Alps. Bryder has argued that generally 'British tuberculosis specialists held that the advantages of special climates had been greatly exaggerated and there was no therapeutic advantage in travelling to the Swiss Alps or the south of Europe'.[91] Nonetheless, she has also noted that climatic conditions were still emphasised in relation to English sanatoria. The Vale of Clwyd Sanatorium was an example of this, as in its advertisement it stated that, 'it has a bracing climate, with a small rainfall and a large amount of sunshine'.[92] Burton-Fanning also wrote that, 'we like the treatment to be carried out in a locality whose air is pure and bracing, and moderately dry'.[93] The height of the institution above sea-level appears to have been important, which could also relate to the supposed efficacy of the Alpine climate.

Sunshine was a particularly important climatic element in relation to non-pulmonary tuberculosis. Sunlight therapy or heliotherapy was popularised by Auguste Rollier in his Alpine clinic in Leysin and was widely adopted by British sanatoria.[94] Sunshine was also described as having psychological as well as physical benefits. In an essay published in the 1930s, Bernard Stacey wrote that, 'there are few people in good health who do not feel the invigorating and cheering influence of a bright, sunny day . . . the warming and cheering influence of sunshine seems to me for this reason alone to be of paramount importance in the treatment of tuberculosis'.[95] The main problem with carrying out this form of therapy in Britain was the natural climatic conditions, which meant that there was little sunshine for much of the year. This led to the development of artificial light treatments in 1925 in Glasgow.[96]

Given the range of sanatoria designed to treat people with tuberculosis, two institutions will be explored in detail here – the famous King Edward VII Sanatorium at Midhurst, West Sussex (opened in 1906), where the gardens were laid out by the well-known garden designer Gertrude Jekyll, and the far less famous Hailey Open-Air Sanatorium, near Wallingford, Oxfordshire (opened c.1890s). Hailey appears to have been established at the end of the nineteenth century and therefore pre-dates the Edward VII Sanatorium. It is listed on the 1901 Census as having sixteen patients, including a post office clerk, a kitchen maid, a parlour maid and a farm manager. They are all described as living off their own means, which establishes that Hailey was a private sanatorium, but given the occupations of the patients, presumably not an expensive one. Hailey was also mentioned in the Ipsden Parish Register of Burials in 1905 and 1907, and this suggests that it was in operation for a period of around ten years. What makes this site of particular interest is that a prospectus illustrated with numerous photographs of the gardens was produced (Figure 34)[97] and that the medical superintendent, Dr Charles Reinhardt, claims to have been the first medical man to describe the open-air method of treatment in England. According to the brochure for the sanatorium written around 1900, his first description was issued by the Popular Publishing Company in September 1895.[98] Whether he was actually the first is open to debate, but he was certainly an early proponent. The prospectus also outlines Reinhardt's visit to Germany and his impressions of the therapeutic benefits of the open-air

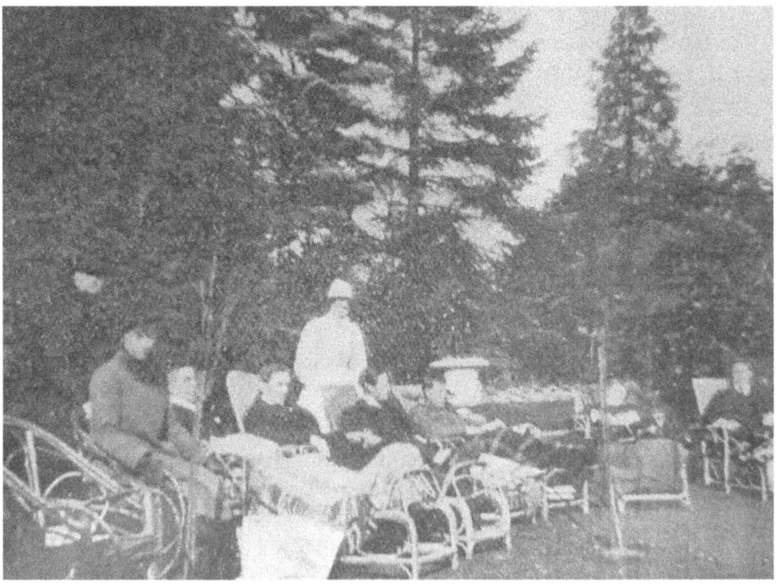

Figure 34 Patients sitting under blankets on the lawns at Hailey Open-Air Sanatorium from Reinhardt's prospectus, c.1900.

system, which firmly establishes that Hailey's regime was based on the German model.[99]

In contrast, the Edward VII Sanatorium was opened as a charitable institution and 'was intended for patients belonging to a class above the poor who could not afford to go to private sanatoria – officers of the Army and Navy, clergy of all denominations, members of professions and the Civil Service, teachers and governesses, clerks in banks and mercantile houses, and the "educated classes generally"'.[100] However, it seems to have taken a similar class of patient to Hailey which suggests there was a cross-over between patients attending private and charitable sanatoria.

The Edward VII Sanatorium is significant because it was designed to promote English sanatoria as an alternative to earlier European counterparts. At the opening of the sanatorium in 1906 it was reported that, 'England may now boast that she is on a level with Continental nations, if not ahead of them, in the means which are being taken to cure and stamp out the insidious disease'.[101] The sanatorium was also promoted as having the most up-to-date scientific approach to the treatment of tuberculosis. According to Linda Bryder, 'Sir William, then Regius Professor of Medicine at Oxford University stated at the opening of Midhurst Sanatorium that he hoped that Midhurst would become a centre for the scientific study of the disease'.[102] The *Liverpool Post* also commented on this scientific element when it reported that the new institution 'possessed "every up-to-date structural and scientific advantage"'.[103]

The design of the hospital was the result of a 1902 essay competition advertised in twenty-two medical papers in Europe and America resulting in 180 entries.[104] According to *The Builder*, mottos for entries included: 'Give him air, he'll straight be well', 'Vis medicatrix naturae' and 'Open air everywhere'.[105] These mottos imply that the open-air method was in the mind of at least some of the architects and must, therefore, have been generally viewed as a modern approach to the treatment of tuberculosis at this time.

The winning entry was written by Arthur Latham, a physician at the Brompton Hospital, in association with an architect, A. William West. Bryder has stated that 'in their essay they stressed spaciousness, airiness . . . and prevention of dust accumulation'.[106] The building was also designed with a step-like façade and *The Builder*[107] commented on how the design allowed patients to obtain the greatest amount of air and sunshine: 'The main idea is that the whole building shall so be arranged as to secure the maximum of sunshine and the maximum of air.'[108] The sanatorium chapel was also designed to be open-air. It is also worth noting that Adams was sent to Germany and Switzerland by the Advisory Committee to study similar sanatoria.[109]

In 1922, John Wilson stated that 'the site to be acquired should provide from one-third to one-half of an acre of land per patient'.[110] The Edward VII Sanatorium was located in 'well-wooded grounds of 150 acres' which, as it was designed for 104 patients, would have meant over an acre per patient.[111] On a smaller scale, Hailey is described by Reinhardt as having grounds that are 'magnificently wooded and very extensive, consisting of 17 acres of parks and a home farm of 35 acres'.[112] The openness of the grounds may have been related to the class of patients. In the case of sanatoria in Ireland, Greta Jones has found that 'in sanatoriums for the upper-class the patients were allowed to go out for walks but the labouring-class they had to keep in by a wall'.[113] One of the arguments for this was the need to keep the poorer classes away from the attractions of any nearby town, and in particular the pubic houses, as these could jeopardise the treatment.[114] At Hailey and the King Edward VII Sanatorium the class of patient would fit the openness model.

Also, in common with earlier asylums, sanatoria were often placed on eminences with far-reaching views. Hailey was no exception and the brochure describes its location in detail:

> Hailey Open Air Sanatorium (on the Chiltern Hills) . . . stands in a beautifully timbered park about two miles in circumference, the highest part being six hundred feet and the lower limit being three hundred feet above sea level. Shelter is afforded on the east and north by upland woods, extending many miles whilst the southern and western aspects are open, offering magnificent views.[115]

The view was also illustrated in the brochure. However, the altitude and cleanliness of the air appears to be of greater importance than the view itself, and sites with these elements would naturally be on eminences with far-reaching views.

Pine woods were a common feature in the grounds of tuberculosis sanatoria, which differentiated their landscapes from other open-air institutions. For example the Edward VII Sanatorium was described as follows:

> The ground slopes gently to the south and is partly clothed with woodland including magnificent pine trees, while the western border consists of open moorland ending in a ravine. The most southerly portion of this property is beautiful park-like ground of considerable extent, and on the upper part of this, backed by a lofty pine grove, at an altitude of 495 feet, the sanatorium has been erected.[116]

Similarly, a pine wood appears to be a feature of Salterley Grange Municipal Sanatorium: *The Medical Officer* described how 'the site chosen is admirably suitable, being 800 feet above sea level, and the chalets are placed on a southern slope, protected on the east by a pine wood'.[117] A photograph in the brochure for Hailey (Figure 34) suggests that pine trees were also a feature of its landscape. In the case of the London Open-Air Sanatorium it was even named 'Pinewood' which establishes the significance of the pine trees in these landscapes.[118]

The popularity of pine trees may have reflected the fact that the original Nordrach institution was located in the coniferous Black Forest and, according to the description of the Edward VII Sanatorium by the Royal Commission on the Historical Monuments of England (RCHME), 'the beneficial effects of the scent of Pines on sufferers of tuberculosis was generally acknowledged'.[119] However, although research for this book has not uncovered any other reference to the therapeutic benefits of the scent of pine trees, woods were seen as beneficial for tuberculosis sufferers because they were believed to help reduce the amount of dust in the air.[120] They also seem to have been seen as helpful in creating shelter.[121] In Dr Latham's essay for the Edward VII design competition of 1903, he explicitly states that 'trees, preferably evergreens, should be arranged near the house so as to give shelter against wind for the more feeble patients, whilst at the same time they allow the free ingress of air and sunlight'.[122]

The gardens at Hailey reflect the design of the domestic gardens of the time, and it is possible that they were already established when the house was acquired as a sanatorium by Reinhardt. The photographs show a number of garden features. One of these is labelled as the 'ornamental gardens', which appear to consist of a round flowerbed, possibly planted with roses, although the photograph is too grainy to be sure, surrounded by turf. It seems to have provided a focus for patients when they sat on the east veranda, which was apparently forty-seven feet in length. There is a photograph of a rustic sun trap, and the sanatorium evidently had productive gardens, as there are photographs of a walled vegetable garden and an orchard with ducks and a bee-hive.

There were also a number of sleeping chalets in the grounds and a tent in the meadow. These were specifically related to the open-air method being practised at Hailey. According to Reinhardt 'Hailey is, with the exception of Alderney Manor, the only British Sanatorium built entirely on the separate chalet or hut principle'.[123] The hut or tent was the ideal structure in which to obtain the greatest benefits from fresh air: 'All that a consumptive requires in the shape of accommodation consists of a hut, which must have windows opening in every direction. In such a contrivance he can breathe air identical with that of the open country, and in no room of a building is this possible.'[124]

The shelters at Hailey were similar to the revolving huts used at the Bristol Homeopathic Hospital, described below, and were a feature of the practice of open-air therapies for tuberculosis.[125] In a design promoted by Burton-Fanning, in his c.1900 text, 'the shelter revolves on a central pivot, and is supported by wheels, which run on a circular rail'.[126] Similarly, verandas were constructed so that patients could sit out of the wind and balconies were created so that patients could be wheeled out on to them without leaving their beds to get some benefit from the fresh air and sunshine. Margaret Campbell has quite rightly argued that these can be seen as similar to the summerhouse, gazebo or shelter that were familiar sights in eighteenth-century landscapes and that they were, as well as being used by institutions, common features of domestic gardens for the use of a sick family member.[127] The choice of designs available reflects this inclusion as part of an aesthetic landscape.[128] There was a competitive market for chalets and huts for domestic use for those who chose to be treated at home, as can be seen in advertisements of the time (Figure 35).[129] Other influences on domestic architecture included the use of balconies and the design of reclining chairs, such as those based on the recliners designed by Alvar Aalto for the Paimio Sanatorium. Campbell also states that 'it cannot be claimed that the introduction of the flat roof, balcony, summer house and recliner chair were the direct result of early treatment methods for tuberculosis, but the popularity of these modernist architectural features in the pursuit of good health and hygiene placed them in the annals of a therapeutic lifestyle that has now been overtaken by new drug therapies and treatment methods'.[130]

In terms of the gardens at the Edward VII Sanatorium, it is hard to separate out the elements that are specifically intended to be therapeutic from those that are common Jekyll design features (Figure 36). For example, David Ottewill has described the gardens as follows:

> Fresh air and outdoor activities were the order of the day, and accordingly the buildings were surrounded by a series of garden enclosures . . . On the south front the canted wings embraced terraced lawns whose retaining walls and steps were built of the lower greensand, quarried on the site.[131]

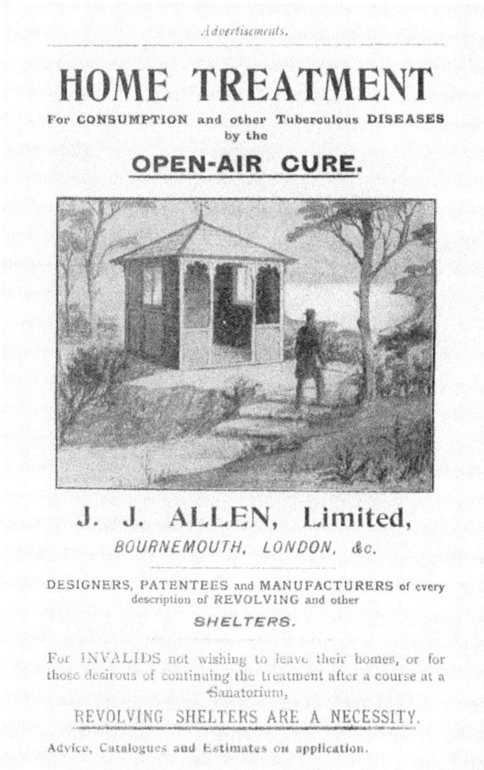

Figure 35 An advertisement from the *British Journal of Tuberculosis* for shelters which could be placed in the domestic garden for use by invalids at home.

The notion of including a series of garden enclosures is one that is common in gardens created in the Arts and Crafts style, such as Hestercombe in Somerset and Sissinghurst in Kent. In the case of the sanatorium, there were seven garden enclosures, and, according to Michael Tooley, each had a distinctive character.

The garden was also laid out in terraces because of its position on a south-facing slope. Kelynack described how 'the large tract in front is beautifully sheltered, and has been laid out as terraced gardens, with croquet lawns and flower borders by the well-known landscape gardener, Miss Jekyll'.[132] This demonstrates that the gardens were of interest to the medical profession but no specifically therapeutic features are described.

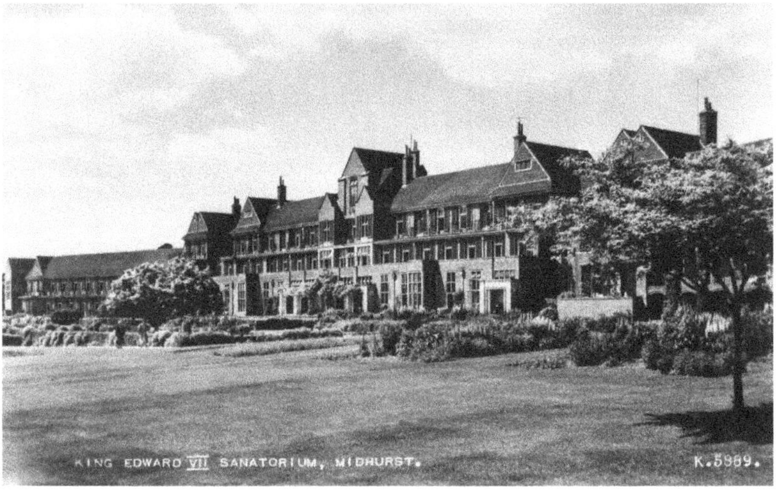

Figure 36 A postcard of unknown date showing the gardens at the King Edward VII Sanatorium as laid out by Gertrude Jekyll.

One of Jekyll's letters implies that the gardens were a combination of therapeutic purpose and her signature designs:

> The garden is laid out on several levels, each level carried by retaining walls built with earth joints for planting. I make out detailed planting plans, and send the plants for each section. There are 1200 feet of the dry walling, and I hope, in a year's time – for nothing shows so quickly as this type of planting – that it will be a good example of wall gardening. It is intended that the garden should provide light and interesting work for the patients and keep them a great deal in the open air. The King takes a great interest in the place and goes there often.[133]

Her gardens were used by some of the patients for light gardening work, using specially constructed light tools.[134] It should also be noted that Reinhardt stated that 'in the open-air method we find that just those things which are pleasant and inviting are more beneficial', which suggests that attractive gardens could be seen as therapeutic in light of the practice of open-air methods.[135]

However, the use of Jekyll at the Edward VII Sanatorium can be explored in terms of her rhetorical value as she was employed, as one of the most popular and well-known garden designers, to design the gardens for the highest-profile hospital in England at that time. The contemporary importance of the hospital can be illustrated by the fact that it was 'unusual for a monarch to be so directly involved with the establishment of a public health institution'.[136] The employment of Jekyll at the sanatorium possibly mirrors the engagement of the Pulham firm at the Homeopathic Hospital in Bristol, to be discussed below. Both hospitals were trying to create the impression that they were the most scientific and up-to-date institution of their kind. Both also wanted to be models for future developments, as well as to attract paying patients, and this may have led them to use contemporary designers to enhance this impression.

At Hailey, Reinhardt appears, from the brochure at least, to have implemented a system based on diet, air and rest. He wrote that the 'amount of exercise taken by each patient is strictly regulated; indeed the whole treatment is eminently a personal one, each patient being visited several times daily'.[137] This seems to be based on the Nordrach system in which exercise is regulated.[138] In his book, *A Handbook of the Open-air Treatment and Life in an Open-air Sanatorium*, Reinhardt described in more detail how he felt exercise should be regulated: 'Speaking generally, slow walking is the best form of activity for tubercular patients, a rate of about two miles an hour being desirable. This strengthens the heart and the circulation without exciting either the cardiac or pulmonary centres unduly.'[139] The 'scientific' assessment of the patient's condition and the carefully planned regime can be viewed as the medicalisation of what is essentially a regime that could be followed in the patient's home. Reinhardt, like many medical men of the period, argued that 'the patient resides in a sanatorium and not in a private house, so that he is isolated from the excitements and distractions of ordinary households. His whole life is subject to medical supervision whilst in the sanatorium.'[140]

Walking, as a form of therapeutic exercise, was also important in many other institutions and the Edward VII Sanatorium was no exception, with walks having been cut through the woods. According to the RCHME description, 'various routes were marked throughout the 150 acres, each graded according to the patient's condition'.[141] Burton-Fanning described the work of Brehmer who 'attached great importance to hill-climbing for the improvement of heart and lungs', and stated that 'most sanatoria have paths of different gradients which the patients systematically use for exercise . . . Towards the end of the "cure", during the "hardening off" stage, the consumptive walks twelve miles, perhaps, during the day'.[142] Other types of exercise included varied forms of recreation. For example, Burton-Fanning recommended that:

> In suitable cases the patient indulges in golf, croquet, fishing, shooting, bicycling or riding on horseback . . . I may say that golf links adjoin the Mundesley Sanatorium, and are constantly used by the patients. Great care has been taken in the selection of patients allowed to play, and in supervision while playing, and no instance of injury from the game has come to the physician's notice.[143]

The RCHME description of the Edward VII Sanatorium mentioned that it once had a golf course to the south of the institution in a clearing below the terraces. Dr Morland argued that being outside could also be encouraged with the inclusion of 'an aquarium, an aviary and an apiary'.[144]

As well as recreational forms of exercise, the Edward VII Sanatorium maintained a regime based on work, although this was most likely to have been aimed at the lower classes of patients admitted into the main sanatorium building, rather than it representing the most scientific form of treatment. According to Bryder:

> Light work in the gardens and grounds of the sanatorium formed part of the regular treatment in place of walking exercise, for both men and women. N.D. Bardswell, medical superintendent of Midhurst Sanatorium in the 1900s, stressed that all 'manual exercise' (he referred to the system as 'manual exercise' rather than 'labour') was carried out under the close supervision of one of the medical officers, and that the patients to whom such work was prescribed were carefully selected.[145]

A more strenuous work regime at the Edward VII Sanatorium was later developed from the work of Marcus Sinclair Paterson, who introduced work as part of the regime for the patients at Frimley Sanatorium, Surrey, after he took charge in 1905.[146] Paterson's desire for patients to be able to return to work immediately after the treatment had been completed suggests that concerns of national efficiency influenced the use of a work-based regime.

This is echoed by the proposal of a work colony to be established in Edinburgh:

> The Committee of the Royal Hospital for Consumptives, Edinburgh, are proposing to open a work colony for convalescents. The employment will be carefully graded according to the state of health of each worker. It is hoped that the undertaking will in time become self-supporting, if not actually a source of revenue. Residence in the colony would afford a transition between the more strictly curative régime of the hospital and the ordinary working existence to which most of the patients must ultimately return.[147]

According to Jones, the concept of work therapy was intended to 'gradually prepare the patient for the return to the world outside and it also served the function of staving off boredom which frequently accompanied long stays in sanatoria'.[148] This idea of work therapy was also practised in psychiatric institutions for similar primary reasons.

There were concerns that once recovering consumptives returned to their previous homes and occupations they would relapse into illness. *The Medical Officer* reported that:

> Dr Augustine Griffith, M.O.H., recently suggested that the Hove Sanatorium grounds should be used to provide work of a beneficial nature for the consumptive patients, and also that the question of employing discharged tuberculosis patients in the various parks, gardens and the golf course should be considered. The health committee have resolved that the superintendent of parks and gardens be instructed to make the necessary arrangements for carrying the proposals into effect.[149]

Similarly, the value of gardens for patients with tuberculosis was described by Dr C. Killick Millard, in his *Annual Report* as the Medical Officer for Health in Leicester, when he wrote that 'nothing is better calculated [than gardens] to counteract the tendency to tuberculosis generated by factory life. The alternative to working in the garden will too often be the crowded place of amusement indoors.'[150] Another writer argued that this was particularly relevant in relation to women and girls where 'the career of a professional gardener is specially attractive, and is certainly one rich in possibilities, not only for health, but for a useful and happy livelihood'.[151] This illustrates the high regard with which gardens and gardening were held by the medical profession at this time and indicates why they were so important in relation to open-air institutions. As will be discussed below, the narrative for patients could be very different. At the root of open-air therapies was the need to keep patients outside in all weathers. Jones has reported that in Ireland it was a challenge to enforce the regime, particularly in bad weather, and there is no reason to believe that English sanatoria would be exempt from the same problems.

Bristol Homeopathic Hospital

Open-air therapies were not restricted to more conventional medical approaches – the Homeopathic Hospital in Bristol also utilised these techniques. The British Homeopathic Society was formed in 1844, and in 1850 the London Homeopathic Hospital opened its doors to patients.[152] Like most general hospitals of the time it was a charitable institution supported by voluntary contributions. According to Phillip Nicholls the 1850s and 60s were a period of optimism and confidence for homeopaths. He says that 'the number of practitioners was growing, new hospitals and dispensaries for the poor were opening, and the new system enjoyed a wide spectrum of public confidence, clerical sympathy and aristocratic patronage'.[153]

However, by the time Mrs Charles of Clifton contributed £1,000 in 1883 towards the founding of a homeopathic hospital in Bristol, interest in homeopathy was declining.[154] In 1882 the *British Journal of Homeopathy* admitted that 'we barely maintain our numbers, and seldom make a convert of any note or weight'.[155] This was due in part to vehement attacks from within the medical profession as well as a decline in heroic surgery and strong doses of drugs, which made conventional medicine more attractive to the public. The use of similar methods by both groups of practitioners also blurred the boundaries between alternative and conventional practice. In particular, natural therapies such as the open-air method were practised in conventional hospitals as well as alternative institutions such as the Homeopathic Hospital in Bristol.

In 1916, Mr Melville Wills, of the Wills tobacco firm, became president of the Homeopathic Hospital. Then, in 1917, he purchased Cotham House and its grounds and presented them 'to the hospital as a site for the new building, which he had already promised to erect as a memorial to his son, Captain Bruce Melville Wills, who was killed in 1915 while serving with H.M. Forces'.[156] Like the original fundraising, the building of the new hospital is indebted to one individual who obviously believed in the importance of homeopathy as an alternative treatment. The hospital was then temporarily moved to Cotham House and, according to the 1921 programme, the 'levelling of mounds in grounds of Cotham House was effected in preparation for erection of the new building'.[157]

Like other institutions, the site was important. In this case, it was described as having, 'the advantage of being on the summit of the hill and slopes towards the south'.[158] The architects for the hospital were Oatley and Lawrence and the hospital was designed so that 'every ward has its own separate sun balcony for open-air treatment'.[159] By 1923, the Building Committee were reporting that 'all Sun Balcony doors and screens are fixed ready for glazing' which establishes that the balconies could be closed off by doors and screens when necessary.[160] HRH Princess Helena Victoria opened the hospital on 20 May 1925.

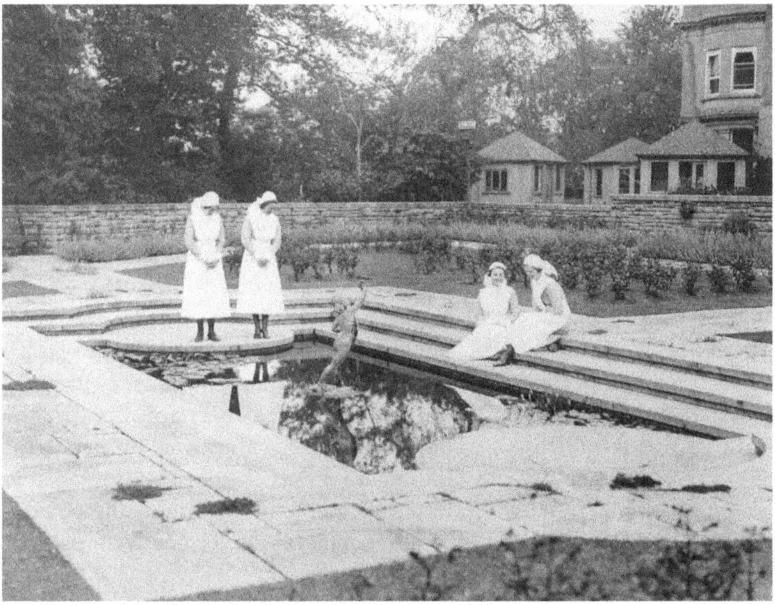

Figure 37 Photograph of nurses around the pond in the rose garden with the revolving shelters in the background at the Homeopathic Hospital, Bristol. This appears to have been taken as part of a photoshoot for an article that was published in *Nursing Times*, 23 August 1941.

From the start, the hospital was intended to be an open-air institution and as well as designing the main building with sun balconies and loggias, open-air shelters in the gardens were also erected (Figure 37). In fact while temporarily resident at Cotham House the hospital had access to four shelters: 'In addition, two open air shelters have been erected recently in the grounds of Cotham House, the open situation – one of the highest points in Bristol – lending itself admirably to the treatment of sufferers from tuberculosis.'[161] Again the situation on a hill was seen as important.

In 1929 it was reported that the shelters had been 'reconstructed' and were now described as 'Châlets', possibly reflecting the Alpine precedent for open-air treatment.

> The open-air Châlets were not available in the earlier months of the year, as they were undergoing reconstruction. All are now in excellent condition,

> and each has been placed on a revolving base, so that it may be turned to take advantage of all the sunshine that our climate allows and to escape cold winds. This provision is greatly appreciated, and the four Châlets are now nearly always occupied and are frequently bespoken for patients weeks in advance.[162]

The design of revolving seats has precedence in garden history. In the eighteenth century, Stephen Switzer described the design of the Windsor seat, which could be moved to avoid the wind or sun.[163]

The chalets in the Homeopathic Hospital garden performed a similar function although in this case they were designed to help the patient capture as much sun as possible whilst sheltering them from the wind. The report also commented that 'opportunities for combined open-air and Homeopathic treatment in the institutions of the country are very few, and the Châlets supply a definite need'.[164] This establishes that the hospital was employing a combination of open-air and homeopathic treatments and saw itself as fulfilling an essential role. The chalets were placed on the terrace on the west side of the building and the circular rails on which they turned can still be seen on the terrace, although the chalets themselves have long since disappeared.

The hospital garden was also important at the Homeopathic Hospital in relation to the practice of open-air treatments. Even before the hospital was completed, the existing grounds of Cotham House were used by the patients and in the 1921 programme, when the hospital was still temporarily based in the house, it was stated that, 'there is accommodation for 25 patients in light and airy wards in pleasant and healthy surroundings, the adjoining grounds providing an inestimable boon to such of the inmates as are able to make use of them, and there enjoy the benefits of fresh air and sunshine'.[165]

Work on the grounds of the new hospital began in 1924. The architect's report within the Building Committee Minutes recorded that jobs remaining to be executed included: 'The Entrance Gates, cleaning of the site, and formation of terraces.'[166] This suggests that, originally, the gardens were to be laid out by the architects Oatley and Lawrence. Sarah Whittingham has stated that, in relation to the design of the gardens, 'it is not known exactly how much involvement Oatley had in the work'.[167] However, in 1925, the Committee reported that, 'in connection with the laying out of the grounds Mr W Melville Wills suggested Messrs Pulham of Broxbourne, Herts might be called in to advise on this, and suggested a Meeting being arranged between them and the Architects who promised to communicate with Messrs Pulham on the subject'.[168] Again the design was heavily influenced by the taste of Melville Wills, and it seems that he was the main benefactor for the hospital. When he suggested employing the Pulham firm there was no comment from the Committee in the recorded minutes, which indicates that his position as president and benefactor allowed him a great deal of influence.

There was a long relationship between Melville Wills and the Pulham firm of garden designers. The Homeopathic Hospital garden was not the first garden he had commissioned them to create. Soon after moving to the newly built Bracken Hill in Leigh woods in 1896 he started developing an extensive garden.[169] According to Rosalind Delaney, 'between c.1900–05, Melville Wills appointed Pulham and Son, one of the most famous landscaping companies of the time, to design and construct a rock and water garden to the north of Bracken Hill; this rock garden was subsequently extended eastwards'.[170] Then between 1908 and 1910, 'Melville Wills gave a further commission to Pulham and Son to lay out the grounds on the opposite side of the North Road. The aim was to form an extension to Bracken Hill's pleasure garden adjacent to the recently erected guest house/estate office.'[171] This has been described by Sally Festing as a particularly elaborate design in terms of the work by the Pulhams during this period. She has outlined its design as including 'archways, gothic pump house, a grotto, recess for a garden seat and five linked pools, one with steps at either end designed for swimming'.[172] Given the fact that Melville Wills appreciated their form of design to such an extent that he employed them for his own domestic gardens, it is perhaps not surprising that he commissioned them to design the gardens at the Homeopathic Hospital. The hospital and garden appear to represent one man's vision.

In 1925, the Building Committee reported that:

> Messrs Pulham's scheme for the lay-out of the Garden has not yet come to hand, but a preliminary suggestion by Mr Rickett of that firm has reached us this morning from Mr Melville Wills, together with a letter upon that subject, in which Mr Wills states that he is most anxious that the garden should be extremely attractive and he does not object to spending a considerable amount of money with this object in view and that this work should be put in hand at once.[173]

It is interesting to note that Melville Wills requested that the 'garden should be extremely attractive'. This perhaps explains why he employed the Pulhams, as they evidently created gardens that suited his taste. It is also clear that he was willing to pay a considerable amount to achieve this.

When the plans were submitted to the Committee it appears that they appreciated the design but were concerned about the cost of maintaining the garden:

> The Committee examined the propositions and liked the scheme very much indeed, but the question of efficient maintenance of such a scheme appeared to require serious consideration . . . The Architect stated under the instructions of the President the scheme was being proceeded with, Messrs Pulham having undertaken to make a start at once, the scheme suggested by Messrs Pulham included the absorption of the Kitchen Garden, this matter to be brought up at the Board meeting, later in the day.[174]

Again the President was very much the driving force and had already instructed the architect that the garden scheme be implemented before the Committee had made a decision about what it thought of it. In the report of that year it is clear how the cost of maintenance was solved – Melville Wills arranged for himself and his wife to maintain the grounds in perpetuity. Like the building, the Wills family also chose to dedicate the garden to one of their sons: Harold Edgar Wills.[175] In the following year, the garden was almost complete and had been extended to include a rock garden:

> The work of converting the Hospital grounds into beautiful gardens, undertaken by the President and Mrs Melville Wills, is now almost completed. Mr Wills decided to extend the original scheme, and has included the laying-out of the western end of the grounds, about the Tennis Courts and Nurse's Home. The rock gardens are one of the most attractive spots in the district and a great boon to the Patients and Staff.[176]

Delaney suggests that 'Melville and Gertrude Wills spent £12,000 on landscaping the hospital gardens in memory of Edgar'.[177]

The idea that the gardens were very much based on the Wills' vision is emphasised by the fact that the design of the hospital gardens was very similar to the design of their own gardens at Bracken Hill, although vestiges of the earlier nineteenth-century garden of Cotham House were retained.[178] The Pulham designs for the hospital included a formal rose garden with a pond (the pond being identical to the one at Bracken Hill), terraces and stone walls.[179] The terraces are Italianate in appearance and reflected the Edwardian interest in such gardens at this time.[180]

The question then remains of why Melville Wills spent so much money on this hospital and its garden. In all the descriptions of the garden in the reports and Committee Minutes there appears to be no reference to any therapeutic benefit the garden may have had for the patients. The only health element mentioned was in relation to the tennis courts, and these were described as for the use of the staff. The chalets were seen to be important, but presumably not the garden itself. Perhaps the key to the value placed on the garden is in this phrase from a pamphlet on the new building produced in 1925: 'The Hospital, therefore, will be one of the most modern, efficiently equipped, and pleasantly situated Institutions to be found in the West of England.'[181] Homeopathy was evidently trying to compete with conventional medical practice and a new building with an attractive garden was perhaps part of the attempt of the homeopathic movement to persuade new patients, presumably of the middle classes and upwards, to be admitted there rather than to a traditional institution. It was trying to appear to be modern and efficient. With the use of open-air therapies, it was also competing on some of the same ground as conventional medicine at a time when homeopathy was losing favour. The amount of money spent on the gardens and building by the Wills suggests that they thought homeopathy was very important and a state of the art building can be very persuasive of a programme's efficacy. There is also perhaps the personal rhetoric of a couple wanting to memorialise their family through the creation of this monument.

Convalescent homes

In addition to the proliferation of specialist medical institutions there was also an increase in the number of convalescent homes. In 1863 John Hilton published a series of lectures entitled, *On the Influence of Mechanical and Physiological Rest in the Treatment of Accidents and Surgical Diseases*. This became the influential book *On Rest and Pain*, which was reprinted continually until the sixth edition in 1950.[182] In this text he provided 'many examples of how Nature ensured rest for damaged tissues so that self-repair could begin; for example, the spasm in the muscle surrounding an inflamed knee joint was evidence for Hilton that Nature was using mechanical means to force rest on the damaged tissue'.[183] This idea led to the bed being seen as therapeutic in itself, and David Armstrong has argued that 'any formal medical intervention was simply additive to this underlying therapeutic agency'.[184] The convalescent home can, therefore, be seen as a place in which patients could rest and allow nature to complete the healing process. The use of bed rest was one approach to this, but graduated exercise and other more active forms of treatment were also used.

From the mid-nineteenth century, convalescent homes and convalescent departments associated with general hospitals began to be built in England, and their number increased rapidly towards the end of the nineteenth century, in line with other specialist institutions. The first specific institution built for convalescent patients was the Metropolitan Convalescent Institution in 1841.[185] The lack of convalescent facilities was soon resolved and, by 1908, Armstrong was able to write that, 'in Great Britain there are 278 such institutions, and thirteen of the London Hospitals have their own convalescent homes'.[186] Although the general hospital was no longer seen as playing a role in patient convalescence, the concept of convalescence itself was still seen as vital. Armstrong explained that he considered convalescing at home to be detrimental for the patient:

> To send a convalescent patient home is to relegate him frequently to an undesirable environment, to inadequate or improper food supply, to the ministration of injudicious relatives or friends, to premature work to earn his support, and each or all of these in the condition of lessened resistance associated with convalescence may divert the latter into a state of permanent invalidism.[187]

From this it appears that one of the factors driving the creation of convalescent institutions was the need for a healthy workforce.

The idea of convalescence was not the sole prerogative of the treatment of physical illnesses; it also became to be seen as important for psychiatric patients. As Stephen Soanes has recently argued, 'psychiatric textbooks published from the 1880s to the 1910s suggest that some alienists [medical superintendents] at least regarded convalescence as a distinctive and significant period in psychiatric treatment. Tonics, nourishment and graduated exercise indicated specifically in these textbooks for recovering patients helped identify recovery itself as a specific phase of asylum care.'[188] This mirrors the convalescent homes for general hospital patients, although in the case of psychiatric care the buildings to house convalescents were often still built on the same site as the asylums. However, 'open spaces and strategically-located trees created a natural barrier and sense of distance devised to shield convalescents' from the central institution.'[189] They were also seen as intrinsically beneficial to recovery: 'inspectors variously highlighted the "very fine views" (Shenley, 1934), "commanding views" (Plymouth, 1937), and "beautiful" situation (Cane Hill, 1936) seen from convalescent villas. Visitors to Plymouth thought the villa "ideally situated" due to its aspect across the surrounding countryside.'[190] This suggests that location and landscape were still important in terms of convalescence in the twentieth century.

One example of a place for physical convalescence was the Blackwell Convalescent Home. It was established for patients who, having undergone surgery, needed time to recover fully before returning to their own homes. The home was developed from the Birmingham Sanatorium, which had been established in 1866 by the Cotton Relief Fund as an establishment to be used specifically for convalescent purposes. Initially the home was based in an existing building but after a few years the fund bought nine acres of land near Blackwell Station from the Midland Railway at a cost of £1250. On this land a new home was built, which opened on 16 April 1873, initially for a maximum of sixty patients. The patients admitted to the home were all referred from a variety of hospitals in the Birmingham area. For example in 1941 there were eighty patients, of whom sixty were male and twenty female. These included one patient from Birmingham Accident Hospital, eight patients from Queen Elizabeth Hospital, two from Selly Oak Hospital, one patient from Dudley Guest Hospital, one private bed case and thirty-four from the Birmingham Eye Hospital.[191]

However, there is an indication that sometimes patients who were in an advanced state of illness were referred to the home, possibly to free up beds in the other surgical hospitals. In the Committee of Management Minute Book there is a record stating that the 'Hon. Secretary was asked to write to the Hospital Authorities requesting them to make certain in future that Patients sent to the Home were not in an advanced state of illness, as the Home could only cater for ordinary Convalescent or Pre-Convalescent Patients'.[192] They do appear to have had a relatively fast turnover at the home as, with only eighty beds available, they treated a total number of 1,625 patients in 1941.[193]

The 1937 Ordnance Survey Map depicts a cluster of open-air and other medical institutions on the west side of Bromsgrove. These are Cropwood Open Air School, Hunters Hill Open Air School, The Uplands (Children's Convalescent Home), Burcot Grange (Birmingham and Midland Eye Hospital) and an institution labelled as the Birmingham and Midland Counties Sanatorium, which is the Blackwell Convalescent Home.[194] There was obviously something about this location that made it suitable for a variety of open-air institutions. One factor was that it was a rural area close to Birmingham and the surrounding towns, and there were good road links from these as well as a railway station near the Convalescent Home. These meant that there was easy access to the area for patients. An undated prospectus for the Home also suggests that its location was important in terms of patient recovery:

> Send your convalescent to Blackwell on the sunny southern slopes of the Lickey Hills to regain health and strength. The Home stands in its own grounds of 12 acres on a gravel soil, high on the S/W foothills of the Lickey Hills, with the ground sloping rapidly away below it. The windows look right over the length and breadth of Worcestershire, across the Severn Valley to the Malvern Hills, 20 miles away, with a view, in clear weather of the Mountains of Wales, from which the prevailing S/W wind blows.[195]

In this text the home links health and strength to its location, which is in some ways similar to the decisions made in relation to the location of hospitals in the nineteenth century, when a rural location was seen as more beneficial for the patients in terms of cleaner air. According to Richardson, 'most convalescent homes were situated in the countryside or by the sea, where rest, graduated exercise, fresh air and wholesome food could help overcome the debility resulting from illness or surgery'.[196] There were also twelve acres of grounds, which suggests that having a large area surrounding the home, possibly designed as gardens, was important.

It is not clear what the therapeutic regime was at the home, but there does appear to be some relation to the open-air principles practised in other similar institutions. According to the *Blackwell Convalescent Home for Birmingham and the Midland Counties Report*, of 1932: 'As the Conservatory was in need of repair a suggestion was put forward that that it should be converted into an Open-Air Ward, which would be of advantage to patients, particularly those received from the Queen's Hospital. This conversion has been carried out and is hoped will be appreciated by and be beneficial to the patients.'[197] There is no way of knowing to what extent open-air therapies were carried out at the home but this shows that they were thought to be important for at least some convalescent patients. The use of the conservatory by patients also reflects earlier institutions such as Brislington House, with a conservatory attached to the main house as well as a smaller one attached to at least one of the cottages, and the grander winter garden with its glass roof at Leeds General Infirmary.

In 1863 Florence Nightingale declared that, 'every hospital should have its convalescent branch, and every county its convalescent home'.[198] She even designed an ideal convalescent home, which was formed from a series of domestic country cottages. The term 'home' itself suggests a domestic situation and this reflects its role as a place that gave patients time to recover before they returned to their own homes. In this context the gardens can be seen as part of the domestic setting, as in the early nineteenth-century asylums. However, they also had a therapeutic role. According to Richardson:

> A fundamental factor governing the design of convalescent homes was the mobility of the patients, who were neither expected, nor encouraged, to remain in their beds during the day. As a result, day-rooms, dining-rooms and attractive grounds were a common features in the earlier homes and, together with a chapel, were often the only features specifically suited to the needs of convalescents, even at the larger institutions.[199]

The grounds appear to have played this kind of therapeutic role at Blackwell Convalescent Home. On the back of a postcard illustrated by a photograph of the home sent to a Mr and Miss Morris on 24 June 1959, is written:

> Have spent three happy weeks here among the 100 patients. This place stands in lovely grounds 15 miles from Worcester overlooking the Malverns. Have spent most of the time sitting in sun lounge and walking or sitting in the grounds. Am feeling much better but cannot walk far yet. Auntie Rose.[200]

This suggests that, as late as 1959, spending time outside either sitting or walking in the grounds formed a central focus of the daily life of the convalescent.

There is little evidence of the design of the grounds but it is possible to establish what some of the features were from two postcards in the Royal Commission on the Historical Monuments of England collection (Figures 38 and 39). Both photographs show the rear of the house. The earlier postcard, which is undated, shows a conservatory adjoining the right side of the house, a steeply sloping garden planted with trees and shrubs and a steep flight of steps that descends to a gate in the foreground of the photograph.[201] On the later photograph, which is the postcard sent by Auntie Rose in 1959, the conservatory was still there but by this time there was also an area with large glass windows in the centre of the building, possibly a day room or dining room. The postcard also shows a flight of steps descending from this new room to a terrace. The steps have a hedge to their left that is cut into an ornamental shape. The ornamental design of the hedge suggests that the gardens were designed to be attractive as well as functional. A structure to the left of the house is also shown in the photograph. This could have been a shelter under

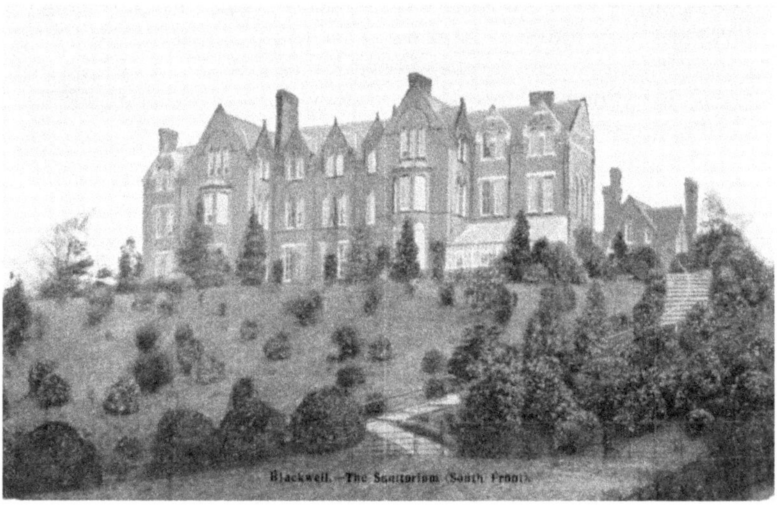

Figure 38 Undated postcard of Blackwell Convalescent Home showing a conservatory and zig-zag steps down into the garden.

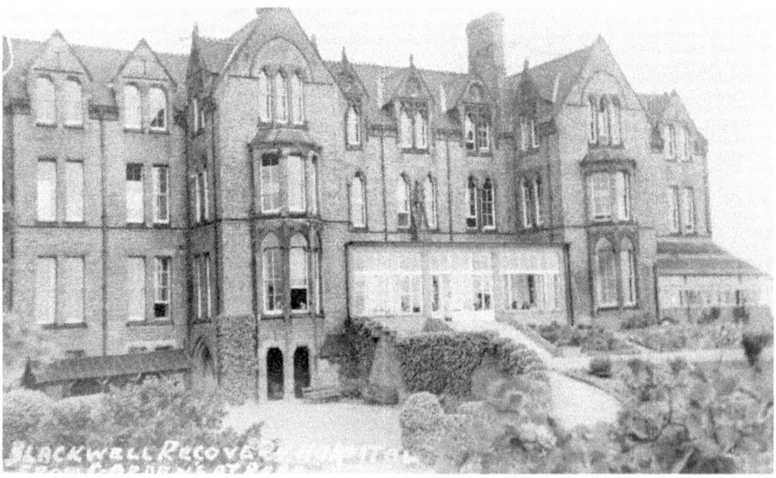

Figure 39 Postcard of Blackwell Convalescent Home from Auntie Rose, dated 1959.

which the patients could sit and take the air. This layout has some similarities to a 1903 garden design to accompany a house designed by W.D. Caröe published in *The Builder*.[202] This latter design appears to have been more complex but it also depicts shelters under which people could sit by the house, a terrace and steps descending to a lower area. This emphasises the domesticity of the home's design. On the Ordnance Survey Map of 1937 there is an avenue of trees running in a diagonal across a field at the base of the steep slope by the home which may have formed part of a wider garden. There is also a footpath marked through the centre of this field that led directly from the home. Part of the convalescent regime included exercise and it is likely that the patients would have been encouraged to walk further than the immediate grounds around the home.

The decline of specialist hospitals, convalescent homes and their gardens

Although the open-air regime was fairly ubiquitous for a range of diseases, it should be remembered that it was not always a pleasant one for the patient. According to Bryder, 'in 1923, a visitor to the Cowley Road Sanatorium, Oxford, found that all the male patients on the verandah, with two exceptions, were soaked with the rain that had fallen in the night, and that without any exception the top blankets on the beds were wet'.[203] Similarly the idea of being made to walk every day, regardless of the weather, in a regimented fashion could have been considered less than pleasant.

By the 1930s there was growing dissent amongst the medical community about the benefits of open-air treatments for children. The county medical officer for Worcestershire, Dr E.G. Hamilton Williams, claimed that the current understanding of the therapeutic basis of open-air schools was 'pure delusion'. He went on to argue that 'we have been led astray by the Continental preventorium schools, and the open-air schools for tuberculous children in Switzerland, to believe that exposure can command energy to combat cold, but we have found not only that cold does not energise, but that it actually produces a state of torpor particularly unbeneficial to the type of sickly children for whom open-air schools are advocated'.[204] Articles such as this were accompanied by growing accounts of children with frozen hands who were too cold to learn. By 1934 one writer was arguing that the fresh-air approach had been 'overdone' and that 'no climate of itself is curative'.[205] This was a huge shift, suggesting that the physical environment was no longer of central importance. Similarly, the *British Journal of Tuberculosis*, which had filled its pages with images of open-air sanatoria, adults and children gardening, and designs for chalets and balconies in the 1900s and 1910s, was taking a different tack by the 1930s. On the re-launch of the journal in 1935 it claimed that it had decided to make it 'more clinical' and it would seem that the open-air cure was starting to fall out of favour.[206]

This move towards a more clinical approach was accompanied by changes in the provision of health care. David Lloyd George, as Prime Minister, was worried about the deterioration of the population and remarked that 'a C3 population would not do for an A1 Empire'.[207] It was this fear, along with the increased demand for medical services, new insurance schemes and fears of the link between poverty and sickness that led to the establishment of the National Health Insurance Act of 1911. This Act was designed to protect the wages of workers who fell ill because Lloyd George, like Edwin Chadwick before him, was particularly bothered about the link between sickness and poverty.[208] In the end a moral element was added so that, in its final form, the Act provided income for the sick and 'access to medical care, the latter conditional on the patient's good character'.[209]

The moral element of 'good character' was not eliminated until the formation of the NHS, and this removal was probably influenced by the two world wars. Granshaw argues that after the First World War there was a further stimulus to hospital development, as all soldiers, 'whatever their rank, expected to be treated in hospital if their injuries necessitated it'.[210] Gradually the old poor law infirmaries became general hospitals and the government began to take control of medical services in Britain. The Local Government Act of 1929 gave authorities 'the power to appropriate poor law institutions and develop them into modern hospitals'.[211]

Before the introduction of the NHS some local authorities had already begun to organise the disparate range of hospitals into a more rational service.[212] There are many political and social issues relating to the formation of the NHS but as they have been discussed in a large number of texts these will not be covered again here.[213] However, in relation to the ideas discussed in this book, it is worth noting that there were a variety of views on the function of the NHS expressed at this time. Some saw the proposed health service as an organisation aimed at dealing with sickness rather than promoting health. For example, in 1944 a writer in *The Lancet* condemned the government's White Paper on the proposed NHS and suggested that:

> A real health service must surely contain itself first with the way people live, with town and country planning, house and open spaces, with diet, with playgrounds, gymnasia, baths and halls for active recreation, with workshops, kitchens, gardens and camps, with the education of every child in the care and use of his body.[214]

These concerns were all prominent during the first part of the twentieth century and the answer to improving the health of the population was often seen to be a combination of educating the individual and improving their access to healthy environments such as parks, gardens and playgrounds.

In 1948, as part of the new Welfare State, the Minister for Health, Aneurin Bevan, established the NHS. It was described as 'comprehensive' in the sense that it was available to all and covered all forms of health care. Under this act nearly all hospitals became the property of the Ministry of Health, although there were some exceptions to this, including the previously discussed St Andrew's Hospital, Northampton. The reorganisation of hospital facilities had been accepted in principle after the Hospital Surveys (1942–45) but it was not until the Hospital Plan of 1962 formulated by Enoch Powell as Minister of Health that this became a national reality.[215] According to Geoffrey Rivett, the goal of this plan was the unification of an area's separate hospitals into one District General Hospital because:

> the waste of consultant time travelling between different hospitals, the difficulty of providing complete training for nurses, the need to bring geriatric and psychiatric services within the curtilage of the DGH [District General Hospital] and the improvement in clinical care possible on a single site made this desirable. It was also essential to bring ophthalmology, chest medicine, paediatrics, obstetrics, accident services and the long-stay specialities alongside general medicine and surgery.[216]

Part of the funding for the new District General Hospitals was raised by closing down old hospitals, such as fever hospitals and tuberculosis sanatoria, as these were no longer considered necessary on medical grounds, along with other specialist hospitals whose services were physically moved to a location within the new District General Hospitals. This resulted in the loss of many of the gardens associated with specialist and convalescent institutions as land was often sold off for housing developments. Examples of hospitals that were affected by this change in thinking include Winford Orthopaedic Hospital, whose services were moved to Southmead Hospital, Bristol, and Blackwell Convalescent Home,

Bromsgrove, which was closed down after the introduction of the 1962 Hospital Plan.

As well as reflecting changes in the provision of health care the decline of gardens associated with specialist hospitals and convalescent homes mirrored the decline of country house estates after the two world wars. Harding and Lambert have suggested that:

> As a result of major social and economic changes, landscape gardening and garden design in Britain suffered a long decline after World War I. Agricultural depression, death duties, scarce and expensive labour and, surprisingly often, the withering of male lineage, have all played a part in the downfall of the country house, its gardens and its landscape park.[217]

Amongst these, the greatest impact on the garden was 'a shortage of labour and its higher price in the wake of the war [which] meant that labour-intensive work was the first to go . . . Flower beds were grassed over . . . Flowering shrubs have replaced labour-intensive herbaceous borders and rose gardens.'[218] This is reflected in the case study of Winford Hospital where the decrease in the number of labourers employed led to the grassing over of flowerbeds and an overall decline in the state of the garden.[219] It appears that, as with the country house, economic restraints played a part in the decline of hospital gardens in the twentieth century. However, the overall loss of gardens associated with specialist institutions and convalescent homes was related to changes in patterns of disease, progress in terms of treatments available and rationalisation within the NHS, which led to the closure of many of these institutions.[220]

Notes

1 From miscellaneous articles on the Edward VII Sanatorium (National Monuments Record Centre (NMRC) Swindon, National Buildings Record Index Number: 101270).

2 Bristowe, *An Introductory Address*, 1862.

3 For more on this see Lindsay Granshaw, 'Fame and fortune by means of bricks and mortar': the medical profession and specialist hospitals in Britain', in Lindsay Granshaw and Roy Porter, eds, *The Hospital in History* (London and New York: Routledge, 1989), 199–220.

4 Roger Cooter, 'Open-air therapy and the rise of open-air hospitals', *Bulletin for the Social History of Medicine*, 35 (1984), 44–6, p. 44.

5 *Ibid.*

6 *Ibid.*, p. 45.

7 F.B. Smith, *The Retreat of Tuberculosis, 1850–1950* (Kent: Croom Helm Ltd, 1988), p. 97.
8 Paul Weindling, 'From infectious to chronic disease: changing patterns of sickness in the nineteenth and twentieth centuries' in Andrew Wear, ed., *Medicine in Society: Historical Essays* (Cambridge: Cambridge University Press, 1992), 303–16, pp. 313–14.
9 Allan Warner, originally a paper given at Leicester, 'Open-air recovery schools', *The Medical Officer* (25 December 1909), p. 469.
10 T.N. Kelynack, ed., *The Year Book of Open-air Schools and Children's Sanatoria* (London: John Bale, Sons and Danielsson, 1915), p. v.
11 C. Muthu, *Pulmonary Tuberculosis and Sanatorium Treatment: A Record of 10 Years' Observation and Work in Open-air Sanatoria* (London: Balliere, Tindall and Cox, 1910), pp. 83–4.
12 *Ibid.*
13 Conway, *People's Parks*, p. 220.
14 Richardson, *Hygeia*, pp. 12–13.
15 Ebenezer Howard, *Garden Cities of Tomorrow*, (1902; this edition edited by F.J. Osborn, 1946) (Northampton, Faber and Faber, 1970), p. 48. For Richardson's influence see in particular Robert Beevers, *The Garden City Utopia: A Critical Biography of Ebenezer Howard* (Abingdon: Olivia Press, 2002), p. 30.
16 *The Medical Officer*, 12 July 1919, p. 11.
17 Muthu, *Pulmonary Tuberculosis*, pp. 192–3.
18 William Morris, *News from Nowhere or an Epoch of Rest, Being Some Chapters from a Utoplan Romance*, first printed serially in the *Commonweal*, 1890, ninth edition (London: Longman Green and Co, 1907), p. 24.
19 *Ibid.*, p. 18.
20 *Ibid.*, p. 29.
21 *Ibid.*
22 *Ibid.*, p. 14.
23 Anne Helmreich, *The English Garden and National Identity: The Competing Styles of Garden Design, 1870–1914* (Cambridge: Cambridge University Press, 2002), p. 10.
24 F.W. Burton-Fanning, *Open-air Treatment of Pulmonary Tuberculosis* (London, Paris, New York and Melbourne: Cassell and Company, c.1900), p. 165.
25 Stewart Harding and David Lambert, *Parks and Gardens of Avon* (Bristol: Avon Gardens Trust, 1994), p. 103.
26 *Ibid.*
27 See John Martin Robinson, *The Country House at War* (London: The Bodley Head, 1989) and Caroline Seebohm, *The Country House: A Wartime History, 1939–1945* (London: Weidenfeld and Nicholson, 1989).

28 Report of the NAPT Architectural Committee, *Design for Sanatoria* (London: NAPT, 1951), p. 11.
29 Taylor, *Hospital and Asylum Architectore*, p. 10.
30 See Sarah M. Whittingham, *Sir George Herbert Oatley (1863–1950): A Nonconformist Architect, a Critical Biography and Catalogue of Works*, PhD Thesis, 3 vols (Bristol: University of Bristol, 2005), pp. 96–9.
31 Jane Brown, *The Art and Architecture of English Gardens: Designs for the Garden from the Collection of the Royal Institute of British Architects 1609 to the Present Day* (London: Weidenfeld and Nicolson, 1989), p. 166.
32 Claire Barrett, 'In peril: Sully Hospital', *Grand Designs*, 2 (2004), p. 112.
33 Jonathan Glancey, *Twentieth-century Architecture* (London: Carlton Books, 1998), p. 169.
34 For more on the links between architecture and tuberculosis sanatoria see Campbell, 'What tuberculosis did for modernism', 463–88.
35 Glancey, *Twentieth-century Architecture*, p. 169.
36 Leslie Patrick Abercrombie, ed., *The Book of the Modern House: A Panoramic Survey of Contemporary Domestic Design* (London: Hodder and Stoughton, 1939), p. xii.
37 Pyrs Gruffudd, '"Science and the stuff of life": modernist health centres in 1930s London', *Journal of Historical Geography*, 27:3 (2001), 395–416, p. 395.
38 Dennis P. Doordan, *Twentieth-century Architecture* (London: Calman & King, 2002), p. 65.
39 David Ottewill, *The Edwardian Garden* (New Haven and London: Yale University Press, 1989).
40 Tim Mowl and Clare Hickman, *Historic Gardens of England: Northamptonshire* (Stroud: Tempus, 2008), p. 162.
41 Gruffudd, 'Science and the stuff of life', p. 395.
42 Clifford Holliday, 'The town house', in Leslie Patrick Abercrombie, ed., *The Book of the Modern House: A Panoramic Survey of Contemporary Domestic Design* (London: Hodder and Stoughton, 1939), 57–100, p. 64.
43 Mark Wigley, *White Walls, Designer Dresses: The Fashioning of Modern Architecture* (Cambridge, Mass. and London: MIT Press, 1995), p. 5.
44 For more on George Oatley's involvement at Winford, see Whittingham, *Sir George Herbert Oatley*, i, p. 99.
45 Winford Hospital, *History*, p. 8.
46 *Ibid.*
47 Programme for the *Foundation Stone Laying of the Open-air Hospital School, Winford, Somerset*, 7 July 1928 (BCLSL: B20807), p. 10. Hereafter referred to as the 1928 Programme.
48 Richardson, *English Hospitals*, p. 117.
49 For a history of orthopaedic surgical techniques see David Le Vay, *The History of Orthopaedics: An Account of the Study and Practice of Orthopaedics from the Earliest Times to the Modern Era* (Carnforth: Parthenon, 1989).

50 Cooter, *Surgery and Society*, p. 20.
51 *Ibid.*, p. 21.
52 1928 Programme, p. 10.
53 'School Gardens', *British Journal of Tuberculosis*, 3:3 (1909), 228–9.
54 G.R. Girdlestone, *The Care and Cure of Crippled Children: The Scheme of the Central Committee for the Care of Cripples* (Bristol: John Wright and Sons, 1925), pp. 26–7.
55 At this point it admitted adult patients under the Emergency Medical Services Scheme. Then in 1941 the Ministry of Health agreed to finance the Occupational Therapy Department and Winford became the first rehabilitation centre in the west of England. When the NHS was formed in 1948, the ownership of Winford was transferred to the Ministry of Health who appointed a new Management Committee.
56 Winford Orthopaedic Hospital, *Sixth Annual Report*, 1936, p. 23 (BCLSL: 14979).
57 *The Charities Register and Digest: Convalescent Section*, third edition (London: Longmans, Green and Co., 1890), p. 64.
58 H.J. Davis, 'The medical inspection of school children: ear, nose and throat affections', *The Medical Officer*, 24 October 1908, 307, p. 307.
59 Smith, *The Retreat of Tuberculosis*, p. 14.
60 Warner, 'Open-air recovery schools', p. 469.
61 Michael Worboys, 'The development of the sanatorium treatment for consumption in Britain, 1880–1914', *Bulletin for the Social History of Medicine*, 35 (1984), 41–3, pp. 41–2.
62 Smith, *The Retreat of Tuberculosis*, p. 14.
63 G.W.S. Brewer, 'School gardening and open-air schools', in T.N. Kelynack, ed., *The Year Book of Open-air Schools* (London: John Bale, Sons and Danielson, 1915), 158–62, p. 162.
64 For more detail on the history of children's gardens, including those related to the Open-Air Movement see Lorna Stacey, 'Gardens for the London child: the utilisation of gardens and nature for the physical, educational and psychological development of children in London', unpublished PhD Thesis (University of Bristol, 2008).
65 Vincent Hooper, 'Architectural ideals and the designing and construction of a children's residential sanatoria', in Kelynack, *The Year Book of Open-air Schools*, 26–31, p. 30.
66 Allan Warner, 'Open-air schools by the seaside', in Kelynack, *The Year Book of Open-air Schools*, 50–62, p. 62.
67 Mrs Joseph Cunning, 'The need for open-air schools for children of the upper and middle classes', in Kelynack, *The Year Book of Open-air Schools*, 65–6, p. 66.
68 James Campbell, 'School gardening in reformatories for boys', in Kelynack, *The Year Book of Open-air Schools*, 90–6, p. 91.

69 Helmreich, *The English Garden*, p. 36.
70 Frances Hodgson Burnett, *The Secret Garden* (1911) (Middlesex: Puffin Books, 1982), p. 239.
71 *Ibid.*, pp. 168–9.
72 Bryder, *Below the Magic Mountain*, p. 1.
73 *Ibid.*, p. 15.
74 *Ibid.*, p. 21.
75 Quoted in Bryder, *Below the Magic Mountain*, p. 21.
76 *Ibid.*
77 *Ibid.*
78 'A short account of Nordrach and the "open-air" treatment of consumption', *St. Thomas's Hospital Gazette*, 10:4 (1900), 73–81, p. 79.
79 *Ibid.*, p. 78.
80 *Ibid.*, p. 79.
81 Thomas Mann, *The Magic Mountain*, 1924, translated by H.T. Lowe-Porter (London: Vintage Books, 1999), p. 721.
82 *Ibid.*, pp. 37–8.
83 *Report on the 'Open-air' Treatment of Consumption at the North London Hospital for Consumption, Mount Vernon, Hampstead*, 1899.
84 Advertisement in *The Medical Officer*, 5 September 1908, p. 41. Doctors suffering from TB would undertake treatment in foreign sanatoria and then bring back to the UK the treatments they had undergone. There was a fairly fluid movement between patients and staff in the sanatorium system.
85 C. Braine Hartnell, *The Prevention and Cure of T.B: An Abstract of a Paper Read before the Worcestershire and Herefordshire Branch of the B.M.A.* (Cheltenham: Norman, Sawyer and Co., c.1900), p. 3.
86 *Ibid.*
87 Richardson, *English Hospitals*, p. 146.
88 *Ibid.*
89 Charles Reinhardt, *A Handbook of the Open-air Treatment and Life in an Open-air Sanatorium*, second edition (London: John Bales, Sons and Danielson, 1902), p. 35.
90 W.J. Fanning, 'Inexpensive sanatoria for working-class patients', *The British Journal of Tuberculosis*, 1 (1907), p. 304.
91 Bryder, *Below the Magic Mountain*, p. 46.
92 Advertisement in *The Medical Officer*, 5 September 1908, p. 41.
93 Burton-Fanning, *Open-air Treatment* p. 160.
94 Bryder, *Below the Magic Mountain*, p. 189.
95 Essay by Dr Bernard Stacey in 'Alpine climate: its physiology and therapeutics', copy of article (held in Bristol University Medical Library) originally published in the *British Journal of Tuberculosis*, (possibly in 1933), 18, p. 18.
96 Bryder, *Below the Magic Mountain*, p. 189.

97 Unfortunately the published images are of poor quality and so only one has been reproduced here.
98 Reinhardt, *Hailey Open Air Sanatorium*, p. 4.
99 *Ibid.*, pp. 8–10.
100 Bryder, *Below the Magic Mountain*, p. 28.
101 From the *Portsmouth Evening Post*, 13 June 1906, quoted in Bryder, *Below the Magic Mountain*, p. 24.
102 Bryder, *Below the Magic Mountain*, p. 26.
103 *Liverpool Post*, 14 June 1906, quoted in Bryder, *Below the Magic Mountain*, p. 49.
104 *Ibid.*, p. 50.
105 From miscellaneous articles on the Edward VII Sanatorium (NMRC Swindon, National Buildings Record Index Number: 101270).
106 Bryder, *Below the Magic Mountain*, p. 50.
107 It is interesting to note that divisions according to class were still being made here, as in the Victorian asylum: 'The better-class patients are housed in a separate block . . . so that as far as possible the residents in these blocks may be free from the feeling of being part of a large institution', *The Builder*, 20 December 1902, p. 582.
108 *Ibid.*
109 *Ibid.*, 23 May 1903, p. 532.
110 John Wilson, 'Notes on the planning of sanatoria, infectious diseases hospitals, and other public health institutions', reprinted from *Journal of the RIBA*, third series, 29:10 (1922) (British Library), p. 2.
111 *Kelly's Directory for Sussex* (1934) (NMRC Swindon, National Buildings Record Index Number: 101270), p. 243.
112 Reinhardt, *A Handbook*, p. 125.
113 Greta Jones, *'Captain of All These Men of Death': The History of Tuberculosis in Nineteenth and Twentieth Century Ireland* (Amsterdam and New York: Rodopi, 2001), p. 167.
114 *Ibid.*
115 Reinhardt, *Hailey Open Air Sanatorium*, p. 3.
116 *Tuberculosis Yearbook 1913–14*, quoted in Bryder, *Below the Magic Mountain*, p. 48.
117 *Medical Officer*, 31 October 1908, p. 326.
118 'The London open-air sanatorium', in *The British Medical Journal*, 2:2116 (1901), 153–4.
119 RCHME, *King Edward VII Hospital (Formerly King Edward VII Sanatorium)*, National Buildings Register no. 101270 (held at National Monuments Record Centre, Swindon).
120 'A short account of Nordrach', p. 74.
121 F. Rufenacht Walters, 'On some German sanatoria for phthsis', *The Lancet*, 14 August 1897, p. 385.

122 Arthur Latham, 'Essay on the erection of a sanatorium for the treatment of tuberculosis in England', *The Lancet*, 3 January 1903, p. 27.
123 Reinhardt, *A Handbook*, p. 123.
124 'The financial aspect of the open air treatment', *Health Resort*, 1903, p. 149, quoted in Campbell, 'What tuberculosis did for modernism', p. 479.
125 For more on the design of this type of hut and their uses see Campbell, 'What tuberculosis did for modernism', pp. 478–81.
126 Burton-Fanning, *Open-air Treatment*, p. 157.
127 Campbell, 'What tuberculosis did for modernism', pp. 478–80.
128 Advertisements for a variety of different architectural styles for open-air huts were published in the *British Journal for Tuberculosis* including Japanese-style buildings. This demonstrates that oriental and decorative themes for gardens could have a medical role and also echoes the Chinese garden buildings at Ticehurst.
129 Campbell, 'What tuberculosis did for modernism', pp. 480–1.
130 *Ibid.*, p. 488.
131 Ottewill, *The Edwardian Garden*, p. 128.
132 *Tuberculosis Yearbook 1913–14*, quoted in Bryder, *Below the Magic Mountain*, p. 48.
133 Letter from Jekyll to an American friend quoted in Ottewill, *The Edwardian Garden*, p. 128.
134 RCHME, *King Edward VII Hospital.*
135 Reinhardt, *A Handbook*, p. 40.
136 RCHME, *King Edward VII Hospital.*
137 Reinhardt, *Hailey Open Air Sanatorium*, p. 7.
138 Burton-Fanning, *Open-air Treatment*, p. 99.
139 Reinhardt, *A Handbook*, p. 65.
140 *Ibid.*, pp. 37–8.
141 RCHME, *King Edward VII Hospital.*
142 Burton-Fanning, *Open-air Treatment*, p. 102.
143 *Ibid.*, pp. 104–5.
144 Geoffrey Morland, 'Essay and plans for the erection of a sanatorium for tuberculosis', *The Lancet*, 3 January 1903, p. 68.
145 Bryder, *Below the Magic Mountain*, p. 62.
146 *Ibid.*, p. 56.
147 *The Medical Officer*, 12 December 1908, p. 453.
148 Jones, '*Captain of All These Men*', p. 173.
149 *The Medical Officer*, 31 May 1919, p. 191.
150 'The value of gardens', *The Medical Officer*, 24 July 1920, p. 30.
151 'Open-air occupations for women', *The British Journal of Tuberculosis*, 3:3 (1909), p. 228. This article is also accompanied by a footnote advertising gardening courses at Warwick's Horticultural College for Women, Studley Castle, Warwickshire.

152 Phillip Nicholls, *Homeopathy and the Medical Profession* (Kent: Croom Helm, 1988), p. 110.
153 *Ibid.*, p. 135.
154 1928 Programme, p. 7.
155 Quoted in Nicholls, *Homeopathy*, p. 182.
156 1928 Programme, p. 8.
157 *Ibid.*
158 *Ibid.*
159 *Ibid.*, p. 11.
160 *Bristol Homeopathic Hospital Building Committee Minutes*, 15 November 1923 (Bristol Record Office (BRO): 36754), hereafter *BCM*.
161 1928 Programme, p. 19.
162 *Bristol Homeopathic Hospital Report*, 1926, p. 15 (BRO: 36754).
163 Stephen Switzer, *Ichongraphia Rustica, or, the Nobelman, Gentleman and Gardener's Recreation, . . .*, 3 vols (London, Printed for D. Browne, B. Barker and C. King, W. Mears and R. Gosling, 1718), iii, pp. 125–6.
164 *Bristol Homeopathic Hospital Report*, 1926, p. 15.
165 1928 Programme, p. 19.
166 *BCM*, 1 October 1924.
167 Whittingham, *Sir George Herbert Oatley*, i, p. 98. For more on Oatley and his involvement with the Homeopathic Hospital, see pp. 96–9.
168 *BCM*, 7 January 1925.
169 Rosalind Delaney, with Gillian Winn, *How Did This Garden Grow? The History of the Botanic Gardens of the University of Bristol* (Bristol: Burleigh Press Ltd., 2002), p. 32.
170 *Ibid.*, p. 40.
171 *Ibid.*
172 Sally Festing, 'Pulham has done his work well', *Garden History*, 25 (1984), 138–58, p. 153. The garden at Bracken Hill, together with the pleasure garden opposite, known as Rayne Thatch, are now listed as Grade II gardens by English Heritage, Delaney, *How Did This Garden Grow?*, p. 44.
173 *BCM*, 4 February 1925.
174 *BCM*, 25 February 1925.
175 *Bristol Homeopathic Hospital Report*, 1925, p. 11 (BRO: 36754).
176 *Bristol Homeopathic Hospital report*, 1926, p. 9.
177 Delaney, *How Did This Garden Grow?*, p. 67.
178 *Ibid.*
179 *Ibid.*
180 For more on this see Ottewill, *The Edwardian Garden*.
181 *Bristol Homeopathic Hospital: The New Building*, 1925, p. 5 (BRO: 36754).
182 John Hilton, *On the Influence of Mechanical and Physiological Rest in the Treatment of Accidents and Surgical Diseases, and the Diagnostic Value of Pain: A Course of Lectures Delivered at the Royal College of Surgeons of*

England, in the Years 1860, 1861, and 1862 (London: Bell and Daldy, 1863) and John Hilton, *On Rest and Pain: A Course of Lectures* (London: George Bell and Sons, 1877).

183 David Armstrong, 'Decline of the hospital: reconstructing institutional dangers', *Sociology of Health and Illness*, 20:4 (1998), 445–57, p. 445.

184 *Ibid.*, p. 448.

185 Richardson, *English Hospitals*, p. 182.

186 Armstrong, 'Decline of the hospital', pp. 1–2.

187 *Ibid.*, p. 3.

188 Stephen Soanes, 'Rest and restitution: convalescence and the public mental hospital in England, 1919–39', unpublished PhD Thesis (Warwick University, 2011), p. 79.

189 *Ibid.*, p. 158.

190 *Ibid.*

191 Blackwell Convalescent Home for Birmingham and the Midland Counties, *Minute Book of the Committee of Management No.15* 1941–45, 16 December 1941 (Worcester Record Office (WRO): b499.8/B.A.10134/20).

192 *Ibid.*, 19 January 1943.

193 *Ibid.*, 16 December 1941.

194 In 1921 it became known as the Blackwell Convalescent Home for Birmingham and the Midland Counties and in 1952 its name changed again to the Blackwell Recovery Hospital.

195 *Prospectus for Blackwell Convalescent Home for Birmingham and the Midland Counties*, stuck in a scrapbook from Blackwell Convalescent Home for Birmingham and the Midland Counties (WRO: b499.8/B.A.10134/20), date unknown.

196 Richardson, *English Hospitals*, p. 183.

197 *Blackwell Convalescent Home for Birmingham and the Midland Counties Report*, 1932, stuck in scrapbook (WRO: b499.8/B.A.10134/20), p. 2.

198 Nightingale, *Notes, Third Edition*, p. 107.

199 Richardson, p. 183.

200 Postcard, 24 June 1959. From Auntie Rose to Mr and Miss Morris (NMRC Swindon, National Buildings Record Index Number 100767).

201 Postcard, undated (NMRC Swindon, National Buildings Record Index Number 100767).

202 'House near Dublin. Architect: Mr W.D. Caröe', *The Builder*, 23 September 1903, p. 322.

203 Bryder, *Below the Magic Mountain*, p. 209.

204 'Open-air schools', *The Medical Officer*, 21 January 1933, p. 23.

205 'The fresh air regime', *The Medical Officer*, 6 October 1934, p. 144.

206 'Our future plans', *British Journal of Tuberculosis*, January 1935, p. 1. For more on changes in relation to tuberculosis in particular see Bryder, *Below the Magic Mountain* and Smith, *The Retreat of Tuberculosis*.

207 Quoted in Jane Lewis, 'Providers, "consumers", the state and the delivery of health-care services in twentieth century Britain', in Andrew Wear, ed., *Medicine in Society* (Cambridge: Cambridge University Press, 1992), 317–45, p. 326.

208 Christopher Lawrence, *Medicine in the Making of Modern Britain, 1700–1920* (London: Routledge, 1994), p. 80.

209 *Ibid.*

210 Lindsay Granshaw, 'The rise of the modern hospital in Britain', in Wear, *Medicine in Society*, 197–218, p. 214.

211 Geoffrey Rivett, *From Cradle to Grave: Fifty Years of the NHS* (London: King's Fund Publishing, 1998), p. 4.

212 *Ibid.*

213 See texts by authors such as Rivett, *From Cradle to Grave*; Lewis 'Providers'; and Charles Webster, ed., *Caring for Health: History and Diversity* (Norwich: Open University, 1993).

214 An urban practitioner, 'The white paper reviewed, VI', *The Lancet*, 1 (1944), 443, p. 443.

215 Rivett, *From Cradle to Grave*, pp. 173–6.

216 *Ibid.*, p. 176.

217 Harding and Lambert, *Parks and Gardens*, p. 110. See also Roy Strong, Marcus Binney and John Harris, *The Destruction of the Country House, 1875–1975* (London: Thames and Hudson, 1974).

218 Harding and Lambert, *Parks and Gardens*, p. 111.

219 In 1962 the hospital minutes recorded that 'it was agreed unanimously that the gardens presented a neglected appearance and this was confirmed on inspection of the grounds'. The head gardener put this down to a lack of staff for the amount of acreage.

220 For more on this see Rivett, *From Cradle to Grave.*

6

Present and future trends in hospital gardens

> Gardens provide restorative nature views and can also improve medical outcomes through other mechanisms, such as promoting access to social support, encouraging exercise, and providing an escape from stressful clinical settings.
>
> Roger Ulrich, 2003[1]

> I have seen, in fevers (and felt, when I was a fever patient myself) the most acute suffering produced from the patient (in a hut) not being able to see out of a window, and the knots in the wood being the only view. I shall never forget the rapture of fever patients over a bunch of bright-coloured flowers. I remember (in my own case) a nosegay of wild flowers being sent me, and from that moment my recovery becoming more rapid. People say the effect is only on the mind. It is no such thing. The effect is on the body too. Little as we know about the way in which we are affected by form, by colour, and light, we do know this, and that they have an actual physical effect.
>
> Florence Nightingale, 1860[2]

With the coalescing of medical services after the establishment of the NHS, the early part of the twentieth century saw a decline in the establishment and maintenance of gardens associated with medical institutions. The need to expand buildings to encompass specialist departments and the increasing number of technological diagnostic and treatment tools, as well as the ever growing need for car-parking space, put pressure on existing hospital gardens and grounds. Any new general hospitals built during this time were predominantly designed with the aim of being clinically effective and most psychiatric hospitals of the Victorian and Edwardian era were eventually closed down in favour of small, specialist units and a shift towards care in the community.

The new ideal of clinical effectiveness was often to the detriment of the overall environment, including gardens. According to Roger Ulrich, who has become one of the most influential voices in hospital design on both sides of the Atlantic:

> healthcare designers and administrators understandably became pre-occupied with creating environments that would succeed as functionally efficient delivery platforms for important new medical technology and science . . . the functional emphasis produced environments that were efficient but often sterile and starkly institutional, and are now considered stressful and otherwise unsuited to the emotional or psychological needs of patients, visitors or staff.[3]

Designs such as that known as the 'matchbox on a muffin', which became popular in the 1950s and consisted of a vertical tower block of wards set on top of a horizontal block for administrative and other functions, left little scope for gardens. Wil Gesler and others suggest that this design 'influenced by office buildings and hospitals built in Europe and the US . . . symbolised modernity, efficiency, and an optimistic attitude towards technology and progress'.[4] The American model of high-rise hospitals, according to Jonathan Hughes, was not lost on hospital architects, who he says were 'swept along by the rhetoric of Harold Wilson's white-hot "scientific revolution". Like Wilson's new Britain, the new NHS hospital was not just to be modern, but more meritocratic, mechanized and efficient.'[5] In 1981 Anthony Cox and Philip Groves were suggesting that the primary requirement of a hospital was that it 'should function with the maximum ease, efficiency and economy in saving human life' reflecting the concern of clinical efficiency over and above that of the environment.[6]

However, this does not mean that hospital gardens were not designed or created in this period. At St Thomas's Hospital, London, a garden was created when the eastern part of the hospital was re-built in the 1960s. The central feature is the Revolving Torsion Fountain (created in 1972–73) by the constructivist sculptor Naum Gabo (Figure 40). The entrance to the hospital on the east side is flanked by trees and shrubs which confer on it a garden-like appearance. Similarly, Charing Cross Hospital, which was built in 1973 on Fulham Palace Road, London, has a pond that people have to cross to enter the hospital. This could be described as resembling a moat, as it provides a physical barrier between the hospital and the outside world. Charing Cross Hospital also has a large grassy area, which was being used by people for sunbathing and picnics

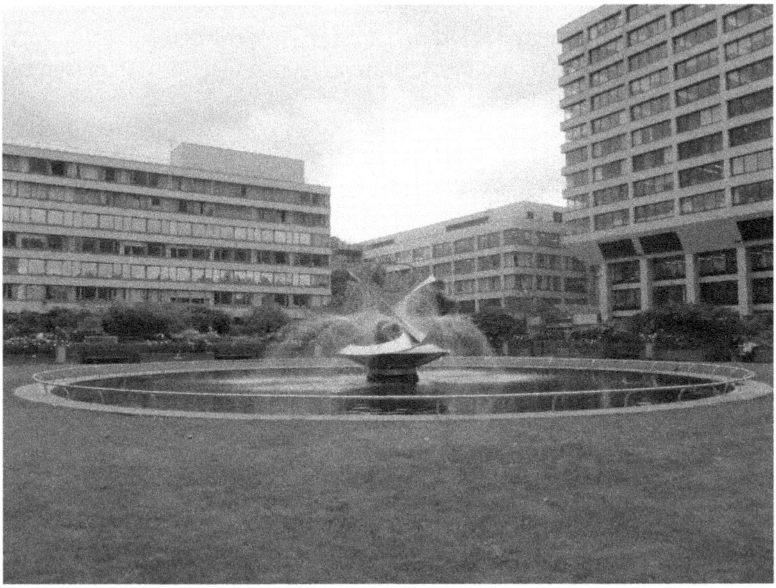

Figure 40 The garden at the east side of St Thomas's Hospital, London, with the Revolving Torsion Fountain by Naum Gabo to demonstrate that some hospital gardens were created during the 1970s.

when it was visited by the author in 2005, and an enclosed garden with a sculpture by Robert Clatworthy that appears to have been designed to be viewed from above (Figure 41). The enclosed area was landscaped in 1995 so provides a recent example of new garden design. It is interesting to note that these late twentieth-century London hospitals, where space was at a premium, still found room for the creation of gardens.

Towards the end of the twentieth century, theories concerning the functions of design began to change. Ruth Richardson has described a conference that took place at the Wellcome Trust in the early 1990s. The topic under discussion was 'deep hospitals' – buildings designed around artificial light and ventilation, with limited access to the external world. Richardson recalls this discussion on 'so-called "deep hospitals" (a favourite idea among architects between the 1960s and 1980s), in which Dr Aileen Adam of Addenbrooke's Hospital memorably spoke out about the disorientating effects of windowless rooms, particularly in intensive care units: "Patients go berserk, everybody goes berserk!"'[7] Richardson

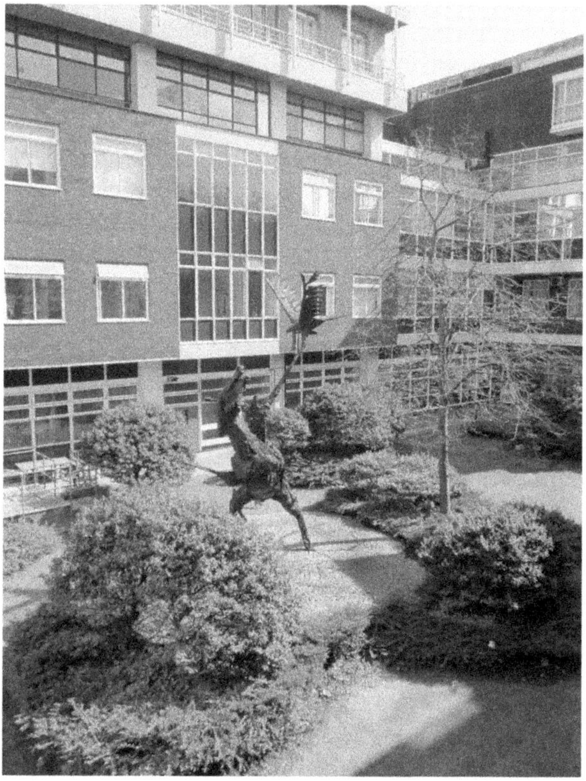

Figure 41 Charing Cross Hospital, London. The sculpture in the foreground is 'Horse and Rider' by Robert Clatworthy, 1983: it is surrounded by beds of shrub planting which look like islands floating in a sea of grass. This garden can be viewed from a number of windows but access is restricted to the ground-floor ward adjacent to it.

also wrote that, 'the therapeutic value of natural fresh air, natural light and natural landscape – particularly for bed-bound patients and sleep-deprived staff – emerged several times during discussion'.[8] These are recurring themes that were prominent in hospital design throughout the nineteenth century and were central concerns of the open-air movement of the late nineteenth and early twentieth centuries. In this way it can be seen as backwards looking, but as it took place on the threshold of the emergence of new ways of thinking about hospital design, it can also be seen as an indicator of future trends.

The discussion described by Richardson is indicative of what Ulrich calls a recently growing awareness of the need to 'create functionally efficient and hygienic environments that also have pleasant, stress reducing characteristics'.[9] He argues that this change is due to mounting scientific evidence from researchers, such as him, on both the positive and detrimental effects that the patient environment can have on patient health outcomes. These include the amount of anxiety experienced, blood pressure levels, the degree of pain the patient feels and length of hospital stay.[10] However, this new interest in hospital environments can also be seen as part of wider cultural changes, particularly the growing consciousness of environmental issues amongst the general public. According to Meredith Veldman, 'the late 1960s and early 1970s witnessed an upsurge of environmental concern in Britain' and this may well have led to an increased awareness of the role of the environment in relation to health.[11]

There is also evidence that gardens are once again being seen as an important part of hospital design. The ideal contemporary healing garden is described in detail by Swedish researchers Ingrid Söderback et al. in an article published in 2004:

> A healing garden seeks to provide maximum influence on health. It should be designed with a plentiful variety of plant materials that flower in different seasons, attract birds and butterflies, with leaves and grass that move with a light breeze, pools that reflect the sky and provide a home for fish. Sculptures and other designs should be unambiguously positive. The design should facilitate visibility (the garden should invite one to visit it), security and physical comfort. The garden should be open to all and give a sense of familiarity. It should be calm and quiet so that its voices (water-splash, birdsong) can be heard. Optimally designed, the gardens facilitate non-discrimination of the participants' age, genus, class, previous occupation, cultural heritage or ethnicity.[12]

This description of the elements in an ideal garden is very detailed and gives a strong impression of the researchers' belief in the potential for well-designed gardens to help improve the healing process. It is also remarkably similar to a description of a healing garden written by the German theorist, Christian Cay Lorenz Hirschfeld in 1785:

> Hospitals are to be situated outside and away from cities, to allow for garden space . . . The garden should be directly connected to the hospital, or even more so, surround it. Because a view from the window into blooming and happy scenes will invigorate the patient, a nearby garden encourages patients to take a walk. The plantings, therefore, should wind along dry paths, which offer benches and chairs. Clusters of trees are preferred to

> alleys of trees, which through the years will mature and meet at the top so air will not circulate . . . Sad conifers should not be used but trees with light and coloured leaves and flowering and fragrant shrubs and flowers. A hospital garden should have everything to enjoy nature and promote a healthy life. It should help forget weakness and worries, and encourage a positive outlook; everything in it should be serene and happy. No scene of melancholy, no memorial to mortality should be permitted to intrude . . . Noisy brooks could run through flowery fields, and merry waterfalls could reach your ear through shady shrubbery. Many plants with fortifying fragrances could be grouped together. Numerous songbirds will be attracted by the shade, peace, and freedom. And their songs will rejoice many weak hearts.[13]

The similarity between these two descriptions of highly sensory and nature-filled gardens suggests that the underlying features of hospital garden design have remained the same. However, the scientific rhetoric that tries to explain why gardens can act as therapeutic spaces has changed.

As the first quotation at the start of this chapter suggests, recent research by Ulrich has found that, 'gardens provide restorative nature views and can also improve medical outcomes'.[14] According to Söderback et al., there are three theories that have been postulated to explain mechanisms by which nature, including gardens, could have a therapeutic effect.[15] The two central ones are 'evolutionary theory' and 'psycho-evolutionary theory'.

The basis of the evolutionary theory, as described by R. and S. Kaplan, is that 'directed attention can be fatigued by overuse'.[16] According to Thomas R. Herzog et al.:

> The consequences of attentional fatigue are a lowered ability to concentrate and solve problems, heightened irritability, and a greater proneness to mistakes or accidents. Recovery for attentional fatigue requires a setting characterized by four features: being away, which implies a setting that is physically or conceptually different from one's everyday environment; extent, which implies a setting sufficiently rich and coherent that it can engage the mind and promote exploration; fascination (or effortless attention), which can come from content (animals, people, water, fire) or process (story telling, gambling, problem solving); and compatibility, which implies a setting that fits with and supports one's inclinations or purposes. Settings that contain these four features in sufficient degree are referred to as restorative environments.[17]

According to Kaplan and Kaplan, these four factors are commonly found at high levels in natural settings and this explains why gardens can act as restorative devices.[18]

Ulrich's psycho-evolutionary theory proposes that nature reduces stress. In this case stress can be described as 'the process by which an individual responds psychologically, physiologically, and often with behaviors, to a situation that challenges or threatens well-being'.[19] This mechanism of stress reduction suggests that the 'restorative influences of nature involve a shift towards a more positively-toned emotional state, positive changes in physiological activity levels, and that these changes are accompanied by sustained attention/intake'.[20]

These theories are both based to some extent on the wide-reaching theory of 'biophilia'. This was first postulated by the biologist Edward O. Wilson in his 1984 book, *Biophilia: The Human Bond With Other Species*, in which he argued that biophilia was 'the innate tendency to focus on life and lifelike processes'.[21] Landscape was one factor identified by Wilson as part of these life processes and he argued that evolutionary development may have influenced the choices made by modern humans in terms of the type of landscape they find most appealing: 'Whenever people are given a free choice, they move to open tree-studded land on prominences overlooking water.'[22] This initial concept has been expanded by later authors who have suggested that 'humans have an innate bond with nature'.[23] According to Howard Frumkin, 'this implies that certain kinds of contact with the natural world may benefit health' so, therefore, biophilia can be viewed as an overarching concept that relates to the scientific theories of Kaplan and Kaplan, Ulrich and others.[24]

In relation to these theories, several studies have found that natural rather than human-made properties are more restorative. For example, in 1991 Terry Hartig and others used data from blood pressure readings and emotional self-reports to establish that both physical and emotional recovery from a stressful experience, such as driving a car through heavy traffic, was greater if after the experience the subjects looked at a nature setting dominated by vegetation rather than a built environment without any natural elements.[25] The idea that viewing nature helps reduce stress is not a recent one. In 1865 Frederick Law Olmsted, an influential American landscape architect and planner, wrote that the enjoyment of scenery 'employs the mind without fatigue and yet exercises it; tranquillizes it and yet enlivens it; and thus, through the influence of the mind over the body, gives the effect of refreshing rest and reinvigoration to the whole system'.[26]

In relation to hospital gardens Ulrich states that, 'there is increasing evidence that gardens foster restoration for stressed patients and family members. Research is also revealing that gardens are used by staff to relax.'[27] The study relating most closely to hospital gardens, and which has been commonly quoted, found that a view of something natural out of a window had a strong positive effect on a group of patients having undergone gall bladder surgery. According to Ulrich, patients that have had surgery often experience considerable anxiety and due to the nature of the operation are confined indoors, so any interaction with the external environment is limited to what they can see through a window.[28] The patients in the study were split into two groups; both had unobstructed views out of their windows but one group looked at a stand of deciduous trees while the other looked at a brown wall. Evidence was only taken during the months when leaves were present on the trees. Ulrich found that the patients 'assigned to rooms with windows looking out on a natural scene had shorter postoperative hospital stays, received fewer negative evaluative comments in nurses' notes, and took fewer potent analgesics' than the patients in similar rooms whose windows faced a brick wall.[29] Although this study is small and is not directly linked to gardens, it can be postulated that the most likely view of something 'natural' in a twenty-first-century hospital will be provided by a garden.

In some ways Ulrich's findings provide evidence for Nightingale's belief in the importance of giving the patient something other than a blank wall to look at. In 1860 she wrote that:

> I have mentioned the cruelty of letting him stare at a dead wall. In many diseases, especially in convalescence from fever, that wall will appear to make all sorts of faces at him; now flowers never do this. Form, colour, will free your patient from his painful idea better than any argument.[30]

Nightingale appears to have believed that something more than a wall to look at would in some way distract the patient from the way that they feel, which reflects the Kaplans' theory that providing fascination in a person's surroundings can prove restorative. This idea is also echoed by Maggie Keswick who described her time as a cancer patient in 1995 stating that 'overhead (sometimes even neon) lighting, interior spaces with no view out and miserable seating against the walls all contribute to extreme mental and physical enervation. Patients who arrive relatively hopeful soon start to wilt.'[31] Nightingale felt equally strongly about the importance of views and suggested that 'it is the seal of ignorance and stupidity just as much on the governors and attendants of the sick if they do not provide the sick-bed with a "view", or with variety of some kind, as if they did not provide the hospital with a kitchen'.[32] One can speculate what she might have thought of the latest wave of NHS hospitals, some of which have been built without kitchens, let alone consideration of the views that patients may or may not have from their beds.

Ulrich's findings on the effect of views on patients are paralleled by results from research conducted in prisons. One study found that cell window views of nature were associated with lower frequencies of prisoner stress symptoms, such as digestive illness and headaches, and with fewer sick calls.[33] This research suggests that views through windows can be of therapeutic importance and Ulrich argues that his findings 'imply that hospital design and siting decisions should take into account the quality of patient window views'.[34]

However, it is worth mentioning that Ulrich does not believe that all gardens are necessarily therapeutic. He argues that, 'considerations include: convenient way-finding to the garden; accessibility; access to privacy; seating that facilitates social interaction; exercise opportunities; and contact with nature'.[35] He goes on to suggest that 'gardens will ameliorate stress effectively if they contain verdant foliage, flowers, non-turbulent water, parklike, or savannalike qualities (grassy spaces with scattered trees), congruent nature sounds (birds, breezes, water), and visible wildlife (birds, squirrels)'.[36] With the exception of water, most of these features were common historically in hospital gardens. On the negative side, Ulrich argues that 'environmental qualities that tend to hinder recovery or even aggravate stress include: predominance of hardscape or starkly built content (concrete, for example); appraised risk or insecurity; crowding; cigarette smoke; intrusive or human-made sounds (for example, traffic, air conditioning equipment, loud aircraft); and ambiguous design features or art works that can be interpreted in multiple ways'.[37] These can be summarised as elements that are associated with contemporary life and he is clearly advocating a return to nature or at least a more rural setting. This is something that nineteenth-century writers would have recognised in terms of improving both moral and physical health.

Ulrich has also written that, 'the use of the term "healing" in the context of healthcare gardens ethically obligates the garden designer to subordinate or align his or her personal tastes to the paramount objective of creating a user-centred, supportive environment'.[38] This leaves little space for the creativity of designers and suggests that he may view Gertrude Jekyll's designs for the King Edward VII Sanatorium, Sussex, as unethical because they strongly reflected her own taste, although they did include many of the elements he has described as therapeutic. American researchers such as Clare Cooper Marcus and Marni Barnes have also become interested in what specific elements make a garden therapeutic and have used recent research to develop detailed guidelines for garden designers on what they believe makes the optimum healing garden.[39]

Although the scientific reasons given for the mechanism by which contact with nature can be therapeutic have changed over time, the design features of the ideal hospital garden and the importance of the external environment in terms of light, views and access to nature appear to have remained current, within the literature at least (apart from a small period after the Second World War to the 1980s). This final chapter is separated into five main themes in order to explore the connections that can be drawn between the past and the present. These are: views; light; the size and accessibility of the landscape; the therapeutic use of the landscape; and contemporary design.

Views, light and the idea of the therapeutic landscape have been flagged up as being of particular importance by the British Medical Association in a briefing document published in January 2011, *The Psychological and Social Needs of Patients.* Within this paper, which draws upon an array of recent journal articles and studies, the BMA states that landscapes 'should be designed with regard to their therapeutic value' and that 'hospital gardens not only provide restorative or calming nature views, but can also reduce stress and improve outcomes through other mechanisms, including fostering access to social interactions and providing opportunities for positive escape and a sense of control with respect to stressful clinical settings'.[40] As this is a current briefing document it highlights the seriousness with which the physical environment is once again being considered by the medical profession and will potentially influence future decisions in relation to the design of healthcare facilities.

Views

Ulrich's work on the benefits of patients having access to views of something natural outside their windows has once again brought the importance of views to the attention of those interested in the therapeutic environment. In the nineteenth century, hospitals, particularly asylums, were often built on eminences, and therefore, patients often had far-reaching views of the surrounding landscape. One contemporary example of a hospital built on an eminence is that of the West Dorset General Hospital, Dorchester, which was officially opened in 1998.

The West Dorset General Hospital has taken the idea of the therapeutic environment seriously, in both its design and practice. As well as being placed on a hill, the hospital is designed around a series of courtyards and has an arts programme based on the theme of 'Bringing the Outside

In'. It is, therefore, not surprising that it has taken the idea of a view out of the window one step further using modern technology. The hospital is currently evaluating the idea of giving patients a virtual view in a project called 'A Room with a View'. It is not always possible to place a patient near a window with a real nature scene, so the project is investigating the benefits of virtual views. Ulrich suggests that in these cases 'simulated nature scenes and even art can be effective alternatives' and has been involved with the project in Dorset.[41] Patients who are unable to leave their rooms or have much contact with the external environment because of their depressed immune systems, leading to a higher risk of infection, such as leukaemia patients, are being given the opportunity to watch a view from three kilometres away that is transmitted via wireless link to an LCD screen in their room. According to Alex Coulter, Arts Co-ordinator for Dorset County Hospital, 'we hope that a live view of nature will allow patients to think about and experience the real world outside their isolation rooms and that this will contribute to their increased well being and quality of life'.[42] The concept of using the latest technology to enhance the patients' environment is also one that has a historical precedent. As previously mentioned, in the nineteenth century, Leeds Infirmary used similar engineering practices to those used to construct the Crystal Palace in order to create a winter garden, and Bristol General Hospital used the newly invented material, asphalt, in order to construct a roof garden for use by patients.[43]

The view being transmitted to the screens would also be familiar to a nineteenth-century audience. The camera is placed on Kingston Maurward House, a former country house, and the view is composed of steps, a lake and parkland. The house is now an agricultural college so during term-time the scene also has flourishes of activity as students walk and sit in the landscape. Therefore, although the mechanism for viewing the landscape is contemporary, there are similarities with the views that could have been experienced from within nineteenth-century hospitals.[44]

Like real views of gardens, Ulrich believes that:

> the live link of the scene will reduce stress and pain because the picture will distract patients. This will relieve depression and has the possibility of speeding up recovery . . . Heart rates and respiration rates will reduce and muscles will relax. The feelings of fear and other negative feelings will reduce and will be replaced by positive ones. It also gives patients control and allows them to see what is going on outside and what the weather is like. The water is important because it is attention holding and mesmerising.[45]

This again emphasises the importance of the interaction, however limited, of the patient with the external environment.

Light

Light was an important factor in the design of pavilion hospitals in the nineteenth century, as well as in twentieth-century sanatoria, with their open-air philosophy. For example, in the pavilion hospital 'the light flooded in from tall windows interspersing the beds'.[46] However, Hughes argues that from the 1950s onwards,

> post-war treatment of such diseases as tuberculosis with streptomycin (rather than light therapy or surgery) and the diminishing length of inpatient stay (partly due to early ambulation) were all contributing to lessen the therapeutic necessity of sunlight. For architects, convenience of planning was now the overriding design consideration, and so balconies, solaria and other such features were rapidly to disappear from post-war hospital architecture.[47]

This led to the design of hospitals that contained wards which received no natural daylight.

Physicians have recently begun using bright light therapy for medical conditions. Most commonly it is used as a treatment for seasonal affective disorder, a condition marked by mild winter depression. Kathleen M. Beauchemin and Peter Hays state that bright lights have also been used successfully alongside pharmacological treatments in other types of depressive illness. In one study Beauchemin and Hays compared patients placed in different rooms. They described how the rooms in their psychiatric inpatient unit 'are so placed that half are bright and sunny and the rest are not'.[48] They go on to say that, 'reasoning that some patients were getting light therapy inadvertently, we compared the lengths of stay of depressed patients in sunny rooms with those of patients in dull rooms. Those in sunny rooms had an average stay of 16.9 days compared to 19.5 days for those in dull rooms, a difference of 2.6 days.'[49] This is a striking piece of research which suggests that something as simple as access to natural daylight can reduce hospital stays.

As well as the ability to reduce depression, part of the role of sunlight is to help the patient feel that they are in contact with the external world. In the design statement for the Callington Road Psychiatric Hospital (opened in 2008) the architects state that they are using natural light and ventilation as much as possible. They argue that:

> This has the benefit of maintaining a human connection between inside and outside as well as reducing the energy requirements over the building's life – and therefore contributing to sustainability. Natural lighting, especially in common and group therapy areas has been maximised to enable users to relate to their outside surroundings and landscape and mitigate, wherever possible, feelings of enclosure, whilst at the same time presenting a feeling of 'openness' to the outside world.[50]

The idea of trying to prevent a feeling of enclosure through design is one that has been discussed in relation to the nineteenth-century asylum. However, asylum superintendents seemed to feel that the best way to access natural light and landscape was to get the patient outside whenever possible. It is also interesting to note that the Callington Road *Design Statement* quotes the financial benefits of using natural light and air as a method of reducing the costs of the building. Again this highlights the focus of these new hospitals on financial considerations. In the design for Callington Road the architects have also orientated the building so that most rooms benefit from direct sun at some point in the day as well as ensuring that the central garden is south facing.[51]

The design profile by Dan Pearson's Studio, headed by popular garden designer Dan Pearson, for the new Maggie's Centre at Charing Cross Hospital, London, also describes how 'the largest of the three courtyards will be light and sun-filled and warm in atmosphere'.[52] This implies that access to natural light is once again being considered as a factor in the design process in contrast to the earlier 'matchbox on a muffin' style of architecture.

Conservatories are also being used to help increase the amount of light that can be accessed by patients. Used as early as 1804 at Brislington House, and recommended by both J.C. Loudon and Humphry Repton, conservatories are being included in new hospital designs.[53] Three new elderly care units owned by Blackpool, Fylde and Wyre Hospitals NHS Trust were opened in 2001 and were designed so that 'each facility . . . contains a conservatory overlooking landscaped grounds'.[54] This incorporates both the availability of light and a garden view.

Another way of bringing light into new hospitals is the use of atria. At Lynfield Mount Hospital, Bradford, 'the use of glass for vertical elements as well as roofing in the form of roof-lights has been of particular importance'.[55] At Daventry Community Hospital, Northamptonshire, opened in 2006, the architects have viewed the atria as similar to the winter garden and included planting in the design: 'The interior atria provide an opportunity to link, vertically through the introduction of high canopy living palms and to orientate and shield space through the introduction of wider architectural form species at a lower level.'[56] In contrast to Nightingale's concept of a winter garden for use by patients, however, they do not mention if this is for the benefit of the people using the building or whether it is simply a design solution.

Size and accessibility of landscape

The main differences between hospital gardens of the nineteenth and early twentieth centuries appear to be scale and accessibility. Although some hospital gardens of the past, such as the roof garden at Bristol General Hospital, were limited in size, many, especially those associated with asylums and open-air hospitals, had wider landscapes of a considerable size.[57] Some new designs do still include extensive grounds like their earlier counterparts. The Callington Road psychiatric facility is described as being on a site of '12 acres of undeveloped land'.[58] A detailed description suggests that there is a mix of landscape types:

> Each of the 16 wards has its own enclosed garden with designs and materials appropriate to the special needs of service users, to contribute to their healing and therapy. Beyond the ward gardens a network of paths create a wandering loop. Therapy spaces for sports and games are provided, as well as seating areas for interaction with wildlife, and a formal water feature providing the relaxing sound of moving water. Rose and herb gardens were requested by service users, and allotment gardens, sheds, greenhouses, cold frames provide opportunities for more active recreation and therapy, which are used enthusiastically.[59]

This mirrors earlier nineteenth-century asylum design as it incorporates both a wider landscape for recreation and individual ward gardens, which can be viewed as similar to airing courts.

Current hospital gardens are more likely to consist of courtyards, balconies and roof gardens with little, or no, wider landscape, because of the pressures of space on many sites. The courtyard is without doubt the most common garden area that is included in contemporary hospital designs. However, like many ideas relating to hospital gardens, it is not a new design solution. As Richardson has written:

> The courtyard and cloister are closely related, and with good reason were favoured features of country houses, as well as Oxbridge colleges and many almshouses. In all these cases (as in monastic cloisters) the enclosed or semi-enclosed space a courtyard creates is a protected space, inward looking, concentrated, secure, fostering privacy within a community, and yet with plenty of light, air and shelter, and a satisfying vista.[60]

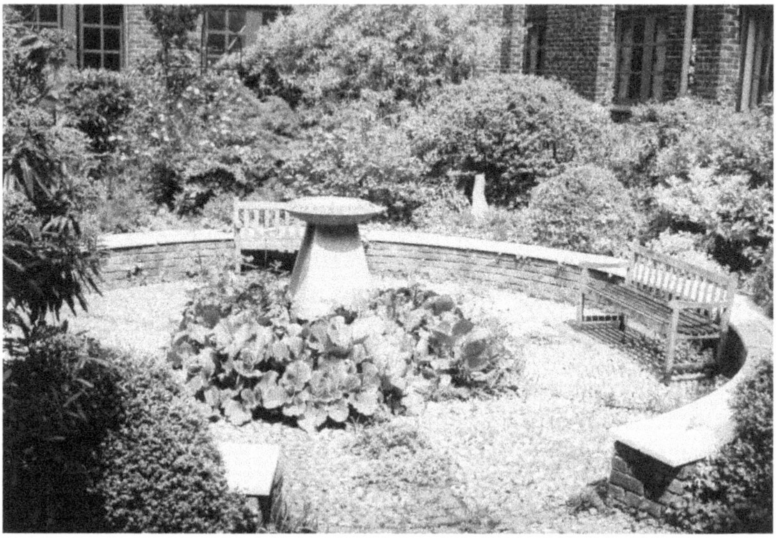

Figure 42 The Bird Garden designed by John Hubbard in 1990 is one of the many courtyards at West Dorset General Hospital.

One example of this in a contemporary context is West Dorset General Hospital. This has been designed to include a number of courtyards which are accessed by different groups as well as providing views from wards, offices and seats in public areas within the hospital (Figure 42). The most public of these spaces is the garden attached to the café, which includes a waterfall as well as exuberant planting, but others are used by specific groups of vulnerable patients, such as the elderly. Similarly, at Northampton General Hospital the stroke ward has a small courtyard (created in 2000) that is for the specific use of patients recovering from strokes as well as their relatives and staff.

A courtyard model was used for the Elderly and Adult Acute Mentally Ill Unit at Southmead Hospital, Bristol, which was built in the 1990s. The unit was created on part of a larger hospital site that had evolved from the original nineteenth-century workhouse. This means that, unlike Callington Road, there is little in the way of a wider landscape as much of the site has been developed. However, there are small garden areas that are accessible to all within the wider site. Sadly, the small courtyard dedicated to the use of patients in the Mentally Ill Unit was further decreased in size in the summer of 2005, due to the extension of some of the hospital buildings. This example is in strong contrast to the vast expanse of gardens and landscape associated with the earlier asylums.

One other contemporary trend is the creation of courtyards that are then inaccessible to any group of patients, relatives or staff. The maintenance plan for Daventry Community Hospital highlights the lack of accessibility to most of its courtyards as the plan states that, 'two main courtyards adjacent to the Listed Building are intended for patient/visitor access and are therefore to be more heavily landscaped in both hard and soft materials. The remaining courtyards are not [their emphasis] accessible except for maintenance.'[61] This implies that the reason for these courtyards being designed as inaccessible spaces is related to the cost of maintaining them. It is worth noting that the Daventry Hospital was built through the Public Finance Initiative which may have influenced the economic aspects of the design.[62]

The cost of maintenance also seems to have determined the design and planting of the courtyards at Daventry. The strategy begins by stating that the 'planting has been selected from shade tolerant varieties with careful consideration of the combination and mixing of varieties to render "all year round" effectiveness. The overall effect in each courtyard is to be of a light, open and cheerful character.'[63] This chimes with earlier theories concerning the creation of a therapeutic landscape and the term 'cheerful' also echoes the desire of the Commissioners for Lunacy in the nineteenth century for gardens to be created for asylums that would help promote 'cheerfulness' amongst the patients. However, the strategy then goes on to demonstrate its primary concern with finance, as it says that:

> Low maintenance is essential and it is envisaged that all planting, once secure, will grow through the gravel mulch layer. Due to intensive draining layout the planting zone is likely to be restricted to the centre of each courtyard. Creeping species have been planted 2.0m from the nearest drain line in all locations. They are to be encouraged to spread over the gravel mulch layers. Limited maintenance is essential. Within the planting zone shrubs of reasonable maturity will be planted where possible with a carpet of ground cover planting spreading towards the edge of the planting area. Changes in height of species and colours are essential in an effort to give these courtyards a degree of interesting variety.[64]

They reiterate the need for low or limited maintenance in this description, in which it is clear that plants are only to be located in the centre of the courtyards. The rest of the area appears to be predominately covered in gravel, which is in contrast to the findings that elements such as plants are more restorative than hard landscaping. The description also suggests that the planting will only offer a small degree of fascination or interest for the viewer and, as they are inaccessible, one wonders if they will add anything to the therapeutic environment.

Therapeutic use of landscape

Hospital gardens have always been used as places for outdoor activities, from exercise, work and recreation outside, which formed a major part of the regime of the Victorian asylum, to occupational therapy using gardening in the twentieth-century psychiatric hospital. Exercise outside was advocated for convalescing patients in the Victorian general hospital, as well as being the central therapeutic method in the open-air institution. Some twenty-first-century designs reflect a continued interest in a more active interaction with the landscape. These range from areas dedicated to exercise, to gardens designed specifically for horticultural therapy.

Again, Ulrich reflects nineteenth-century ideas when he argues that exercise is important for patients:

> Physical activity and mild exercise are associated with a spectrum of physical health benefits and play a critical role in rehabilitation following illness and injury. Activity and mild exercise are also very important for improving emotional well-being, tending to be especially beneficial with respect to alleviating depression.[65]

He goes on to argue that gardens can play a role in this:

> Because depression is a widespread and serious problem among patients, healthcare facilities should be provided, for instance, with pleasant gardens or art display spaces to serve as pleasant accessible trip destinations that motivate increased walking or wheelchair movement.[66]

Callington Road has been designed with specific 'therapeutic activity areas in gardens'.[67] These include basketball courts for use by patients, which are a more modern version of the fives court, cricket pitch and bowling green found at Brislington House in the early nineteenth century. The new facility also has 'a network of pedestrian paths' that 'will link all facilities on site and will offer service users, staff and visitors the potential to walk around the site'.[68] This again is similar to the walks laid out around the wider landscape at Brislington. These facilities are not only geographically close; it also appears that they are close in terms of design.

Dan Pearson has stated that his garden at the Evelina Children's Hospital at St Thomas's Hospital, London, is designed so that 'the roof terrace can be divided into two main areas, each creating a different version of the beach landscape, which allows for different kinds of usage from simply stepping out to breathe in the fresh air and contemplate the surroundings, to taking a short walk, sitting privately, relaxing, reading or playing around with the children'.[69] This is a more modern description of the use of general hospital gardens by convalescents in the nineteenth century.

A word should also be said about horticultural therapy but this area will not be covered in detail here as it is specialist field of its own.[70] This term became common in the health sciences during the 1980s and, according to Söderback et al., it can be described as follows:[71]

> Horticultural therapy includes interventions mediated by nature-oriented views and spaces such as gardens and everything associated with them, the plants and material related to them, garden tools and garden occupations performed among disabled people for healing and for restoring or improving health and well-being or for rehabilitation or simply general benefit.[72]

This term takes on board passive as well as active participation in the garden and has developed, via occupational therapy, from the use of gardening as part of the regime in early asylums.

Research conducted in the UK by Loughborough University in association with Thrive concluded that:[73]

> Garden projects offer clients the opportunity to engage in regular, structured forms of outdoor physical activity. Many of the tasks, such as digging or hard landscaping, require the exertion of substantial effort. Clients reported that they felt better, both physically and psychologically, when attending projects and attributed this to their participation.[74]

This suggests that physical interaction with the environment can be important in patient recovery as well as in the maintenance of physical health. Research from Loughborough also looked at the current state of horticultural therapy in the UK. Although little evidence was found of current hospital gardens being used for horticultural therapy during the research for this book,[75] in 2003 Loughborough found that fourteen per cent of all current therapeutic garden projects were associated with hospitals or set in their grounds.[76] Again this points to the fact that hospital gardens are once more being viewed as important places for active, as well as passive, interaction with nature. As the Loughborough team discovered, it is the association with nature, and not just being outdoors, that is important: 'Evidence from the study shows that there was not only a sense of escape from the "inside" and its associated restrictions, but a desire to be in the natural environment. The natural, green environment was preferred to the outdoor city environment.'[77] However, as Parr's work has demonstrated, gardening-based projects can have limitations. For example, as with the Victorian asylum, green space can cause issues of spatial isolation from the wider community and a lack of social interaction can mean that the integration and inclusion of users is limited.

Contemporary design

Another recurring element is the use of contemporary garden design and materials in the creation of hospital gardens. Garden designers such as the Pulham firm (Bristol Homeopathic Hospital, 1925) and Gertrude Jekyll (Edward VII Hospital, Midhurst, 1906) created gardens that were full of contemporary design references and reflected their own styles. Even gardens designed by doctors, such as those at Brislington House, appear to have followed popular aesthetic movements. Similarly, new technologies were used to create the Leeds General Infirmary Winter Garden and the roof garden at Bristol General Hospital. It seems therefore fitting that one of today's popular garden designers, Dan Pearson, has been employed to create three gardens associated with hospitals in London. Two of these will be looked at in detail in this section, in terms of their contemporary design and materials as well as in relation to the therapeutic ethos behind them.[78] They are the designs for a roof-terrace garden at the Evelina Children's Hospital, and the wider landscape and inner courtyards for the Maggie's Centre at Charing Cross Hospital.

Pearson, who was trained at both the Royal Horticultural Society's garden, Wisley, and at the Royal Botanic Garden at Kew, has risen to public prominence through his weekly column on gardening in the *Daily Telegraph* and through a number of television programmes. His personal views on the therapeutic benefits of parks and gardens make him an obvious choice as a designer of hospital gardens. As a signatory of the Commission for Architecture and the Built Environment (CABE) Space's Manifesto for Better Public Spaces he said that:

> However small, a park which takes the needs of local people into consideration provides an engaging, restorative, therapeutic and educational

> environment of benefit to all who use it. A well-designed public park should be an aesthetic place for contemplation, relaxation, and physical activity which allows us to cope with the stresses of urban/modern life while also teaching us about our relationship with nature and the environment.[79]

Similarly, in *The Essential Garden Design Book*, written with Terence Conran, he stated that:

> At the most basic level, comfort and a sense of peace can be achieved by creating a garden that is pleasing to the eye: a palette of pastel colours, a seat nestling among a bank of grasses or a well-placed piece of garden sculpture might encourage meditation or simply banish everyday worries.[80]

These views suggest that he is sympathetic to the potential of hospital gardens as therapeutic spaces and his approach to the design for the Evelina Children's Hospital roof terrace seems to further prove this.[81]

The Evelina Hospital has been designed in consultation with children and 'in order to create an accessible and friendly environment for children each floor of the hospital is themed. The theme of the 3rd floor is "The Beach"'.[82] It is from this floor that the garden is accessed so Pearson has taken this theme and broken the garden into two separate areas: the Islands and the Jetty/Pier. The concept takes a very sensory approach and states that:

> The aim of the garden is to provide an outside space that will encourage people using this floor of the hospital to move outside and experience a change of environment. The garden will be a healing space where adult visitors can spend thoughtful time, but children will also be encouraged to use it, to be exposed to daylight, the fresh air and the fun of being in a playful landscape on the third floor of a building. The dialysis wing looks out onto the roof terrace and this demands that there is constant visual interest, as patients are confined for many hours at a time in this area. However, this requirement will be carefully balanced with the need for it to be a restful and contemplative environment for those needing a calm reflective space. The Beach theme of this floor will be developed into a magical treatment for the roof garden. A coastal environment will be conjured up through the choice of hard and soft landscaping materials, while the airiness and exposure of the beach will be captured with elements that both stimulate the sense and soothe the mind. Light, movement, scent, texture and sound will all play a part in this extension to the floor and will provide a completely absorbing environment for those who use it.[83]

He is also concerned about the function of noise in his designs for the Maggie's Centre: 'The corridor created by the peripheral wall of the building has at its focal point a large rough stone into which a shallow dish has been cut that contains moving water. The sound of water and lofty bamboo that forms the full stop to the corridor will add a calming effect to the entrance area and hold your attention until the front door becomes visible.'[84] This further suggests that he has taken a strong sensory approach for these designs.

It is clear from the plans that, without losing sight of the various needs of different patients, such as it being 'magical' for the children and having some element of visual interest for the dialysis patients, and visitors, Pearson has maintained specific characteristics associated with his designs. For example, the 'Islands' at Evelina are constructed out of grassy mounds that are contained within curved benches. According to Pearson, 'The islands will be gently mounded so that they appear to rise naturally out of the space. The mounds will be soft and sensuous with a dense planting of grasses, which will capture the wind. The larger of the two islands will be planted with two craggy, wind tolerant Tamarisk, a small, flowering tree native to coastal areas.'[85] Pearson has previously used mounds of grass in his designs for fourteen roof gardens for the Roppongi Hills development in Tokyo, Japan and grasses also feature in the public garden created with James Fraser at Bonnington Square, Vauxhall, London.[86] He has also previously used the design concept of the beach in the creation of a garden for Worthing Hospital, Sussex, which, like his other designs, incorporated grasses.[87] This suggests that, like Jekyll at the Edward VII Sanatorium, Pearson is bringing his own design signature to these hospital garden designs.

Other contemporary design concepts used at the Maggie's Centre (Figure 43) include the idea of wrapping the new building with birch trees and the use of naturalistic planting. For example, 'a bound-gravel path will wind its way between the trunks of the established plane trees and through a woodland planting of low ground covering perennials. Wood sedge, *Luzula sylvatica*, sweet woodruff, *Galium odoratum* and ferns will help to create a soothing mood as one approaches the entrance courtyard and informal drifts of bulbs will be injected into the planting for spring.'[88] This use of natural planting is also something associated with Pearson's designs as his studio website states that as a team they 'are committed to making better environments for wildlife and people and making as gentle a mark on the land as possible'.[89]

Another influence on his designs appears to come from Japan. In the area directly in front of the Maggie's Centre there are stands of magnolias, a large boulder and a diagonal paving pattern which 'refers to the

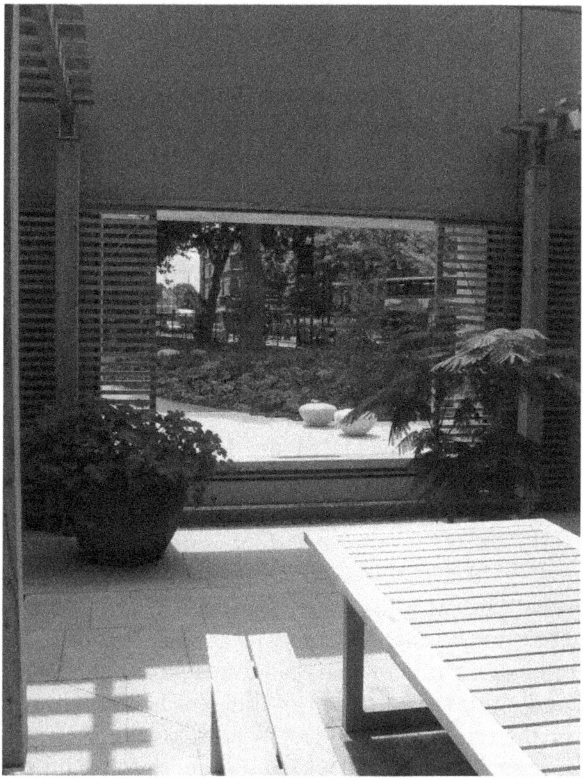

Figure 43 The central table and view of the garden at the Maggie's Cancer Centre designed by the Richard Rogers Partnership at Charing Cross Hospital, with Japanese-influenced planting by Dan Pearson's Studio.

Japanese tradition of creating certain paths that change direction so that devils, which [can only] travel in a straight line, are unable to use them'. Similarly he has used the concept of 'borrowed landscape' in the design for Evelina, by including views of Archbishop's Park: 'There is a sensation of being in the trees on this level and the immediacy of the busy road below is eclipsed by the expansive green horizon. This restful backdrop will become the borrowed scenery for the roof-garden.'[90] This idea of 'borrowing' the landscape can either be seen as an eighteenth-century English concept or as following the Japanese tradition of incorporating the wider landscape into the design of a garden. Again, the use of

Japanese elements into the design is perhaps more associated with Pearson's approach to design than the specific concept of a therapeutic garden.

This approach of incorporating contemporary elements into hospital gardens is part of a tradition in England. However, as well as financial constraints, designers can also face difficulties when trying to please a variety of medical personnel. According to Sally Court:

> All too often each therapeutic department tries to whittle away at the concept and turn it into something to suit its own needs. It then becomes a compromise that loses its purpose and identity. A place where patients can grow their own seedlings all too frequently becomes too much for staff and patients alike, and then the garden becomes neglected. Nothing is worse that these sad apologies for gardens.[91]

A further pressure may be placed on designers if hospitals demand gardens based predominantly on Ulrich's ideas concerning the elements that are needed to create a therapeutic garden. This combined effect could be to the detriment of new and interesting design approaches.

One modern idea that sets Pearson's garden designs apart from earlier hospital gardens is the use of lighting. He and Conran state that 'electricity has transformed the modern garden' because it 'brings the garden to life at night'.[92] In the Island area of the children's hospital garden design, there are a number of different lighting ideas. The most dramatic of these is the creation of lighting in the shape of a cloud: 'Above the largest island a cloud will be suspended to complete the beach landscape. The cloud will be formed from a mass of twisted stainless steel wire that will glimmer in sunshine. At night, fibre optic cables woven into the form will transform the space by throwing down a gentle glow onto the islands.'[93] In the jetty area he also has lighting at 'ground level to trace the textured ribbon in the paving'.[94] He goes on to suggest that 'the lights could take the form of multiple LED's which pinprick the ribbon along its length. Alternatively, a countersunk fibre optic cable could be set alongside the ribbon, with the possibility of one or two slabs along the length of the jetty being touch sensitive so that children can change the colour of the fibre optic cable.'[95] This use of lighting will give the garden a very contemporary feel and would make it a product of the time in which it was designed, like earlier hospital gardens.

Less dramatic is the more 'delicate and functional' lighting that he has suggested for the Maggie's Centre: 'The internal courtyards will be lit with subtlety, the plants being lit from below so that stems are made into sculptural forms and in the largest courtyard low level lighting will be fixed into the pergola to throw light onto the bench below.'[96] He has also made use of the roof areas, in the form of terraces, for the design of the Maggie's Centre. In this way Pearson is bringing contemporary garden design concepts and technology into hospital garden design, something that the Victorians would have recognised.

Notes

1 Roger Ulrich, 'Workshop summary: research on building design and patient outcomes', in NHS Estates, *Exploring the Patient Environment: An NHS Workshop* (Norwich: The Stationery Office, 2003), 4–6, p. 5.
2 Florence Nightingale, *Notes on Nursing: What It Is And What It Is Not* (London: Harrison, 1860), p. 84.
3 Roger Ulrich, 'Effects of gardens on health outcomes: theory and research', in Cooper Marcus and Barnes, *Healing Gardens*, 27–86, p. 27.
4 Gesler et al., 'Therapy by design', p. 122.
5 Jonathan Hughes, 'The "matchbox on a muffin": the design of hospitals in the early NHS', *Medical History*, 44 (2000), 21–56, p. 41.
6 Anthony Cox and Philip Groves, *Design for Health Care*, The Butterworth Design Series for Architects and Planners (London: Butterworth and Co., 1981), p. 35.
7 Ruth Richardson, 'Building healing environments: an historical perspective', in Deborah Kirklin and Ruth Richardson eds, *The Healing Environment: Without and Within* (London: Royal College of Physicians, 2003), 25–40, p. 34.
8 *Ibid.*, pp. 35–6.
9 Roger Ulrich, 'Health benefits of gardens in hospitals', Paper for conference: Plants for People, International Exhibition Floriade 2002, http://greenplantsforgreenbuildings.org/attachments/contentmanagers/25/HealthSettingsUlrich.pdf (accessed 4 March 2012).
10 Ulrich, 'Effects of gardens', p. 28.
11 Meredith Veldman, *Fantasy, the Bomb, and the Greening of Britain: Romantic Protest, 1945–1980* (New York: Cambridge University Press, 1994), p. 208.
12 Ingrid Söderback, Marianne Söderström and Elizabeth Schälander, 'Horticultural therapy: the "healing garden" and gardening in rehabilitation measures at Danderyd Hospital Rehabilitation Clinic, Sweden', *Pediatric Rehabilitation*, 7 (2004), 245–60, p. 246.
13 Christian Cay Lorenz Hirschfeld, 1785, quoted in Gerlach-Spriggs et al., *Restorative Gardens*, p. 18.
14 Ulrich, 'Workshop summary', p. 5.
15 Ingrid Söderback et al., 'Horticultural therapy'.

16 Thomas R. Herzog, Andrea M. Black, Kimberlee A. Fountaine and Deborah J. Knotts, 'Reflection and attentional recovery as distinctive benefits of restorative environments', *Journal of Environmental Psychology*, 17 (1997), 165–70, p. 165.
17 *Ibid.*
18 Terry Hartig, Gary W. Evans, Larry D. Jamner, Deborah S. Davis and Tommy Garling, 'Tracking restoration in natural and urban field settings', *Journal of Environmental Psychology*, 23 (2003), 109–23, p. 110.
19 Roger S. Ulrich, Robert F. Simons, Barbara D. Losito, Evelyn Fiorito, Mark A. Miles and Michael Zelson, 'Stress recovery during exposure to natural and urban environments', *Journal of Environmental Psychology*, 11 (1991), 201–30, p. 202.
20 Ulrich et al., 'Stress recovery', p. 201.
21 Edward O. Wilson, *Biophilia: The Human Bond with Other Species* (Cambridge, Mass. and London, England: Harvard University Press, 1984), p. 1.
22 *Ibid.*, p. 110.
23 Howard Frumkin, 'Beyond toxicity: human health and the natural environment', *American Journal of Preventive Medicine*, 20:3 (2001), 234–40, p. 234.
24 *Ibid.*
25 Described by Ulrich in 'Health benefits of gardens'.
26 Frederick Law Olmsted (1865), reprinted as 'The value and care of parks' in Roderick Frazier Nash, ed., *American Environmentalism: Readings in Conservation History*, third edition (New York: Mc-Graw Hill, 1990), 45–51, p. 48.
27 Ulrich, 'Workshop summary', p. 6.
28 Ulrich, 'View through a window', p. 420.
29 *Ibid.*, p. 420.
30 Nightingale, *Notes on Nursing*, p. 86.
31 Maggie Keswick, *A View from the Front Line*, ed. Marcia Blakenham (Maggie's Centres Booklet, 1995), p. 21.
32 *Ibid.*, p. 87.
33 Ulrich et al., 'Stress recovery', p. 204.
34 Ulrich, 'View through a window', p. 421.
35 Ulrich, 'Effects of gardens', p. 74.
36 *Ibid.*, pp. 74–5.
37 *Ibid.*, p. 75.
38 *Ibid.*, 1999, p. 30.
39 Cooper Marcus and Barnes, *Healing Gardens*, 1999.
40 BMA, *The Psychological and Social Needs of Patients* (2011), p. 14.
41 Kathleen A. O'Shaughnessy, 'Environmental psychology: the science behind virtual windows', *ADVANCE for Radiologic Science Professionals* (15 November 1999), p. 19.
42 *Ibid.*

43 See Chapter 4.
44 For example, see the parkland at Derbyshire Royal Infirmary, Chapter 4.
45 Quoted in Trimedia Broadcast, 'Hospital room with a view' posted 12 November 2004, www.trimedia.co.uk/articles.asp (accessed 20 October 2005).
46 Richardson, *English Hospitals*, p. 37.
47 Hughes, 'The matchbox on a muffin', p. 32.
48 Kathleen M. Beauchemin and Peter Hays, 'Sunny hospital rooms expedite recovery from severe and refractory depressions', *Journal of Affective Disorders*, 40 (1996), 49–51, p. 49.
49 *Ibid.*
50 Avon and Wiltshire Mental Health Parternship NHS Trust, *Callington Road Campus, Bristol: Design Statement to Support Planning Application* (Bristol City Council Planning Office: 03/0/029/M/E), p. 10.
51 *Ibid.*, p. 12.
52 The Maggie's Centres are built and run by a charitable organisation set up by Maggie Keswick Jencks when she was suffering from cancer. They provide non-institutional buildings that provide a drop-in service for people with cancer and their carers. The Maggie's Centre at Charing Cross is being designed by the Richard Rogers Partnership. The charity chooses leading architects because it also believes that environment is important and that the buildings should be attractive, comfortable, supportive and stimulating. Dan Pearson Design Studio, 'The design – southern winter garden', *Maggie's Centre Charing Cross; Landscape Design Concept* (January 2005), Compact Disc supplied by studio.
53 See Chapter 2.
54 Department of Health and NHS Estates, *A New Generation of Healthcare Facilities* (2003), p. 10.
55 NHS design portfolio, Lynfield Mount Hospital.
56 Aedas Architects, *Daventry Community Hospital: Project Design Statement* (Leeds), received at Daventry District Council (DDC) Nov. 2004. DDC File 1 DA/2004/1499.
57 For more on the Bristol General Hospital roof garden see Chapter 4.
58 *Planning Report in Support of Reserved Matter of Application: Erection of a New Mental Healthcare Hospital: Land at Callington Road, Bristol*, 19 March 2003 (Bristol City Council Planning Office 03/0/029/M/E), p. 5.
59 Online case study, www.landscapeinstitute.org/casestudies/casestudy.php?id=110 (accessed 13 August 2011).
60 Richardson, *English Hospitals*, p. 36.
61 Aedas Landscape and Environment, 'Landscape design concept', in *Daventry Hospital PFI – Landscape Maintenance and Management Strategy* (Huddersfield). Received at DDC Nov 2004. DDC File 1 DA/2004/1499, p. 8.
62 In an online article Clare Cooper Marcus has described how 'many otherwise attractive hospital gardens are kept locked at all times to prevent use. This

has specifically been observed at Private Finance Initiative (PFI) hospitals in the UK. One assumes this is so because the owners do not wish to pay for upkeep.' www.worldhealthdesign.com/Patient-specific-Healing-Gardens.aspx (accessed 27 September 2011).

63 Aedas, 'Landscape design concept', p. 8.

64 *Ibid.*

65 Roger Ulrich, 'Appendix one: research on building design and patient outcomes', in *Exploring the Patient Environment: An NHS Workshop* (Norwich: The Stationery Office, 2003), p. 14.

66 *Ibid.*

67 Avon and Wiltshire Mental Health Partnership, *Callington Road Campus*, p. 14.

68 *Planning report . . . Callington Road*, p. 8.

69 Dan Pearson Studio, 'Part 4.1: the design – the plan', *Evelina Children's Hospital.*

70 A good basic history, 'Horticultural therapy', has been written by Ingrid Söderback et al.

71 *Ibid.*, p. 245.

72 *Ibid.*

73 Thrive is a UK-based national charity which aims to enable positive change in the lives of disabled and disadvantaged people through the use of gardening and horticulture.

74 Joe Sempik, Jo Aldridge and Saul Becker, *Health, Well-being and Social Inclusion: Therapeutic Horticulture in the UK. Executive Summary* (Loughborough University in association with Thrive, 2005), p. 7.

75 One exception was the garden for stroke patients at Northampton General Hospital.

76 Joe Sempik, Jo Aldridge and Louise Finnis, 'Social and therapeutic horticulture: the state of practice in the UK', A paper for the Centre of Child and Family Research, *Evidence*, 8 (2004).

77 Joe Sempik et al., *Health, well-being and Social Inclusion.*

78 The third garden is a re-landscaping of the memorial garden at Guy's Hospital, Southwark, London. As this is a public area with a number of functions unrelated to the therapeutic role of the hospital it is not being discussed in this chapter.

79 CABE, *Press Release*, www.cabe.org.uk/news/press/showPRelease.asp?id=674 (accessed 24 October 2005).

80 Terence Conran and Dan Pearson, *The Essential Garden Design Book* (London: Conran Octopus Ltd., 1998), p. 20.

81 Opened in October, 2005 by Guy's and St Thomas's NHS Foundation Trust, Evelina Children's Hospital is London's first new children's hospital for more than 100 years.

82 Dan Pearson Studio, 'Part 1', *Evelina Children's Hospital.*

83 Dan Pearson Studio, 'Part 3: the concept – the beach', *Evelina Children's Hospital.*

84 Dan Pearson Studio, 'The design – the entrance', *Maggie's Centre Charing Cross.*
85 Dan Pearson Studio, 'Part 4.2: the islands – plan', *Evelina Children's Hospital.*
86 Dan Pearson showed photographs of his work in Tokyo as part of a lecture at the British Library, February 2005. One of the gardens had large mounds of grass that people could touch.
87 Sally Court, *The Modern Garden Makers* (London: Cardinal Publishing, 1999), p. 112.
88 Dan Pearson Studio, 'The design – the shady entrance', *Maggie's Centre Charing Cross.*
89 From Dan Pearson Studio, *About*, www.danpearsonstudio.com (accessed 10 November 2005).
90 Dan Pearson Studio, 'Part 2: the analysis', *Evelina Children's Hospital.*
91 Court, *The Modern Garden Makers*, p. 112.
92 Conran and Pearson, *Essential Garden Design*, p. 70.
93 Dan Pearson Studio, 'Part 4.5: the design – the cloud', *Evelina Children's Hospital.*
94 Dan Pearson Studio, 'Part 5.2: light concept – the pier/jetty', *Evelina Children's Hospital.*
95 *Ibid.*
96 Dan Pearson Studio, 'The design – the lighting', *Maggie's Centre Charing Cross.*

Conclusion

In an article on how to design contemporary hospital gardens published in November 2005, Clare Cooper Marcus argued that 'appealing, soothing and accessible spaces in hospitals are simply essential not dispensable'.[1] This article was aimed at landscape architects, and demonstrates the growing rhetoric for the importance of designed spaces in hospitals. As Gesler and others have suggested, this increasing awareness of the role of the environment in patient recovery means that the new generation of UK hospitals is 'thus informed by a number of design goals which include new understandings of hospitals as therapeutic environments as well as more traditional ideas of hospitals as efficient clinical spaces, spaces that are integrated with their surroundings and spaces that are accessible and responsive to patients' needs'.[2] This points the way towards a wider concept of a therapeutic environment being more than clinical efficiency and one that could include the garden as an important element. This, plus the commissioning of such a prominent designer as Pearson to work at two London hospitals, points to a positive future, where gardens can once again be given an important status within hospitals.

However, there is the conflicting problem of the considerable cost of designing and maintaining such gardens. Pearson's designs for the Evelina Hospital have been paid for by the Guy's and St Thomas's Hospital Charity and those for the Maggie's Centre have been funded by the Maggie's Centre Charity; they are, therefore, not affected by the costing considerations that concern the NHS. Within an NHS that is struggling to finance essentials such as new buildings, therapeutic interventions, technological developments and staff, gardens may well be viewed in the future as luxuries rather than important structural elements that should be integral to the design of hospitals. The locking of courtyards to save on maintenance costs is just one example of how financial restraints may affect hospital gardens in the future. Even if they are created in the first place, if gardens are not maintained they will wind up repeating the story of decline and neglect at hospitals in the middle of the twentieth century, such as that at the Winford Orthopaedic Hospital where insufficient staff were retained to manage the up-keep of the gardens.[3]

Whether finance or theory will be the main factor in determining the design and creation of hospital gardens in the future remains to be seen. The constraints on space mean that there will not be a return to the large landscapes of nineteenth-century institutions and early twentieth-century open-air hospitals. However, the fact that in the twenty-first century new and exciting designs, albeit for small gardens in restricted spaces, have been produced by such designers as Pearson suggests that, if the money is available, the future for hospital gardens might be bright, and their role in the therapeutic regime could be as influential as in the past.

The Maggie's Cancer Care Centres are also developing a new architectural language for medical and health care buildings. Charles Jencks has described them as a 'kind of non-type. It is like a house which is not a home, a collective hospital which is not an institution, a church which is not religious, and an art gallery which is not a museum'.[4] In this way I believe he is echoing earlier centuries when efforts were made to grapple with the need to create something which was functional as well as domestic in style, and he describes the particular influence of the Hospices de Beaune built in Burgundy in 1443.[5] I would suggest there are also later connections. Like the York Retreat, where the centrality of the kitchen reflected Quaker domestic principles, the kitchen table in the Maggie's Centres acts as a type of informal reception area.[6] Similarly Jencks has stated his hope 'that works of art and landscape become as important to the programme as the architecture'.[7] Here there is an attempt to see the landscape as an active agent once more and to incorporate it into the overall design. The gardens designed by Dan Pearson's Studio at the Charing Cross Maggie's Centre certainly seem like part of the coherent whole and an essential part of the building's fabric. So it seems that there is some future for gardens as therapeutic spaces and that their current relationship with specialist, charitable centres might act as an impetus for larger institutions if green spaces can once again be viewed as intrinsically important for staff, visitors and patients alike.

In the United States, where there is a mixed provision of health care, the wealthier hospitals already have a variety of associated hospital gardens.

The interest this has sparked has led to courses in health care garden design[8] and even a network of people interested in the subject, called the Therapeutic Landscapes Network, which was founded by Naomi Sachs in 1999. In the UK it seems that those gardens which are being created now often belong to charitable organisations, such as those attached to the Maggie's Centres.

The Penny Brohn Cancer Centre on the outskirts of Bristol, near Pill, seems like the perfect site on which to conclude as it reflects many of the themes discussed within the book. It represents the cross-over between the domestic and the institutional as well as the continuity of sites for health care. The initial building on the site was a domestic manor house built in the early eighteenth century by the Meyler family and then passed through marriage to Henry Bright who developed the gardens in 1750–70.[9] The location, up on the hill and away from the growing city of Bristol, may have originally been chosen for its healthy air.

During his time Bright created a pleasure ground with a gazebo and riverside water gate, known as the 'Adam and Eve folly', as well as the ubiquitous ha-ha. It was evidently a site suited to an eighteenth-century domestic residence with its views across the Avon River. In the late nineteenth century, the land was acquired for the establishment of Ham Green Hospital. Demonstrating the suitability of sites for both domestic and institutional residences, the hospital took on the 99 acres of land and built new ward blocks for patients suffering from infectious diseases. Medical services remained on the site throughout the twentieth century, although much of the farmland was sold off after rationalisation following the formation of the NHS. Finally the NHS sold the remainder of the site to Penny Brohn Cancer Care in 2002.

Now the gardens have been redesigned and revitalised in a new type of health care setting. According to the Brohn Centre's own history, even the eighteenth century perambulation has been restored as a new pathway to be used by those visiting the centre. They describe how the inner courtyard in particular offers a safe space which can 'help people take the quiet, reflective time often needed following a diagnosis'.[10] This centre, as well as the Maggie's Centres, seems to offer new approaches to health care placed within the type of mixed domestic and institutional setting that earlier generations also felt was essential.

Hospital gardens can act as important marginal spaces between the institution and the wider world. They allow people to spend time in a recognisable setting and can provide privacy and space away from the often crowded and noisy internal spaces. These elements all seem to be important whether you are a patient yourself, you are visiting someone or you work there. It may be hard to quantify statistically, although researchers are building up strong evidence as the previous chapter has shown, but there is certainly a qualitative response to accessible green space and in the past this has been valued and proved influential in hospital design. In conclusion I would argue that it is time such spaces were seen once again as important features in their own right rather than as inconsequential adjuncts to the associated medical institution.

Notes

1 Clare Cooper Marcus, 'Help with healing', *Green Places*, 20 (2005), 26–9, p. 29.
2 Gesler et al., 'Therapy by design', p. 118.
3 See Chapter 5.
4 Charles Jencks and Edwin Heathcote, *The Architecture of Hope: Maggie's Cancer Caring Centres* (London: Francis Lincoln, 2010), p. 14.
5 *Ibid.*, p. 16.
6 *Ibid.*, p. 50 and Ann-Marie Akehurst, 'The York Retreat: "a vernacular of equality"', in Pater Guillery, ed., *Built From Below: British Architecture and the Vernacular* (London: Routledge, 2010), 73–98, p. 89.
7 Jencks and Heathcote, *The Architecture of Hope*, p. 29.
8 Including a Certificate Programme in Healthcare Garden Design at the Chicago Botanic Garden, US.
9 The history of Ham Green House is taken primarily from James Russell, 'Mr Bright's pleasure ground at Hung Road: the gardens of Ham Green House, Easton-in-Gordano', *Avon Gardens Trust Journal*, 3 (2008), 4–19.
10 'A short history of Penny Brohn Cancer Care's Home'; undated leaflet.

Select bibliography

Primary sources

Main archives consulted

Borthwick Institute for Archives, University of York
Bristol Central Library
Bristol Record Office
Daventry District Council Planning Department, Northamptonshire
Kings College London Archives
National Monuments Record Centre, Swindon
Northampton Local Studies Library
Northampton Record Office
St Andrew's Healthcare Archives
Somerset Heritage Centre
Tyne & Wear Archives, Newcastle
Wellcome Library and Archives
West Yorkshire Archive Service, Leeds
Worcester Record Office

Reports, pamphlets, lectures, essays, speeches and parliamentary papers

Bristowe, John Syer, *An Introductory Address Delivered at St Thomas's Hospital on the Occasion of the Opening of the Session of its Medical and Surgical College*, 1 October 1858 (Southwark: E. Billing and Son, 1858)

Bristowe, John Syer, *An Introductory Address on the Future of St Thomas's Hospital, Delivered at the Hospital in the Surrey Gardens on the Occasion of the Opening of the Session of its Medical and Surgical College*, 1 October 1862 (London: J.W. Roche, 1862)

Bristowe, John Syer and Holmes, Timothy, 'Report on the hospitals of the United Kingdom', appendix 15 to the Sixth Report of the Medical Officer of the Privy Council, 1863, *British Parliamentary Papers*, xxviii (1864)

Foster, Edward, *An Essay on Hospitals, or, Succinct Directions for the Situation, Construction, and Administration of Country Hospitals* (Dublin: Printed for the author by W.G. Jones, 1768)

Further Report of the Commissioners in Lunacy to the Lord Chancellor (London: Shaw and Sons, 1847)

Galton, Douglas, *An Address on the General Principles which Should be Observed in the Construction of Hospitals*, delivered to the British Medical Association at Leeds, 29 July 1869 (London: Macmillan and Co., 1869)

General Regulations of the Bethel Hospital Norwich (Norwich: Jarrold and Sons Printers, 1861)

Hartnell, C. Braine, *The Prevention and Cure of T.B: An Abstract of a Paper Read before the Worcestershire and Herefordshire Branch of the B.M.A.* (Cheltenham: Norman, Sawyer and Co., c.1900)

Lawson, Bryan, 'ASPECT Evidence-based tool: Focusing on patient and staff environments', in *The Environment for Care: An NHS Estates Symposium* (2004)

NHS Estates and King's Fund, *Improving the Patient Experience: Evaluation of the King's Fund's Enhancing the Healing Environment Programme* (Norwich: The Stationery Office, 2003)

Reinhardt, Dr Charles, *Hailey Open Air Sanatorium for the Treatment of Consumption and Other Tuberculosis Diseases* (Stratford: Cole and Clark Printers, c.1900)

Report of the NAPT Architectural Committee, *Design for Sanatoria* (London: NAPT, 1951)

Report on the 'Open-air' Treatment of Consumption at the North London Hospital for Consumption, Mount Vernon, Hampstead, 1899

Robins, E.C., *Modern Hospital Construction* (London: Printed for the Council of the Parkes Museum, 1883)

Sempik, Joe, Aldridge, Jo and Becker, Saul, *Health, Well-being and Social Inclusion: Therapeutic Horticulture in the UK. Executive Summary* (Loughborough University in association with Thrive, 2005)

Sempik, Joe, Aldridge, Jo and Finnis, Louise, 'Social and therapeutic horticulture: the state of practice in the UK', A paper for the Centre of Child and Family Research, *Evidence*, 8 (2004)

The New Regulations of Wonford House Hospital for the Insane Near Exeter, Adopted at a General Court of Governors held on 11 February 1880 (Exeter: William Pollard Printer, 1880)

Ulrich, Roger, 'Appendix one: research on building design and patient outcomes', in *Exploring the Patient Environment: An NHS Workshop* (Norwich: The Stationery Office, 2003)

Ulrich, Roger, 'Workshop summary: research on building design and patient outcomes', in NHS Estates, *Exploring the Patient Environment: An NHS Workshop* (Norwich: The Stationery Office, 2003), 4–6

Wells-Thorpe, John, 'The Maggie's Centres project', in NHS Estates, *The Environment for Care: An NHS Estates Symposium* (2004)

Articles

Journals consulted regularly include: *British Medical Journal*, *British Journal of Tuberculosis*, *The Builder*, *The Lancet*, *The Medical Officer*

'A short account of Nordrach and the "open air" treatment of consumption', *St Thomas's Hospital Gazette*, 10:4 (1900), 73–81

'Account of Leeds Infirmary', *The British Medical Journal* (31 July 1869)

Armstrong, David, 'Decline of the hospital: reconstructing institutional dangers', *Sociology of Health and Illness*, 20:4 (1998), 445–57

Armstrong, S.T., 'The need of care for the convalescent from the hospital standpoint', reprinted from *New York Medical Journal* (7 March 1908) (British Library)

Asher, R.A.J., 'The dangers of going to bed', *British Medical Journal*, 1 (1947), 967–8

Barrett, Claire, 'In peril: Sully Hospital', *Grand Designs*, 2 (2004), 112

Beauchemin, Kathleen M. and Hays, Peter, 'Sunny hospital rooms expedite recovery from severe and refractory depressions', *Journal of Affective Disorders*, 40 (1996), 49–51

Campbell, Margaret, 'What tuberculosis did for modernism: the influence of a curative environment on modernist design and architecture', *Medical History*, 49:4 (2005), 463–88

Cook, G.C., 'Henry Currey FRIBA (1820–1900): leading Victorian hospital architect, and early exponent of the "pavilion principle"', *Postgraduate Medical Journal*, 78:920 (2002), 352–9

Cooper Marcus, Clare, 'Help with healing', *Green Places*, 20 (2005), 26–9

Cooter, Roger, 'Open-air therapy and the rise of open-air hospitals', *Bulletin for the Social History of Medicine*, 35 (1984), 44–6

Edginton, Barry, 'Moral architecture: the influence of the York Retreat on asylum design', *Health and Place*, 3:2 (1997), 91–9

Festing, Sally, 'Pulham has done his work well', *Garden History*, 25 (1984), 138–58

Frumkin, Howard, 'Beyond toxicity: human health and the natural environment', *American Journal of Preventive Medicine*, 20:3 (2001), 234–40

Gesler, Wil, Bell, Morag, Curtis, Sarah, Hubbard, Phil and Francis, Susan, 'Therapy by design: evaluating the UK hospital building program', *Health & Place*, 10:2 (2004), 117–28

Goldin, Grace, 'Building a hospital of air', *Bulletin of the History of Medicine*, 49 (1975), 512–35

Gruffudd, Pyrs, '"Science and the stuff of life": modernist health centres in 1930s London', *Journal of Historical Geography*, 27:3 (2001), 395–416

Hartig, Terry, Evans, Gary W., Jamner, Larry D., Davis, Deborah S. and Garling, Tommy, 'Tracking restoration in natural and urban field settings', *Journal of Environmental Psychology*, 23 (2003), 109–23

Herzog, Thomas R., Black, Andrea M., Fountaine, Kimberlee A. and Knotts, Deborah J., 'Reflection and attentional recovery as distinctive benefits of restorative environments', *Journal of Environmental Psychology*, 17 (1997), 165–70

Hickman, Clare, 'The "Picturesque" at Brislington House: the role of landscape in relation to the treatment of mental illness in the early nineteenth-century asylum', *Garden History*, 33:1 (2005), 47–60

Hickman, Clare, 'Cheerful prospects and tranquil restoration: the visual experience of landscape as part of the therapeutic regime of the British asylum, 1800–1860', *History of Psychiatry*, 20:4 (2009), 425–41

Hughes, Jonathan, 'The "matchbox on a muffin": the design of hospitals in the early NHS', *Medical History*, 44 (2000), 21–56

King, Antony, 'Hospital planning: revised thoughts on the origin of the pavilion principle in England', *Medical History*, 10:4 (1966), 360–73

O'Shaughnessy, Kathleen A., 'Environmental psychology: the science behind virtual windows', *ADVANCE for Radiologic Science Professionals* (15 November 1999), 19

Porter, Roy, '"All madness for writing": John Clare and the asylum', in Hugh Haughton, Adam Phillips and Geoffrey Summerfield, eds, *John Clare in Context* (Cambridge: Cambridge University Press, 1994), 259–78

Smith, Tony, 'Convalescence', *Medical Journal*, 312 (1996), 383

Söderback, Ingrid, Söderström, Marianne and Schälander, Elizabeth, 'Horticultural therapy: the "healing garden" and gardening in rehabilitation measures at Danderyd Hospital Rehabilitation Clinic, Sweden', *Paediatric Rehabilitation*, 7 (2004), 245–60

Ulrich, Roger S., 'View through a window may influence recovery from surgery', *Science*, 224:4647 (1984), 420–1

Ulrich, Roger S., Simons, Robert F., Losito, Barbara D., Fiorito, Evelyn, Miles, Mark A. and Zelson, Michael, 'Stress recovery during exposure to natural and urban environments', *Journal of Environmental Psychology*, 11 (1991), 201–30

Wilson, John, 'Notes on the planning of sanatoria, infectious diseases hospitals, and other public health institutions', reprinted from *Journal of RIBA*, third series, 29:10 (1922) (British Library)

Worboys, Michael, 'The development of the sanatorium treatment for consumption in Britain, 1880–1914', *Bulletin for the Social History of Medicine*, 35 (1984), 41–3

Books

Abercrombie, Leslie Patrick, ed., *The Book of the Modern House: A Panoramic Survey of Contemporary Domestic Design* (London: Hodder and Stoughton, 1939)

Alison, Archibald, *Essays on the Nature and Principles of Taste* (Edinburgh: Printed for J.J.G. and G. Robinson, London and Bell and Bradgate, Edinburgh, 1790)

Andrews, Jonathan, *The History of Bethlem* (London: Routledge, 1997)

Anning, S.T., *The General Infirmary at Leeds*, 2 vols (Edinburgh and London: E. & S. Livingstone, 1963/66)

Ayres, Henrietta, *A Changing Community: The Brief History of St Crispin Hospital, Duston, Northampton, 1876–1976* (Northampton: The Northamptonshire Area Health Authority, 1976)

Barnes, Rachel, *The Pre-Raphaelites and Their World* (London: Tate Gallery Publishing, 1998)

Barrell, John, *The Dark Side of the Landscape: The Rural Poor in English Paintings, 1730–1840* (Cambridge: Cambridge University Press, 1980)

Bartell, Edmund, *Hints for Picturesque Improvements in Ornamented Cottages and Their Scenery* (1804) (reprinted Farnborough: Gregg International Publishers, 1971)

Bate, Jonathan, *John Clare: A Biography* (London: Picador, 2003)

Batey, Mavis, *Regency Gardens* (Buckinghamshire: Shire Publications, 1995)

Battie, William, *A Treatise on Madness by William Battie, M.D. and Remarks on Dr. Battie's Treatise on Madness by John Monro M.D.* (1758), introduced and annotated by Richard Hunter and Ida Macalpine (London: Dawsons of Pall Mall, 1962)

Beeton, Samuel Orchart, *The Beeton Book of Garden Management* (originally published as *Beeton's Illustrated Book of the Garden* in 1889–91) (facsimile reprinted Hertfordshire: Omega Books, 1985)

Bermingham, Ann, *Landscape and Ideology: The English Rustic Tradition 1740–1860* (London: Thames and Hudson, 1987)

Brantley, Richard, E., *Wordsworth's 'Natural Methodism'* (New York: Yale University, 1975)

Brown, Jane, *The Art and Architecture of English Gardens: Designs for the Garden from the Collection of the Royal Institute of British Architects 1609 to the Present Day* (London: Weidenfeld and Nicolson, 1989)

Browne, W.A.F., *What Asylums Are, Were and Ought To Be* (1837), ed. with an introduction by Andrew Scull in *The Asylum as Utopia* (London and New York: Routledge, 1991)

Bryder, Linda, *Below the Magic Mountain: A Social History of Tuberculosis in Twentieth-century Britain* (Oxford: Clarendon Press, 1988)

Burdett, Henry, *Hospitals and Asylums of the World: Their Origin, History, Construction, Administration, Management and Legislation*, 4 vols (London: Churchill, 1893)

Burke, Edmund, *A Philosophical Enquiry into the Origin of our Ideas of the Sublime and Beautiful* (London: Printed for A. Robertson, 1824)

Burton, Robert, *The Anatomy of Melancholy* (1621), ed. T.C. Faulkner, N.K. Kiessling and R.L. Blair (Oxford: Clarendon Press, 1990)

Burton-Fanning, F.W., *Open-air Treatment of Pulmonary Tuberculosis* (London, Paris, New York and Melbourne: Cassell and Company, c.1900)

Bynum, W.F., *Science and the Practice of Medicine in the Nineteenth Century* (Cambridge: Cambridge University Press, 1994)

Bynum, W.F. and Porter, Roy, eds, *The Companion Encyclopedia of the History of Medicine*, 2 vols (London and New York: Routledge, 1993)

Bynum, William F., Porter, Roy and Shepherd, Michael, eds, *The Anatomy of Madness: Essays in the History of Psychiatry*, 3 vols (Cambridge: Cambridge University Press, 1985)

Chadwick, Edwin, *Great Britain Poor Law Commissioners: Report on the Sanitary Condition of the Labouring Population of Great Britain, 1842*, ed. with an introduction by M.W. Flinn (Edinburgh: Edinburgh University Press, 1965)

Chadwick, George F., *The Park and the Town: Public Landscapes in the Nineteenth and Twentieth Centuries* (London: Architectural Press, 1966)

Coates, Peter, *Nature: Western Attitudes Since Ancient Times* (Cambridge: Polity Press in association with Blackwell, 1998)

Coleridge, Samuel Taylor, *Selected Poems*, ed. with an introduction by Richard Holmes (London: Penguin Books, 1996)

Connolly, John, *Treatment of the Insane Without Mechanical Restraints* (1856), ed. with an introduction by Richard Hunter and Ida Macalpine (Folkestone and London: Dawsons of Pall Mall, 1973)

Conrad, Lawrence. I., Neve, Michael, Nutton, Vivian, Porter, Roy and Wear, Andrew, *The Western Medical Tradition: 800 BC to AD 1800* (Cambridge: Cambridge University Press, 1995)

Conran, Terence and Pearson, Dan, *The Essential Garden Design Book* (London: Conran Octopus Ltd., 1998)

Conway, Hazel, *People's Parks: The Design and Development of Victorian Parks in Britain* (Cambridge: Cambridge University Press, 1991)

Cooper, Anthony Ashley, 3rd Earl of Shaftesbury, *Characteristicks*, 3 vols (Glasgow: R. Foulis, 1743–45)

Cooper Marcus, Clare and Barnes, Marni, eds, *Healing Gardens: Therapeutic Benefits and Design Recommendations* (New York and Chichester: John Wiley and Sons, 1999)

Cooter, Roger, *Surgery and Society in Peace and War: Orthopaedics and the Organization of Modern Medicine, 1880–1948* (Basingstoke and London: Macmillan Press, 1993)

Court, Sally, *The Modern Garden Makers* (London: Cardinal Publishing, 1999)

Cox, Anthony and Groves, Philip, *Design for Health Care*, The Butterworth Design Series for Architects and Planners (London: Butterworth and Co., 1981)

Dawson, Jennifer, *The Ha-Ha* (London: Virago, 1961)

Delaney, Rosalind with Winn, Gillian, *How Did This Garden Grow? The History of the Botanic Gardens of the University of Bristol* (Bristol: Burleigh Press Ltd., 2002)

Doordan, Dennis P., *Twentieth-century Architecture* (London: Calman & King, 2002)

Drabble, Margaret, *Wordsworth* (London: Evans Bros, 1966)
Elliott, Brent, *Victorian Gardens* (London: Batsford, 1986)
Foss, Arthur and Trick, Kerith, *St Andrew's Hospital, Northampton: The First One Hundred and Fifty Years, 1839–1988* (Cambridge: Granta Editions, 1989)
Foucault, Michel, *Discipline and Punish: The Birth of the Prison* (1975), translated by Alan Sheridan (New York: Random House, 1979)
Foucault, Michel, *Madness and Civilization: A History of Madness in the Age of Reason* (1961), translated by Richard Howard (Cambridge: Routledge, 1995)
Gaskell, Ronald, *Wordsworth's Poem of the Mind: An Essay on the Prelude* (Edinburgh: Edinburgh University Press, 1991)
Gerlach-Spriggs, Nancy, Kaufman, Richard Enoch and Warner, Sam Bass, *Restorative Gardens: The Healing Landscape* (New Haven and London: Yale University Press, 1998)
Gittins, Diana, *Madness in its Place: Narratives of Severalls Hospital, 1913–1997* (London: Routledge, 1998)
Glancey, Jonathan, *Twentieth-century Architecture* (London: Carlton Books, 1998)
Golby, Fred, *A History of Upton and Berrywood* (Warwick: Warwick Printing Company Limited, 1994)
Granshaw, Lindsay, *St Thomas' Hospital, London, 1850–1900*, PhD Thesis (Bryn Mawr: Bryn Mawr College, 1981)
Granshaw, Lindsay and Porter, Roy, eds, *The Hospital in History* (London and New York: Routledge, 1989)
Hall, Peter, *Cities of Tomorrow*, third edition (Malden, USA, Oxford, UK and Victoria, Australia: Blackwell, 2005)
Hall, Peter and Brockington, Ian F., eds, *The Closure of Mental Hospitals* (London: Royal College of Psychiatrists, 1991)
Hamlyn, Edward, *The Healing Art of Homeopathy: The Organon of Samuel Hahnemann* (Buckinghamshire: Beaconsfield Publishers, 1979)
Harding, Stewart and Lambert, David, *Parks and Gardens of Avon* (Bristol: Avon Gardens Trust, 1994)
Harvey, W.J. and Gravil, Richard, eds, *Wordsworth, The Prelude: A Casebook* (London: Macmillan, 1972)
Helmreich, Anne, *The English Garden and National Identity: The Competing Styles of Garden Design, 1870–1914* (Cambridge: Cambridge University Press, 2002)
Hilton, John, *On the Influence of Mechanical and Physiological Rest in the Treatment of Accidents and Surgical Diseases, and the Diagnostic Value of Pain: A Course of Lectures Delivered at the Royal College of Surgeons of England, in the Years 1860, 1861, and 1862* (London: Bell and Daldy, 1863)
Hilton, John, *On Rest and Pain: A Course of Lectures* (London: George Bell and Sons, 1877)
Hodgson Burnett, Frances, *The Secret Garden* (1911) (Middlesex: Puffin Books, 1982)

Horsfield, T.W., *The History, Antiquities and Topography of the County of Sussex*, 2 vols (Lewes: Sussex Press, 1835)

Howard, Ebenezer, *Garden Cities of Tomorrow* (1902; this edition edited by F.J. Osborn, 1946) (Northampton: Faber and Faber, 1970)

Hudson, Bernard, *Alpine Climate and Tuberculosis* (Davos-Platz: Davos Printing Company, c.1920s)

Hunt, J.D. and Willis, Peter, *The Genius of the Place: The English Landscape Garden 1620–1820* (Cambridge, Mass. and London: MIT Press, 1988)

Jacobi, Maximilian, *On the Construction and Management of Hospitals for the Insane with a Particular Notice of the Institution at Siegburg*, translated by John Kitching and with introductory observations by Samuel Tuke (London: John Churchill, 1841)

Jellicoe, Geoffrey et al., eds, *The Oxford Companion to Gardens* (New York: Oxford University Press, 2001)

Jones, Katheleen, *Asylums and After: A Revised History of the Mental Health Services, from the Early Eighteenth Century to the 1990s* (London: Athlone Press, 1993)

Kelynack, T.N., ed., *The Year Book of Open-air Schools and Children's Sanatoria* (London: John Bale, Sons and Danielsson, 1915)

Kilvert, Francis, *Kilvert's Diary: Selections from the Diary of the Reverend Francis Kilvert 1870–1879*, ed. with an introduction by William Plomer (London: J. Cape, 1944)

Kirkbride, Thomas, *On the Construction, Organization and General Arrangements of Hospitals for the Insane* (Philadelphia: Lindsay and Blakiston, 1854)

Kirklin, Deborah and Richardson, Ruth, eds, *The Healing Environment: Without and Within* (London: Royal College of Physicians, 2003)

Lane, Joan, *A Social History of Medicine: Health, Healing and Disease in England 1750–1950* (London: Routledge, 2001)

Langley, John, *Illustrated Guide to Abington Manor and Church* (Northampton: Lingsprint, 1991)

Lawrence, Christopher, *Medicine in the Making of Modern Britain, 1700–1920* (London: Routledge, 1994)

Le Vay, David, *The History of Orthopaedics: An Account of the Study and Practice of Orthopaedics from the Earliest Times to the Modern Era* (Carnforth: Parthenon, 1989)

Liversidge, Michael and Edwards, Catherine, eds, *Imagining Rome: British Artists and Rome in the Nineteenth Century* (London: Merrell Holberton, 1996)

Livingstone, R., *Homeopathy, Born 1810 – Still Going Strong* (London: The British Homeopathic Association, 1973)

Locke, J., *An Essay Concerning Human Understanding* (1690) ed. Roger Woolhouse (London: Penguin, 1997)

Loudon, J.C., *An Encyclopaedia of Gardening* (London: Printed for Longman, Rees, Orme, Brown, Green and Longman, 1834)

Loudon, J.C., *The Suburban Gardener and Villa Companion* (1838), reprinted in The English Landscape Garden Series (New York and London: Garland Publishing, 1982)

Massingham, Betty, *Miss Jekyll: Portrait of a Great Gardener* (Newton Abbot: David and Charles, 1973)

McInnes, E.M., *St Thomas' Hospital* (London: George Allen and Unwin Ltd, 1963)

Midgley, Kenneth, *Garden Design* (Harmondsworth, Middlesex: Penguin, 1966)

MIND, *Hospital Land: A Resource for the Future* (MIND: July 1975)

Mingay, G.E., ed., *The Victorian Countryside*, 2 vols (London: Routledge and Kegan Paul, 1981)

Moore, Norman, *The History of St Bartholomew's Hospital*, 2 vols (London: C. Arthur Pearson Ltd., 1918)

Morley, John, *Regency Design 1790–1840* (London: Zwemmer, 1993)

Morris, William, *News from Nowhere or an Epoch of Rest, Being Some Chapters from a Utopian Romance*, first printed serially in the *Commonweal*, 1890, ninth edition (London: Longmans Green and Co., 1907)

Mouat, Frederic J. and Snell, Saxon H., *Hospital Construction and Management* (London: J. & A. Churchill and Co., 1883)

Mowl, Tim, *Historic Gardens of Gloucestershire* (Stroud: Tempus, 2002)

Muthu, C., *Pulmonary Tuberculosis and Sanatorium Treatment: A Record of 10 Years' Observation and Work in Open-air Sanatoria* (London: Balliere, Tindall and Cox, 1910)

Nash, Roderick Frazier, ed., *American Environmentalism: Readings in Conservation History*, third edition (New York: Mc-Graw Hill, 1990)

Nicholls, Phillip A., *Homeopathy and the Medical Profession* (Kent: Croom Helm, 1988)

Nightingale, Florence, *Notes on Hospitals; Being Two Papers Read Before the National Association for the Promotion of Social Science, at Liverpool, in October, 1858 with Evidence Given to the Royal Commissioners on the State of the Army in 1857*, second edition (London: John W. Parker and Son, 1859)

Nightingale, Florence, *Notes on Nursing: What It Is and What It Is Not* (London: Harrison, 1860)

Nightingale, Florence, *Notes on Hospitals, Third Edition: Enlarged and For the Most Part Re-written* (London: Longman, Green, Longman, Roberts and Green, 1863)

Northampton Country Lunatic Asylum, Berrywood: How it was Established and a Sketch of its History from its Opening to March, 1913 (Northampton: Jos. Tebbutt, 1913)

Northampton Public Libraries, *Old Northampton: A Selection of Old Photographs, Prints and Drawings of Historical Interest* (Northampton: Northampton Public Libraries, 1973)

Ottewill, David, *The Edwardian Garden* (New Haven and London: Yale University Press, 1989)

Papworth, J.B., *Rural Residences, Consisting of a Series of Designs for Cottages, Decorated Cottages, Small Villas and Other Ornamented Buildings* (London: Sedding and Turtle, 1832)

Parissien, Steven, *Regency Style* (London: Phaidon Press, 1992)

Parr, Hester, *Mental Health and Social Space: Towards Inculsionary Geographies?* (Malden: Blackwell, 2008)

Parry-Jones, William Llewellyn, *The Trade in Lunacy: A Study of Private Madhouses in England in the Eighteenth and Nineteenth Centuries* (London: Routledge and Kegan Paul, 1972)

Payne, Christiana, *Toil and Plenty: Images of the Agricultural Landscape in England 1780–1890* (New Haven and London: Yale University Press, 1993)

Perceval, John, *Perceval's Narrative: A Patient's Account of his Psychosis, 1830–1832*, ed. Gregory Bateson (London: Hogarth Press, 1962)

Philo, C., *A Geographical History of Institutional Provision for the Insane from Medieval Times to the 1860s in England and Wales: The Space Reserved for Insanity* (Lewiston and Queenston, USA and Lampeter, Wales: Edwin Mellen Press, 2004)

Porter, Roy, *Mind Forg'd Manacles: A History of Madness in England from the Restoration to the Regency* (London: Penguin Books, 1987)

Porter, Roy, *The Greatest Benefit to Mankind: A Medical History of Humanity from Antiquity to the Present* (London: Fontana Press, 1997)

Porter, Roy, ed., *The Cambridge Illustrated History of Medicine* (Cambridge: Cambridge University Press, 1996)

Pringle, John Bart, *Observations on the Diseases of the Army in Camp and Garrison . . . With an Appendix, Containing Some Papers of Experiments, Read at Several Meetings of the Royal Society* (London: 1752)

Raphael, Winifred, *Psychiatric Hospitals Viewed by their Patients*, second edition (London: King Edward's Hospital Fund for London, 1977)

Reinhardt, Charles, *A Handbook of the Open-air Treatment and Life in an Open-air Sanatorium*, second edition (London: John Bales, Sons and Danielson, 1902)

Repton, Humphry, 'Fragments on the theory and practice of landscape gardening' (1816), reprinted in *Aesthetics and the Picturesque*, ed. and introduced by Gavin Budge (Bristol: Thoemmes, 2001)

Richardson, Harriet, ed., *English Hospitals 1660–1948: A Survey of Their Architecture and Design* (Swindon: RCHME, 1998)

Rivett, Geoffrey, *From Cradle to Grave: Fifty Years of the NHS* (London: King's Fund Publishing, 1998)

Rosenthal, Michael, *British Landscape Painting* (Oxford: Phaidon, 1982)

Rutherford, S., *The Landscapes of Public Lunatic Asylums in England, 1808–1914*, PhD Thesis, 3 vols (Leicester: De Montfort University, 2003)

Scull, Andrew, *The Most Solitary of Afflictions: Madness and Society in Britain 1700–1900* (New Haven and London: Yale University Press, 1993)

Seebohm, Caroline, *The Country House: A Wartime History, 1939–1945* (London: Weidenfeld and Nicholson, 1989)

Shortt, S.E.D., *Victorian Lunacy: Richard M. Bucke and the Practice of Late Nineteenth-century Psychiatry* (Cambridge: Cambridge University Press, 1986)

Showalter, Elaine, *The Female Malady: Women, Madness and English Culture, 1830–1980* (London: Virago Press, 1987)

Smiles, Sam, *The Image of Antiquity: Ancient Britain and the Romantic Imagination* (New Haven and London: Yale University Press, 1994)

Smith, F.B., *The Retreat of Tuberculosis, 1850–1950* (Kent: Croom Helm Ltd, 1988)

St Andrew's Hospital, *150 years of Progress, Saint Andrew's Hospital* (Northampton: St Andrew's Hospital, 1988)

St Crispin Hospital Management Committee, *Review of the Hospital During the First Ten Years of the National Health Service* (Northampton: St Crispin Hospital, 1958)

Stevenson, Christine, *Medicine and Magnificence: British Hospital and Asylum Architecture, 1660–1815* (New Haven and London: Yale University Press, 2000)

Stuart, David, *The Garden Triumphant: A Victorian Legacy* (London: Viking, 1988)

Switzer, Stephen, *Ichongraphia Rustica, or, the Nobelman, Gentleman and Gardener's Recreation, . . .* , 3 vols (London: Printed for D. Browne, B. Barker and C. King, W. Mears and R. Gosling, 1718)

Symes, J. Odery, *A Short History of the Bristol General Hospital* (Bristol: John Wright and Sons Ltd, 1932)

Tankard, Judith B., *Gardens of the Arts and Crafts Movement: Reality and Imagination* (New York: Harry N. Abrams, 2004)

Taylor, Jeremy, *Hospital and Asylum Architecture in England, 1840–1914; Building for Health Care* (London: Mansell, 1991)

Taylor, Jeremy, *The Architect and the Pavilion Hospital: Dialogue and Design Creativity in England, 1850–1914* (London and New York: Leicester University Press, 1997)

The Charities Register and Digest: Convalescent Section, third edition (London: Longmans, Green and Co., 1890)

Thompson, J.D. and Goldin, Grace, *The Hospital: A Social and Architectural History* (New Haven and London: Yale University Press, 1975)

Tooley, Michael and Arnander, Primrose, eds, *Gertrude Jekyll: Essays on the Life of a Working Amateur* (Witton-le-Wear: Michaelmas Books, 1995)

Tuke, Samuel, *Description of The Retreat: An Institution Near York for Insane Persons of the Society of Friends* (1813), reprinted with an introduction by Richard Hunter and Ida Macalpine (London: Dawsons of Pall Mall, 1964)

Veldman, Meredith, *Fantasy, The Bomb, and the Greening of Britain: Romantic Protest, 1945–1980* (New York: Cambridge University Press, 1994)

Way, Twigs, ed., *Picturing Paradise: Studies in Eighteenth to Twentieth-Century Gardens and Garden Design* (Cambridge: University of Cambridge, 2003)

Waymark, Janet, *Modern Garden Design: Innovation Since 1900* (London: Thames and Hudson, 2003)

Wear, Andrew, ed., *Medicine in Society: Historical Essays* (Cambridge: Cambridge University Press, 1992)

Webster, Charles, ed., *Caring for Health: History and Diversity* (Norwich: Open University, 1993)

Whittingham, Sarah M., *Sir George Herbert Oatley (1863–1950): A Nonconformist Architect, a Critical Biography and Catalogue of Works*, PhD Thesis, 3 vols (Bristol: University of Bristol, 2005)

Wigley, Mark, *White Walls, Designer Dresses: The Fashioning of Modern Architecture* (Cambridge, Mass. and London: MIT Press, 1995)

Wilson, Edward O., *Biophilia: The Human Bond with Other Species* (Cambridge, Mass. and London, England: Harvard University Press, 1984)

Winford Hospital, *History of Winford Orthopaedic Hospital: A Hundred Years of Orthopaedic Care, 1876 to 1976* (Winford, Bristol: Winford Orthopaedic Hospital, 1976)

Woodbridge, Kenneth, *The Making of Stourhead: Henry Hoare's Paradise* (London: National Trust, 1965)

Woodring, Carl, *Nature into Art: Cultural Transformations in Nineteenth Century Britain* (Cambridge, Mass.: Harvard University Press, 1989)

Wordsworth, William, *The Prelude: A Parallel Text* (1850), ed. with an introduction by J.C. Maxwell (New Haven and London: Yale University Press, 1971)

Wordsworth, William, *Complete Poetical Works*, ed. Thomas Hotchinson, revised by Ernest de Selincourt (Oxford: Oxford University Press, 1973)

Worsley, Giles, *Architectural Drawings of the Regency Period, 1790–1837* (London: Andre Deutsch, 1992)

Yeo, Geoffrey, *Images of Bart's: An Illustrated History of St Bartholomew's Hospital in the City of London* (London: Historical Publications Ltd. in association with the Archives Department St Bartholomew's Hospital, 1992)

Index

Page numbers in *italic* refer to illustrations.
Literary works can be found under authors' names.

EU authorised representative for GPSR:
Easy Access System Europe, Mustamäe tee 50,
10621 Tallinn, Estonia
gpsr.requests@easproject.com

www.ingramcontent.com/pod-product-compliance
Ingram Content Group UK Ltd.
Pitfield, Milton Keynes, MK11 3LW, UK
UKHW021834100926
8556IPUK00004B/330

* 9 7 8 0 7 1 9 0 8 6 6 0 1 *